Assessing Competence in Medicine and Other Health Professions

Assessing Competence in Medicine and Other Health Professions

Claudio Violato

Professor and Assistant Dean
University of Minnesota Medical School

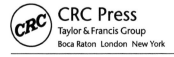

CRC Press
Taylor & Francis Group
Boca Raton London New York

CRC Press is an imprint of the
Taylor & Francis Group, an **informa** business

CRC Press
Taylor & Francis Group
6000 Broken Sound Parkway NW, Suite 300
Boca Raton, FL 33487-2742

International Standard Book Number-13: 978-1-138-59634-4 (Hardback)
International Standard Book Number-13: 978-1-4987-8508-2 (Paperback)

Library of Congress Cataloging-in-Publication Data

Names: Violato, Claudio, author.
Title: Assessing competence in medicine and other health professions / by Claudio Violato.
Description: Boca Raton : Florida : CRC Press, [2019] | Includes bibliographical references and index.
Identifiers: LCCN 2018032562 | ISBN 9781138596344 (hardback : alk. paper) | ISBN 9781498785082 (pbk. : alk. paper) | ISBN 9780429426728 (e-book)
Subjects: | MESH: Clinical Competence | Professional Competence | Educational Measurement | Formative Feedback.
Classification: LCC RA399.A1 | NLM W 21 | DDC 616—dc23
LC record available at https://lccn.loc.gov/2018032562

Visit the Taylor & Francis Web site at
http://www.taylorandfrancis.com

and the CRC Press Web site at
http://www.crcpress.com

Dedication

LeRoy Douglas Travis (October 14, 1940–August 9, 2017)
A dear friend and inspirational teacher

Contents

Preface

Assessing competence in medicine and other health professions continues to be a challenge. The assessment and evaluation of competence and learning have their origins in antiquity but are only now beginning to emerge as a unified field. This is due to developments in statistical and mathematical theory, test theory, and advances in computer hardware and software, as well as the developing internet. Testing and assessment are the acts of quantifying an educational or psychological dimension or assigning a numerical value to it. Evaluation requires a value judgment to be made based on the measurement. While the history of testing dates back two millennia, it has emerged on a large scale only in the 20th century, coincidental with mass education.

The current status of testing is paradoxical: it is on the increase and receives overwhelming public support, and yet most teachers, instructors, and professors (who construct, administer, and interpret the vast majority of tests) have little or no formal education in testing. Tests can be used to motivate students, enhance learning, provide feedback, evaluate educational programs, and for research. Other functions include curriculum revisions, selection and screening, certification, and guidance and counselling. Tests can be used in a variety of ways and for several evaluation functions. Testing is likely to expand in modern society. The improvement of healthcare professional competence depends, in part, on the improvement of testing and assessment of medical competence. The alarming rate of medical errors that currently result in death or negative outcomes may be reduced.

My purpose in writing this book is to provide a resource for teachers, assessors, administrators, pedagogues, generally, and students in health professions education for understanding, implementing, and critically evaluating testing, assessment, and evaluation. This is a comprehensive book on how to assess competence in medicine, medical education, and healthcare throughout the clinician's career. It is organized into three main sections: (1) Foundations, (2) Validity and reliability, and (3) Test construction and evaluation consisting of 16 chapters. Each chapter begins with an advanced organizer and contains summaries, reflections, and exercises.

The book also contains a glossary of testing and statistical terms—e.g., reliability, validity, standard error of measurement, biserial correlation, problems, and data. Fundamental problems will be presented—e.g., calculating reliability, conducting item analyses, running confirmatory factor analyses; here appropriate software (e.g., SPSS, Iteman, EQS), and examples of its use are demonstrated.

There are several titles on assessment and evaluation in the health professions, but none is a single-authored textbook. All are edited, multi-authored books. When dealing with a discipline (e.g., biology, assessment), edited multi-authored books are not generally regarded as "textbooks" by professors and students. These edited collections suffer from the problems of such books: the emphasis is skewed (doesn't represent the curriculum) by selection of contributors, the writing is uneven for the same reason; they lack the "authoritativeness" that a recognized single author of a textbook does. Additionally, they lack the clarity and comprehensiveness (partly because of the multi-authorship) that a textbook in the field requires. Currently, none of the existing books in this area or the field are textbooks in the real sense. Therefore, I have tried to write a usable, a balanced, a well-written, and an authoritative textbook for assessing competence in medicine and other health professions.

Author

Claudio Violato, PhD, is Professor and Assistant Dean, Assessment, Evaluation and Research at the University of Minnesota Medical School. He has taught at and held leadership positions at Wake Forest School of Medicine, the University of Calgary, University of British Columbia, University of Victoria, Kwantlen University, and the University of Alberta.

Dr. Violato's publications in medical education include competency-based assessment, psychometrics, research methods, leadership, and clinical reasoning and cognition. In addition to 10 books, Dr. Violato has published more than 300 scientific and technical articles, abstracts, and reports in major journals such as *Academic Medicine, Medical Education, British Medical Journal, Canadian Medical Association Journal*, and the *Lancet*. He has received millions of dollars in research funding from various institutions.

Some of Dr. Violato's recent honors and awards include the "Outstanding Achievement Award" from the Medical Council of Canada "For Excellence in the Evaluation of Clinical Competence" and the "Innovation Award for the development of the Physician Achievement Review Program," from the Royal College of Physicians and Surgeons of Canada.

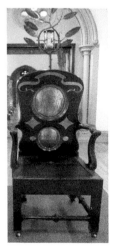 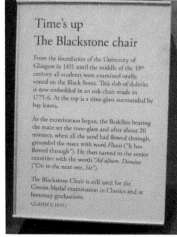

SECTION I

Foundations

The Foundations section consists of four chapters. Chapter 1 introduces the need for testing and assessment; deals with questions of "what are testing, assessment, measurement, and evaluation?"; provides a brief history of testing; describes the common types of tests and assessments; and summarizes the uses of tests. While the history of testing dates back two millennia, it has emerged on a large scale only in the 20th century, coincidental with mass education.

The current status of testing is paradoxical: it is on the increase and receives overwhelming public support and yet most professionals who construct, administer, and interpret the vast majority of tests have little or no formal education in testing. Testing is likely to expand in modern society. The improvement of healthcare professional competence depends, in part, on the improvement of testing and assessment of medical competence. The alarming rate of medical errors that currently result in death or negative outcomes may be reduced.

In Chapter 2, the somewhat controversial topic of competence in medicine is discussed. This chapter deals with the definition of competence, controversies surrounding it, and its multiple forms. In this chapter, there is a discussion of the various methods of assessing competence over the career span.

Competence and professionalism are complex, interrelated, multidimensional constructs commonly based on three primary components: knowledge, skills, and attitudes. Entrustable professional activities (EPAs) are clinical actions that require the use and integration of several competencies and milestones critical to safe and effective clinical performance. To assess the competence of physicians for EPAs requires complex and comprehensive assessments.

The present views define medical competence and professionalism as the ability to meet the relationship-centered expectations required to practice medicine competently. For Asian countries, professionalism is a Western concept without a precise equivalent in Asian cultures. Instruments and procedures that are designed to measure competence and professionalism are challenged on validity, reliability, and practicality.

A variety of professional organizations have recently weighed in on the constructs of competence and professionalism. The Canadian Medical Education Directions for Specialists (CanMEDS) framework consists of seven roles: manager, communicator, professional, scholar, expert, health advocate, and collaborator and has been used as the theoretical underpinnings of physician competencies.

Chapter 3 deals with somewhat more technical content, the basic statistics in testing. It includes descriptive statistics, standard scores, and graphical analyses. The understanding of statistics and data analysis allows for a greater appreciation of the differences and similarities between learners and also helps the teacher better organize and interpret test scores and other educational measures. The normal curve is a particularly important distribution as are skewed, bimodal, and rectangular distributions with the characteristic of many frequency distributions of their central tendency—the scores tend to cluster around the center. There are three measures of central tendency or average: the mode, median, and mean. Other descriptions include measures of dispersion, the range, and standard deviation. Norms and standard scores are an important aspect of test score interpretation and reporting. There are four types of standard scores: z-scores, T-scores, stanines, and percentiles.

Correlational techniques—indispensable methods in testing—are presented, detailed, and discussed in Chapter 4. The correlation is a statistical technique to study the relationship between and among variables. Several other statistical techniques have evolved based on the original Pearson's r: rank-order correlation, biserial correlation, regression analyses, factor analysis, discriminant analysis, and cluster analysis.

The correlation coefficient, r, must always take on values between +1.0 and −1.0 since it has been standardized to fit into this range. The sign indicates the direction of the relationship (i.e., either positive or negative), the magnitude indicates the strength of the relationship (weak as r approaches 0; strong as r increases and approaches +1.0 or −1.0), and the coefficient of determination (r^2) which is an indicator of the variance accounted for in y by x.

The following major correlational techniques are presented: Pearson product–moment, Spearman rank-order, biserial, point biserial, regression, multiple regression (linear, logistic), factor analysis (exploratory factor analyses [EFA], confirmatory factor analyses [CFA]), structural equation modelling, and hierarchical linear modelling.

Introduction

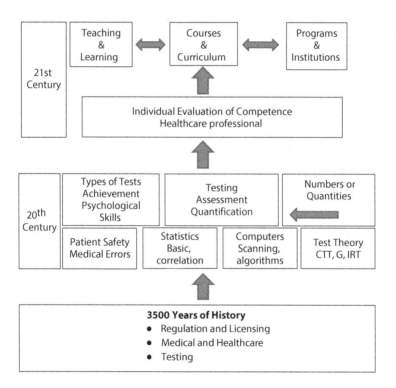

ASSESSMENT OF MEDICAL AND HEALTHCARE COMPETENCE

The assessment of medical and healthcare competence continues to be one of the most challenging aspects of the education, training, licensing, and regulation of healthcare professionals such as doctors, nurses, dentists, optometrists, and other allied healthcare workers. The report *To Err Is Human: Building a Safer Health System*,[1] of the Institute of Medicine of the National Academy of Sciences in the United States, made some staggering claims: nearly 100,000 people die annually in American hospitals as the result of medical mistakes. Subsequent commentators have suggested that this is an underestimate and the actual mortality rate is much higher. Some argue that the number of medical mistakes is much higher than is commonly accepted because most of the errors are not reported. A recent report by leading American researchers, employing more detailed and advanced methods than previously, has estimated that a conservative estimate of the real death rate due to medical error is more than 250,000 per year. It is the third most common cause of death in the United States after heart disease and cancer but ahead of chronic obstructive pulmonary disease, suicide, firearms, and motor vehicle accidents.[2]

An international report on adults' healthcare experiences in seven countries (New Zealand, the United Kingdom, the United States, Australia, Canada, Germany, and the Netherlands) indicated that 12%–20% of adults experienced at least one medical error in the 2 years of the study.[3] These findings have triggered international discussion, concerns, and controversies about patient injuries in healthcare. The major factors underlying medical errors are thought to be system-based factors (e.g., miscommunication on the ward) as well as person factors resulting in drug overdoses or interactions, misdiagnoses, surgical mistakes, incorrect medications, and simple carelessness. Patient safety, a topic that had previously been little understood and even less discussed in healthcare systems, has become a public concern in most Western countries.

Patient safety has now become a mantra of modern medical practice. Despite this, thousands of people are injured or die from medical errors and adverse events (incapacitation, serious injury, or death) each year. Worldwide, this figure may run into millions. Leaders in the healthcare systems have emphasized the need to reduce medical errors as a high priority. Doctors, as main participants, have been called upon to address the underlying systems causes of medical error and harm. Unfortunately, several studies[4] have shown that more than half of the hospital doctors surveyed haven't even heard of the report *To Err Is Human*. The magnitude of the problem is thought to be similar in the United Kingdom, Canada, and elsewhere in the world.[2]

While both system-based factors as well as person factors are at the root of medical errors, it is now believed that the impact of some person factors has been underestimated: physician carelessness, lack of knowledge, lack of professionalism, physician exhaustion and sleeplessness, and poor self-assessment, particularly of personal limitations in medical skills.[5,6] There is concern that the preferred tendency to put the emphasis on systems but not holding individuals responsible for errors will weaken accountability for physician performance. Failure to identify individual factors may contribute significantly to the risk of adverse events and may lead to a focus of patient safety away from the clinician to a systems-based approach. The assessment of the competence of individual healthcare professionals looms larger than ever.

Assessment is also commonly known as testing. Testing has its roots in antiquity and has undergone rapid advances in the later part of the 20th and the first part of the 21st century. This is because some necessary developments in its emergence—statistical and mathematical theories, advances in test theory, and computer technology and optical readers, online testing, social and political policy—have come only in the last several decades. Currently, the field is undergoing rapid development and change bringing exciting possibilities and challenges. Before describing the current status of testing and its history, however, we must describe and distinguish testing, assessment, and evaluation.

BOX 1.1: Licensing physicians throughout the ages

Prior to systematic testing as in modern times, the licensing of physicians has nevertheless been regulated. Control of the medical marketplace through licensing, prosecutions, and penalties has a long history and is not unique to modern society. Several cases illustrate the practices in the past several hundred years.

Jacoba Felicie paced nervously in her room glancing through her notes a final time before she set out for the court house.[7] Powerful forces including the Dean and Faculty of Medicine at the University of Paris were allied against her. This was Paris in 1322, and the physician guilds and university faculty had increased in power and control of the medical marketplace. They were seeking to consolidate their regulation of medical practice. They decided that Jacoba was a particularly good case to prosecute as she was a woman practicing medicine. The Dean and Faculty of Medicine were determined to put a stop to the illegal practice of medicine.

For some time now, the Parisian faculty wanted to gain stronger control over various practitioners of medicine such as surgeons, barbers, and empirics, whether male or female. The Dean and the Faculty of Medicine charged Jacoba with illegally visiting the sick, examining their limbs, bodies, urine and pulse, prescribing drugs, and collecting fees. The Dean and Faculty were most outraged because she actually cured some patients, frequently after conventional physicians had failed to do so.

The Dean and Faculty of Medicine who prosecuted her did not deny her skill or even that she cured patients. They argued that Jacoba had not read the proper texts; medicine was a science to be acquired through proper reading of texts such as Galen and lectures and discourses based on the written word. Medicine was not a craft to be learned empirically.

Jacoba argued in court that the intent of the law was to forbid the practice of medicine by ignorant and dangerous quacks and charlatans but that this did not apply to her as she was both knowledgeable and skillful. She also argued that she was fulfilling a particular need with female diseases because conventional modesty precluded male practitioners from dealing with these. Many of Jacoba's patients came to court that

(Continued)

BOX 1.1 (*Continued*): Licensing physicians throughout the ages

day to testify to her skill, knowledge, and caring. Jacoba must have been crushed when the court ruled in favor of the Dean and Faculty of Medicine that she was not legally constituted to practice medicine in Paris. She was therefore prohibited from practicing medicine in the future on penalty of imprisonment. The court acknowledged her patients' positive testimonies, but this was not deemed relevant to her legal status as a medical practitioner. Thus, the case of Jacoba ended, and we have no further historical record of her. Perhaps, she left Paris to practice medicine.

The French medical establishment continued to battle with illegal practitioners of medicine including the famous skirmishes with Louis Pasteur in the mid-19th century,[8] some 500 years after the case of Jacoba. One incensed physician even challenged Pasteur to a duel. Louis Pasteur, primarily a chemist and microbiologist, is one of the main founders of the germ theory of disease. Although his discoveries reduced mortality from puerperal fever, created the first vaccine for rabies and anthrax, and eventually revolutionized medical practice, the medical establishment in France was hostile to him as an unlicensed interloper.

THE RENAISSANCE AND THE CASE OF LEONARDO FIORAVANTI

The Milanese physicians had been plotting against him since his arrival from Venice in 1572. Fioravanti had been arrested and imprisoned by officers of the Public Health Board in Milan on the sketchy charge of not medicating in the accepted way.[9] After 8 days in prison, Fioravanti was becoming increasingly outraged by the indignity he was suffering. The Milan medical establishment considered him an outsider, an alien, and an unwelcome intruder. They finally were able to have him incarcerated.

Fioravanti was not a conventional medical charlatan hawking his nostrums in the piazza and then moving on. Nor was he a run-of-the-mill barber-surgeon. He had practiced medicine for years in Bologna, Rome, Sicily, Venice, and Spain. He had an MD from the University of Bologna, had published several medical texts, had developed many medicines, and was a severe critic of much of conventional medical practice. The Milan physicians were not welcoming and considered him a foreign doctor.

A prison guard provided pen-and-paper for Fioravanti, and in his most elegant and formal language, he addressed it to Milan's public health minister from "Leonardo Fioravanti of Bologna, Doctor of Arts and Medicine, and Knight." He asked to be released from prison and to "medicate freely as a legitimate doctor." A paid messenger delivered the letter to the health office located in the Piazza del Duomo.

(Continued)

> ## BOX 1.1 (*Continued*): Licensing physicians throughout the ages
>
> The health minister, Niccolo Boldoni, was responsible for overseeing every aspect of medical practice in Milan, from examining midwives, barber-surgeons, and physicians, to collecting fees, imposing fines, inspecting apothecaries, and ruling on appeals. The letter from the doctor and knight, Leonardo Fioravanti, claimed that the Milan physicians were in a plot to stop him from providing care and cures to the sick of Milan. Moreover, he claimed that the Milan physicians were a menace to their patients and did more harm than good with quack treatments, poisonous medicines, and careless and arrogant behaviors. Fioravanti challenged the minister to provide 25 of the sickest patients to him and an equal number to Milan doctors that the minister selected and that he—Fioravanti—would cure his patients quicker and better than the other doctors. It is unlikely that this early clinical trial ever occurred as there is no historical record of it, but Boldoni and the Milan court set Fioravanti free.

ASSESSMENT, TESTING, AND EVALUATION

Assessment involves the assignment of numbers, quantities, or characteristics to some dimension. Evaluation is the process of interpreting or judging the value of the assessment. Testing as used in the usual sense is a subset of assessment: in the classroom, in the clinic, or on the ward, it is assessment of educational outcomes. In recent years, the focus for classroom, clinic, or ward-based assessment has been on *performance assessment* (also called authentic, direct, or alternative assessment). This sort of assessment involves "real life," open-ended activities that are intended to measure aspects of higher-order thinking and professional conduct which together can be referred to as competence.[10]

In psychology and health sciences education, assessment instruments include examples such as intelligence tests, achievement tests, personality inventories, biomedical tests, and any classroom tests that you have taken in school, college, and medical school. All of these are measurement instruments because they attempt to quantify (assign a number to) some dimension whether it is length (ruler), time (clock), intelligence (IQ test), or scholastic aptitude for medical school (Medical School Admission Test—MCAT). Each assigns a number to one of a physical (length), psychological (intelligence), or educational/achievement/aptitude dimension (MCAT).

In addition to the MCAT, another very important test in medicine is the United States Medical Licensing Examination (USMLE), which is given in steps, reflecting emerging competence over time in the physician's development.

Step 1 assesses understanding and application of important concepts of the sciences basic to the practice of medicine. Here the focus is on principles and mechanisms underlying health, disease, and modes of therapy. Step 2 assesses the application of medical knowledge, skills, and understanding of clinical science essential for the provision of patient care under supervision. Step 3, the final examination, assesses the application of medical knowledge and understanding of biomedical and clinical science essential for the unsupervised, independent practice of medicine, with emphasis on patient management in ambulatory settings. In all cases, scores or numbers are derived from these tests. Tests and assessment devices, therefore, are measurement instruments in education and psychology. Long before systematic or standardized testing in the United States and Europe, however, physician licensing has been rigorously practiced (see Box 1.1 for historical examples).

Evaluation involves value judgments. To make an evaluation, you interpret a measurement according to some value system. A measurement may be a clinical teacher reporting Jason's score on a procedural skills test, such as intubation, as 19. If the teacher interprets this score and concludes that Jason is excellent at intubation, then this is an evaluation.

Assessment = assigning a number

Measurement = assigning a number

Testing = assigning a number

Evaluation = assessment or measurement or testing + a value judgment

Test scores generally serve as measurements or attempts to quantify some aspect of student or clinician educational functioning. The letter grades (A, B, C, D, F) or adjective descriptions (Excellent, Fair, Poor) associated with these numbers are evaluations based on these test scores. In some medical schools, students are provided with a class ranking, which is a type of evaluation, because the higher the rank, the *better* the standing. Evaluation, therefore, is measurement plus value judgments. The quality of the evaluation depends on both the quality of the measurement and the care with which this result is interpreted. A careless interpretation of good quality data is likely to lead to a poor evaluation just as a careful interpretation of shoddy data would. Evaluations by professors (or others) of student performance that are based on little or no data (that is, subjective evaluations) are likely to be of very poor quality. One of the main aims of this book, therefore, is to help course professors, clinical teachers, assessment experts, licensing authorities, and others to develop good-quality assessments (measurement instruments) and to conduct careful interpretations of the results. Thus, their evaluation of student and clinician performance will be enhanced.

BRIEF HISTORY OF TESTING

Modern testing of physicians and other healthcare professionals is well established and rely on scientific processes and procedures encompassed in the field of psychometrics. While the science of testing and assessment for the purpose of certification and licensure has developed in the past century or so, the regulation of medical and healthcare practice has its roots in antiquity (see Box 1.2 for its origins).[11]

According to the *Book of Judges*, the tribe of Gilead defeated the invading tribe of Ephraim (around 1370–1070 BCE). The Gileadites captured the fords of the Jordan opposite Ephraim. When any of the fugitives of Ephraim asked to cross-over to return home, they were given a test. To discern whether the request was to be allowed, the requester was asked to pronounce the word "Shibboleth."

> The men of Gilead would say to him, "Are you an Ephraimite?" If he said, "No," then they would say to him, "Say now, 'Shibboleth.'" But he said, "Sibboleth," for he could not pronounce it correctly. Then they seized him and slew him at the fords of the Jordan. Thus there fell at that time 42,000 of Ephraim.[12]

This was a *final* exam indeed!

The first country in the world to implement standardized testing on a broad scale was Ancient China. Called the imperial examination, the main purpose of the test was to select candidates for specific jobs in the government.[13] The imperial examination was established during the Sui Dynasty in 605 AD. It lasted for 1,300 years and was abolished in 1905 during the Qing Dynasty.[14] During the period of use, the imperial examination system played a central role in the Chinese imperial government. It served as a tool for the political and ideological control, functioned as a proxy for education, produced an elite social class, and became a dominant culture in traditional Chinese society.[15] The examination system was an attempt to recruit candidates on the basis of merit rather than on the basis of family or political connection. The texts studied for the examination were the Confucian classics. After a period of emphasis on memorization, without practical application and a narrow scope, the exam underwent change (circa 960), stressing the understanding of underlying ideas and the ability to apply classical insights to contemporary problems. Students sometimes spent 20–30 years memorizing the classics in preparation for a series of up to eight examinations in philosophy, poetry, mathematics, and so on.

By the 20th century, the imperial examination was considered outdated and inadequate. Meanwhile, an examination system modelled on the Chinese imperial exam was adopted in England in 1806. Its purpose was to select specific candidates for positions in Her Majesty's Civil Service. This system was later applied to education and influenced testing in the United States as it became a model of standardized tests. These practices include using standard conditions for the test (e.g., quiet setting, proctors supervising), standard scoring procedures (e.g. using exam scorers who were blinded to the candidates' identity), and protocols (e.g., scoring rubrics).

BOX 1.2: Regulation of medical practice since antiquity

MEDICAL PRACTICE IN ANTIQUITY

A set of laws, known as the Code of Hammurabi (circa 1740 BC), have come down to us from the Babylonians after its namesake, the founder of the Babylonian empire.[16] These 282 statutes or common laws governed nearly all aspects of social, political, economic, and professional life including those pertaining to physicians, surgeons, veterinarians, midwifes, and wet nurses. Carefully conscribed details were devoted to specifying the relationship between patients and practitioners, including fees and penalties. Problems of "internal medicine" were dealt with by physicians of the priestly class who saw to internal disorders caused by supernatural factors.

The surgeon who dealt with physical problems, however, was accountable for both remuneration and liability to earthly courts. If a doctor performed surgery, generally with a bronze knife, and saved the life or eyesight of an upper class citizen, he was to be paid 10 shekels of silver. A similar outcome for a commoner was worth 5 shekels and only 2 shekels for a slave. If the outcome for the upper class citizen was bad (blindness or death), the doctor's hand was amputated. If a slave died because of the surgery, the doctor had to provide a replacement but had to pay only half the value in silver, if the slave was blinded. The code provided further detail for many procedures including those of the veterinarians ("doctor of an ox or ass").

Probably, the most famous physician of all time and the founder of clinical medicine is Hippocrates (circa 460–360 BCE) of Greek antiquity, the putative author of the *Corpus Hippocraticum*. Upon graduation from medical school, many modern physicians continue to take the Hippocratic Oath, the model of the ideal physician. Many historians question whether Hippocrates actually wrote this oath or even the essays attributed to him. Some even question whether Hippocrates was a real person or was a composite created later by Greek and Roman scholars. Nonetheless, even in antiquity, there were rules, policies, and regulations on how to behave as a physician.

After Hippocrates, Galen is probably the next most famous physician in history. His works and texts continued to be studied by medical students and scholars for hundreds of years after his death. When Galen ventured to Rome in 161 AD., he was met with hostility by the medical establishment. For 5 years, he was able to continue to practice medicine, lecture, and conduct public discussions under the protection of the powerful Emperor Marcus Aurelius who named him the "first of physicians and philosophers."[17] Eventually, Galen returned to Greece complaining that he had been driven out of Rome by the medical establishment who saw him as an interloper. Galen did subsequently return to Rome honoring a request from Marcus Aurelius. He remained there for the rest of his life.

(Continued)

BOX 1.2 (*Continued*): Regulation of medical practice since antiquity

MODERN REGULATIONS AND PROCEDURES FOR
LICENSING PHYSICIANS

The modern rules, policies, and regulations governing the practice of medicine today are well established. In most jurisdictions—the United States, Canada, Europe—like the Code of Hammurabi, regulations govern nearly every aspect of the patient–physician relationship, clinical guidelines, best practices, evidence-based medicine, fees, collegiality, and so forth. In the United States, for example, a number of organizations, such as the American Board of Internal Medicine (ABIM), American Board of Medical Specialties (ABMS), and the state licensing authorities (e.g. Medical Board of California), as well as doctor organizations such as the American Medical Association (AMA), are all involved in governing the assessment, licensing, and behavior of physicians.

Nearly all jurisdictions in the world nowadays require physicians to be university educated and earn an MD (medical doctor degree) or other approved degrees (e.g., MBBS, MBChB). In many jurisdictions, students who have earned a medical degree are required to undergo further postgraduate supervised clinical training. In the United States and Canada, this is called residency, also called a house officer or senior house officer in the United Kingdom and several Commonwealth countries. Depending on the medical specialty and jurisdiction, residency can be 1–6 years in duration. Once a doctor has passed all relevant examinations and qualifying procedures, the physician may be granted a license in a specified jurisdiction to practice medicine without direct supervision.

TRADITIONAL METHODS OF TESTING

In the United States, written tests to assess students were not generally used until Horace Mann introduced them in 1845. This was seen as a radical and controversial innovation when American educators adopted them in the late 1800s. Testing quickly became an important element in America's modern public school system as well as in postsecondary education including medical schools.

THE FLEXNER REPORT

In 1910, Abraham Flexner produced the now famous Flexner Report, *Medical Education in the United States and Canada: A Report to the Carnegie Foundation for the Advancement of Teaching* that was commissioned by the Carnegie Foundation.[18] At that time, there were approximately 157 medical schools that

BOX 1.3: History of licensure and regulation in the United States

Timeline of Medical Licensure and Regulation: Adapted from AM Last Page: History of Medical Licensure and Regulation, David Johnson and Amy Gerald, Federation of State Medical Boards, *Academic Medicine*: 2014; 89: 953 doi: 10.1097/ACM.000000000000260

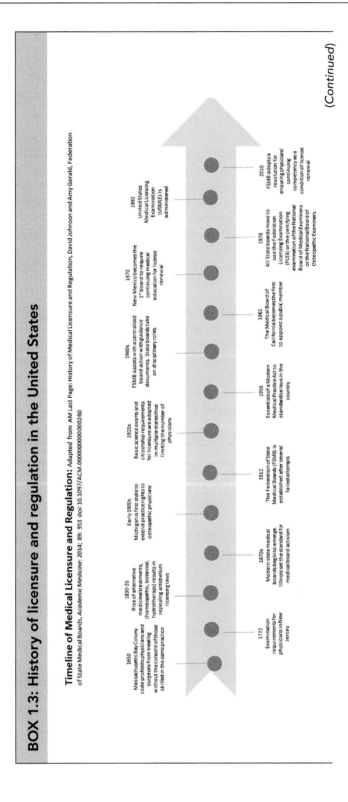

1650
Massachusetts Bay Colony code prohibits physicians and surgeons from treating without the consent of those skilled in the same practice

1830-35
Rise of alternative medicinal treatments, (homeopathic, botanical, hydrotherapy) results in repealing antebellum licensing laws

Early 1900s
Michigan is first state to extend practice rights to osteopathic physicians

1920s
Basic science exams and citizenship requirements for licensure are adopted in multiple states thus limiting the number of physicians

1960s
FSMB assists with a centralized board action with guidance documents. State boards take on disciplinary roles

1970
New Mexico becomes the 1st board to require continuing medical education for license renewal

1992
United States Medical Licensing Examination (USMLE) is administered

1772
Examination requirements for physicians in New Jersey

1870s
Modern state medical boards begin to emerge. Illinois set the standard for medical board activism

1912
The Federation of State Medical Boards (FSMB) is established after several failed attempts

1955
Essentials of a Modern Medical Practice Act to standardize laws in the country

1961
The Medical Board of California becomes the first to appoint a public member

1978
All State boards move to use the Federation Licensing Examination (FLEX) or the certifying examination of the National Board of Medical Examiners or the National Board of Osteopathic Examiners.

2010
FSMB adopts a resolution for ensuring physicians' continuing competency as a condition of license renewal

(Continued)

BOX 1.3 (*Continued*): History of licensure and regulation in the United States

Flexner provided a review of medical education and medical institutions and reviewed the economic and social factors that had an impact on the delivery of medicine of that era. He concluded that the situation was untenable and that medical education needed to be radically transformed. Today, with a few rare exceptions, medical school organization in the United States and Canada consists of four years, the first two preclinical or laboratory sciences consisting of foundational knowledge in anatomy, physiology, pharmacology, and pathology, followed by 2 years of clinical sciences experiences. The Flexner Report also contained arguments for evidence-based and scientific-based medicine. It has had an impact on the medical school admissions process, the learning environment, the qualifications and expectations of medical teachers, and the need for standardized licensure exams. The Flexner Report has been pivotal to most of modern medical education including the development of standardized testing and assessment in medicine.

Meanwhile, developments in large-scale standardized testing were taking place in Europe and the United States largely as a consequence of World War I. Large-scale testing in Germany for army inductees had been in progress since 1905. Alfred Binet and Theodore Simon had discussed the application intelligence testing for the French army in 1910. In the United States, Lewis Terman had completed the revision and standardization of the Binet scales in 1917, and these principles of mass testing were soon applied to the American military effort resulting in the Army Alpha and Beta Tests of intelligence. Nearly 2 million recruits were tested with these instruments before the end of World War I.[19] This testing was seen as so successful that, after the war, large-scale standardized testing swept the American school systems. The major types of test used throughout the 20th century were pencil-and-paper multiple-choice questions (MCQs).

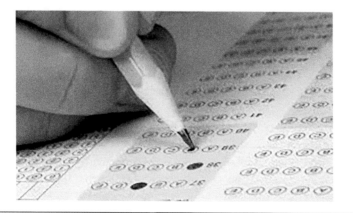

were loosely affiliated with educational institutions, and the education of physicians was primarily a for-profit business. The knowledge and skills of the graduating physicians was highly variable, resulting in an over-production of poorly educated medical practitioners.

STATISTICAL AND MATHEMATICAL THEORIES

Another important development that underlay this widespread testing was the development of modern statistics. The large databases that were generated from this prodigious testing required improvements in statistical methods. Beginning in the late 19th century, there were a series of statistical and mathematical initiatives. The major contributors to the field have been Sir Francis Galton (polymath, correlation), Sir Ronald Fisher (analysis of variance), Karl Pearson (mathematical statistics, correlation), Charles Spearman (measurement of intelligence, factor analysis), EL Thorndike (educational measurement), Fredrick Kuder (reliability), Lee J Cronbach (reliability, generalizability theory), George Rasch (item response theory), Fredric M Lord (item response theory), Karl Joreskog (confirmatory factor analysis), Peter Bentler (structural equation modelling), and many others.

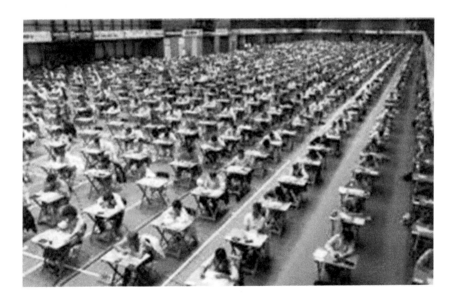

Group-administered final exams

TEST THEORY

There are three major interrelated test theories today: (1) classical test theory (CTT), (2) generalizability theory (G-theory), and (3) item response theory (IRT). All three theories are fundamental to the field of psychometrics: the theory and technique of psychological and educational measurement. This includes the objective measurement of attitudes, personality traits, skills and knowledge, abilities, and educational achievement. Psychometric researchers focus on the construction and validation of assessment instruments such as questionnaires, tests, raters' judgments, and personality tests as well as statistical research relevant to the measurement theories.

CTT is so-called because it was developed first in psychometrics. The premise is simple: any observed score (e.g., a test score) is composed of the "real" score or true score plus error of measurement: X (Observed score) = T (True score) + e (error of measurement). The early foundational work of scholars like Karl Pearson, Charles Spearman, EL Thorndike, and Fredrick Kuder was based on this idea.

G-theory was developed by Cronbach et al.[20] as an advance over CTT. In CTT, each observed score has a single true score and has a single source of error of measurement. G-theory is a statistical framework for conceptualizing and investigating multiple sources of variability in measurement. An advantage of G-theory is that researchers can estimate what proportion of the variation in test scores is due to factors that often vary in assessment, such as raters, setting, time, and items. Anyone who has watched Olympic diving has observed the effect of different sources of variance: the divers' scores vary based on particular differences in performance, by the different raters (judges), and the items (components of the dive). The variation in scores, therefore, comes from multiple sources. In healthcare assessment, the same situation obtains when the student performs skills which are rated by two or more judges or raters. Both CTT and G-theory continue to play a role in testing and measurement. Both of these theories and their applications will be discussed in subsequent chapters (Chapters 8 and 9).

The third major theory, IRT, is also known as latent trait theory. Like CTT and G-theory, it can be used for the design, analysis, and scoring of tests, questionnaires, and assessments measuring abilities, attitudes, or other variables. IRT is based on mathematical modelling of candidates' response to questions or test items in contrast to the test-level focus of CTT and G-theory. This model is widely used with MCQs (that are scored right or wrong) but can also be used on a rating scale, patient symptoms (scored present or absent), or diagnostic information in disease.

In IRT, it is assumed that the probability of a response to an item is a mathematical function of the person and item characteristics. The person is conceptualized as a latent trait such as aptitude, achievement, extraversion, and sociability. The item characteristics consist of difficulty, discrimination (how they distinguish between people), and guessing (e.g., on multiple-choice items). All three psychometric theories—CTT, G-theory, and IRT—have their relative advantages and disadvantages and will be further discussed in later chapters (Chapters 8 and 9).

COMPUTERS

The advent of computers has played a large role in the expansion and evolution of testing in the last 60 or so years. Many of the complex statistical techniques that have been applied to testing, such as correlational and factor analysis and test theories like IRT have only been possible with the use of computers. As large mainframe computers became commonplace in universities and some other institutions during the 1960s, large databases from testing programs could be stored and the data analyzed with software programs. At the same time, software programs that could be installed into the computers also became available. Prior to this, users had to write their own software from scratch. Data could be entered into the computers (e.g., with punch cards, optical scanning sheets, bubble sheets, keyboards) and analyzed, and reports generated for individual test-takers. By the 1980s, optical reading scanning machines (reading bubble sheets marked with pencils) had been more-or-less perfected and matched to desktop computers. Large numbers of bubble sheets (e.g., 1,000) can be quickly and efficiently entered into a desktop computer where sophisticated software can quickly analyze the test results and produce individual reports and psychometric results of the test.

The next evolutionary step that began in the 1990s was the elimination of pencil-and-paper (i.e., bubble sheets) so that students could take a test directly on a computer. This is called computer-based testing (CBT). The main advantage of CBT historically has been for report generation and quick feedback. With the advent of the personal computer, CBT functions primarily for the computer-administered versions of paper-and-pencil tests. These provided some advantages over paper-and-pencil in test administration and item innovation. Some disadvantages include the need for latest hardware and software and large test centers to accommodate large group testing.

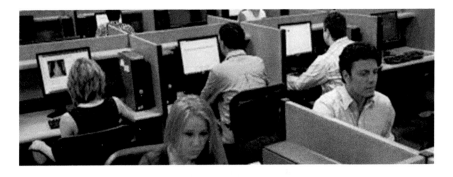

Taking the USMLE, Step 1

CBT can be innovative allowing flexible scoring of items. Test items can use sound or video to create multimedia items. An item may contain a 40-s video and audio sequence of a doctor performing a focused physical exam on the left lower quadrant of the abdomen for example. This can be followed by a series of MCQs to the student. Content innovation also relates to the use of dynamic item types such as drag-and-drop, point-and-click, or hovering over hot-spots. Future developments in CBT are likely to focus on item innovation that measure complex cognitive outcomes such as clinical judgment and professionalism.

ONLINE TESTING

Online testing refers to the delivery of tests via the internet. This approach also provides a new medium for distribution of test materials, reports, and practice manuals and also for the automated collection of data. Even traditional paper-and-pencil materials can be delivered online as PDF format files using e-book publishing technologies. Theoretically, anyone with an internet connection could take a test at anytime from anywhere in the world. Such an approach provides much more flexibility in testing than has been possible in the past. Online testing highlights a whole set of issues: confidentiality, cheating, test-taker identification, hacking, breaching the test bank, and so on.

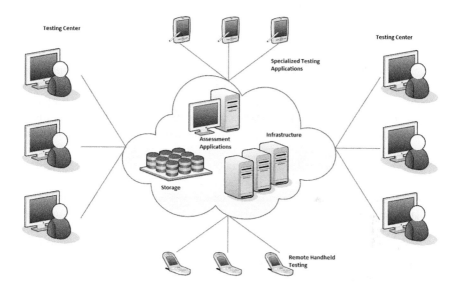

CURRENT STATUS OF TESTING

The current status of testing is paradoxical. On the one hand, rapid advances in computer technology, statistics, and test theory have brought impressive new capabilities to assessment of learning and performance. On the other hand, most classroom testing is still very primitive. In education in general, there are probably 500 million or so tests given in the United States in classrooms every year, the vast majority would not meet even minimal standards of appropriate tests. How can this be?

The main reason for the poor quality of tests in most classrooms is that teachers have little knowledge of basic educational measurement or test construction principles. Teachers (including professors) receive almost no education whatsoever in these theories and practices in their university programs. In the United States, most of the 50 states require no explicit training in measurement and assessment as part of teacher certification. Most states simply require completion of an accredited teacher education program. A majority of teacher education programs, however, have neither a compulsory nor an optional course in educational measurement and assessment. Indeed, many programs have no course offering in these areas at all. Most American teachers have no education in this subject.

For those that teach in post-secondary institutions and medical schools (i.e., instructors, professors) the situation is even worse. Not only do the instructors, clinical teachers, and professors have no education in testing and assessment, they have no instruction of basic pedagogical principles or learning theories. The situation is similar throughout most of the world.

There is a further irony to the situation. While as we have seen testing is on the increase and teachers, instructors, and professors as well as university administrators know little about it, the general public is very much in favor of increased testing in schools[21] including post-secondary institutions. A majority (>80%) of the American public is in favor of using standardized testing in their community for core subjects (English, Math, Science, History, and Geography), favor it for problem-solving skills, and favor it for the ability to write. Finally, more than half of Americans are in favor of having students repeat their grade based solely on standardized national achievement test performance. To sum up the current situation in the educational institutions, then, the public overwhelmingly supports testing, as does the current political climate, but most teachers who are the primary constructors and administrators of tests know little about appropriate testing practices and standards. The situation is similar in post-secondary education, including medical schools. Testing and assessment is likely to increase in the future, but most instructors and professors know little about appropriate testing practice and standards.

The demands of assessment are currently rigorous and are likely to become even more so. Professors and instructors may spend as much as 20% or 30% of their professional educational time in assessment-related activities. These include designing, developing, selecting, administering, scoring, recording, evaluating and revising tests, and assignments. Healthcare instructors, professors, and medical education leaders such as ES Holmboe, DS Ward, RK Reznick, and others[22] are very concerned about the quality of tests and measurements and lack confidence in them.

Currently, medical education is under pressure to adopt competency-based approaches that emphasize outcomes. This shift in emphasis requires more effective evaluation and feedback by professors and instructors than is currently the case. The existing faculty is not fully prepared for this task for traditional competencies of medical knowledge, clinical skills, and professionalism, never mind for the newer competencies of interdisciplinary teamwork, quality improvement, evidence-based practice, and systems. Medical and healthcare faculty welcomes relevant and useful training or assistance in measurement and assessment, but they feel frustrated by their lack of training and support.[19]

THE ROLE OF ASSESSMENT IN TEACHING, LEARNING, AND EDUCATION

There are essentially four categories in which testing and assessment play a role: (1) teaching and learning, (2) program evaluation and research, (3) guidance and counselling, and (4) administration. While these are interrelated and test results can be used in several categories, they are described in turn.

Teaching and learning

All teaching has some goal or objective as its purpose. The objective may be implicit or explicit (see Chapter 10 for a discussion of objectives). Teaching, then, is for the purpose of having students reach some intended learning outcome (objective). The only sound means by which a teacher can determine the extent to which students have achieved the objectives is to assess performance. The outcome of the testing, therefore, is an evaluation of not only student performance but the effectiveness of the teaching itself as well. A main function of testing is to measure the extent to which the instructional objectives have been met.

Here are some examples of learning objectives that can be measured by testing or assessment, including direct observation with a checklist:

1. The student will be able to describe in writing the interaction of tRNA and mRNA in protein synthesis.
2. At the conclusion of the neurology course, students can write a cost-effective approach to the initial evaluation and management of patients with dementia.
3. At the conclusion of internal medicine clerkship, third-year medical students will be proficient in the diagnosis and management of hyperlipidemia, hypertension, diabetes, chronic obstructive pulmonary disease, angina, and asymptomatic HIV.
4. Student nurses will demonstrate proper handwashing technique prior to changing a dressing on a patient.

Tests also have a number of other functions in teaching and learning.

MOTIVATION AND ENGAGEMENT

Tests motivate students to work and study harder than they might otherwise. With the many demands made on medical students and other healthcare students, tests can motivate students to set a high priority on material that will be tested. Also, frequent short testing will motivate students to sustain a consistently higher effort than long-term infrequent tests. Few things can motivate students to read a scientific article, a chapter, or a whole textbook as a forthcoming test can. Any technique that teachers can use to motivate students is desirable.

In a recent study, researchers were able to definitively demonstrate the impact of testing on medical student effort. Employing an online curriculum system by first-year medical students, researchers were able track activities through logons, amount of time engaged, and areas and content of use.[23] As illustrated in Figure 1.1, the data on Digital-Space (D-Space) use is summarized on a weekly basis for 114 first-year medical students. The dates for the seven first-year course examinations are also indicated on the figure with drop-down arrows and identified by a corresponding course name.

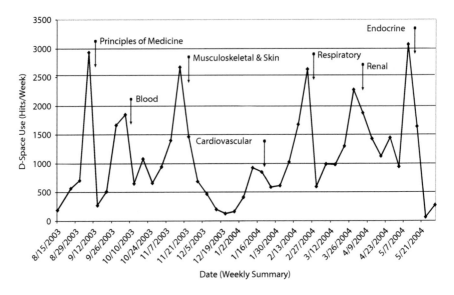

Figure 1.1 Summary of 2003/2004 D-Space use and course examination schedule for the class of 2006 first-year medical students.

As is depicted by the fluctuations in the use of course materials and resources online, the medical students as a class show a dramatic increase in academic engaged time 1 or 2 weeks before a scheduled examination. In preparation for the "Principles of Medicine" course examination, for example, students in the week ending September 8 recorded a total of 531 D-Space hits. In the week ending September 15, the day of the scheduled examination, the students' recorded an over five-fold increase in D-Space usage at 2,865 hits. The week that followed the course examination, the students' use dropped ten-fold to a baseline low of 238 hits. This similar pattern of online use of course materials and resources is repeated both on an individual student basis and for the class as a whole throughout the year. The same pattern of academic engaged time seen for "Principles of Medicine" was obtained for all seven of the scheduled course examinations. In particular, the frequency of D-Space use based on the number of recorded hits the weeks just before and after a course examination varied from two- to ten-fold. Student effort, motivation, and academic engaged time are determined by the examinations and engagement peaks just prior to the examinations and drops to near zero just after the examination.

ENHANCE LEARNING

Increasing student motivation to work and academic engagement will also increase their learning. When students anticipate a forthcoming test, they will attend to material more closely, increase their study time, and work harder to learn the relevant material than they otherwise would. Also the anticipation of a test improves students' learning set so that they increase their memory capacities for the material (through rehearsal, elaboration, organization). Students will make a conscious effort to improve their knowledge and understanding of material when they anticipate a test as opposed to when they do not.

Testing also promotes overlearning which occurs when you systematically study and prepare for a test. Of course some of the material learned for the test will be forgotten afterwards (hence the term overlearning) but more material will be retained in the longrun than if overlearning had not occurred. This "forgotten" material is much easier to recall or relearn even years later than if it had to be acquired without prior knowledge. Thus, testing promotes not only learning in the immediate future but results in longer more stable learning as well.

FEEDBACK

Test scores provide feedback for both the faculty and student. The professor can evaluate the efficacy of instruction based on the students' performance. If, for example, no student in the class was able to correctly diagnose endometriosis on a case presented on the test, then the professor can conclude that his teaching of clinical presentation of endometriosis failed. Similarly, if students are unable to describe the interaction of tRNA and mRNA in protein synthesis on a test, this indicates that the teaching of this material failed. These outcomes also indicate the need for review of this material.

Feedback can also be provided directly to the student. Based on performance, the student can evaluate progress as a whole or in specific sub-areas measured by the test. If in the class presented in Figure 1.1, a student performed well on six of the tests but scored poorly on "Endocrine," this is clear and diagnostic information to the student. Upon a closer look, the student discovered that he did particularly poorly on the reproductive sections of "Endocrine," this provides even more precise diagnosis of learning required. This information can also provide insights for the student about effort. The test may indicate that effort had been adequate or that it may have to be increased.

TEACHING

Giving a test itself is a form of teaching. Students may learn substantially merely from writing a test, since they will have to formulate answers to questions. In a study, Foos and Fisher[24] gave students a short essay about the American Civil War to read. Half of the students were then given an initial test and half were not. Two days later, all the students took a final common exam: those students who took the initial test generally did better than those who did not. It may very well be that the act of retrieving the information for the original test may have altered and strengthened it. In the Foos and Fisher study, then, actually taking the initial test may have taught the students about the Civil War. This is called the "forward effect of testing."

These findings can be applied in medical courses as well.[25] A professor may give a test in obstetrics and gynecology two weeks before the final exam. The main purpose of this test is to help students learn and organize the material as they will need to formulate answers to the test. A secondary purpose of the test is to provide feedback to the students on their current performance before the final exam. Taking the test will teach students about obstetrics and gynecology, capitalizing on the forward effect of testing.

Program evaluation and research

Tests can also be useful to evaluate educational programs and to conduct basic research. One of the most widely evaluated and researched educational programs in medicine is problem-based learning (PBL) approaches. PBL generally consists of the following characteristics[26]: (1) medical problems (e.g., case presentation of acute abdominal pain in a 28-year-old woman) are used as a trigger for learning, (2) lectures are used sparingly, (3) learning is facilitated by a tutor, (4) learning is student initiated, (5) students collaborate in small groups for part of the time, and (6) the curriculum includes ample time for self-study.

Many of the program evaluation studies have used test data (e.g., course examinations in pediatrics, USMLE Step 1, etc.) to compare performance between students in PBL versus those in more conventional curricula (e.g., lectures focused on systems). These curriculum comparison studies have been reviewed extensively over the past 25 years with mixed results: sometimes students in PBL curricula outperform comparison groups in conventional curricula and sometimes they do not.

Schmidt et al.[26] went beyond simple program evaluation to some basic theoretical aspects of PBL from a careful review of the PBL findings. They concluded that PBL works. This is because it encourages the activation of prior knowledge in the small-group setting and provides opportunities for elaboration on that knowledge. Activation of prior knowledge results in the understanding of new information related to the problem and facilitates transfer to long-term memory. Real problems (e.g., myocardial infarction) as presented in PBL arouse interest that motivates learning. Skilled tutors permit flexibility in cognitive organization compared to rigid structures in worksheets or questions added to problems. Although initially students do not study much beyond the learning issues required, the self-study focus increases the development of self-directed learning. The extent of learning in PBL results come from both group collaboration and individual knowledge acquisition.

In another evaluation study, researchers[27] studied the relationship between basic biomedical knowledge and clinical reasoning outcome in a clinical presentation curriculum. They hypothesized a model of medical students' knowledge as a function of their aptitude for medical school, basic science achievement, and clinical competency. A variety of models through an explicit representation of a distinct number of observed and latent variables were tested using sophisticated statistical application—structural equation modelling—that allows researchers to test the goodness-of-fit of various models. The models included the knowledge encapsulation theory and the emphasis on clinical knowledge. Consideration was given to an alternative model that includes both the basic science knowledge and clinical knowledge components as contributing independently to the diagnostic or clinical reasoning skills (CRS) of medical students.

Test data were collected from a total of 589 students (292 males, 49.6%; 297 females, 50.4%) who completed medical school. The data consisted of the following medical students' aptitude, achievement, and performance measures: (1) the MCAT subtests (verbal reasoning [VR], biological sciences [BS], physical sciences [PS], and writing sample [WS])*; (2) undergraduate grade point Average (UGPA) at admission; (3) basic science achievement in the first 2 years of medical school (Y1, Y2); (4) clinical performance in the medical school's single clerkship year (Y3); and (5) the Medical Council of Canada's (MCC) Part I test, which consists of a seven-section, 196 multiple-choice question (MCQ) examination on declarative knowledge (e.g., medicine, pediatrics, psychiatry), and an approximately 60-case or 80-item CRS test designed to assess problem-solving and clinical decision-making abilities.

Figure 1.2 shows the final three latent variable model with respective parameter estimates and goodness-of-fit index values for CFI, SRMR, and RMSEA (Chapter 7, pp. 164–172). In this maximum likelihood model fit, the theoretical structure of the model is supported with the existence of covariance between the aptitude for medical school and basic science achievement latent variables. In this model, the combination rules of cutoff score values are achieved for the CFI at .905 and are close to the criteria set for robustness and non-robustness conditions with $n > 250$ and values of SRMR at .054 and RMSEA at .105. In comparison, the test values obtained for the knowledge encapsulation and emphasis on clinical knowledge

Model: CFI = .905, SRMR = .054, RMSEA = .105

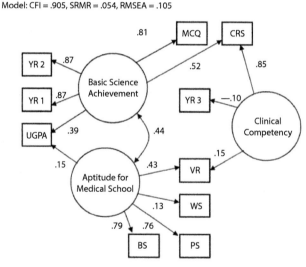

VR = Verbal Reasoning, BS = Biological Sciences, PS = Physical Sciences, WS = Writing Sample
UGPA = Undergraduate Grade Point Average, YR 1 = Year 1, YR 2 = Year 2, YR 3 = Year 3,
MCQ = MCC Part I: Multiple-Choice Question Exam, CRS = MCC Part I: Clinical Reasoning Skills Exam

☐ measured/observed variables   ⟶ paths with coefficient

◯ latent variables   ⌒ correlation coefficient

Figure 1.2 A model of relationship between basic science achievement, aptitude for medical school, and clinical competency.

* A new version of the MCAT (2015) has been implemented since this research was conducted. This is discussed in detail in Chapter 5.

models were found to be less than the minimum 0.90 cutoff CFI values at 0.81 and 0.82, respectively.

The clinical competency latent variable was found to have a large path coefficient value of .85, accounting for 72% of the variance, with the MCC Part I—CRS subtest. The MCAT–VR subtest has a small positive (.15) path coefficient on the clinical competency latent variable and may reflect the importance of verbal proficiency in the clerkship year. The Y3 variable, however, has a small negative (–.10) path coefficient on the clinical competency latent variable that may demonstrate the variability of clinical performance measures obtained from medical students during their different clerkship rotations. As anticipated, the aptitude for medical school latent variable is related to the MCAT subtest and UGPA proximal measures obtained at the beginning of students' medical school experience.

These findings support an integrated medical school curriculum that would nurture the inherent connection between the basic sciences and clinical competency in the further development of CRS in medical students. The results of this program evaluation and research study, therefore, have implications for curriculum design and delivery in developing medical reasoning skills. With this study, then, the researchers were able to not only make an evaluation of the effects of curriculum content but to explore a basic research problem as well.

Administration monitoring

Administrative decisions about education from university administrators to government officials can be informed and improved by test results. Standardized test results such as the USMLE data, for example, might be used by a dean to monitor the medical school's overall performance and take appropriate action if any is required. Suppose that such results indicated that the students in a given medical school were performing poorly in renal compared to other similar schools and relative to their own performance in cardiology, this might suggest to the dean a need for a revamping of the renal curriculum. Similarly, associations of medical schools might monitor the whole country's performance. A national picture may be provided with test data that shows inadequate knowledge of anatomy of beginning physicians. This might suggest the need for administrative action in educational policy on a national scale.

CURRICULUM DECISIONS

Results on a standardized basic skills test (such as the Medical Council of Canada Examinations—MCCE) might show that students in a medical school are achieving better scores with basic science curriculum A (e.g., PBL) than other students with basic science curriculum B (e.g., systems). The administration and faculty of the medical school may decide to adopt curriculum A as a standard. A dean of a medical school may discover that students who take an elective advanced clinical skills course score 15 points higher on the MCCE than students who do not take the course. She might decide to expand the course offering thereby providing other students this advantage on the MCCE.

SELECTION AND SCREENING

Tests are used to improve selection and screening decisions. Selection decisions for programs for the gifted are frequently made on the basis of test data (e.g. IQ and achievement). Screening for admission to college can be based, at least in part, on the Scholastic Achievement Test (SAT), for medical school on the Medical College Admission Test (MCAT), and for law school on the Law School Admission Test (LSAT). Similarly, the Graduate Record Entrance exam (GRE) is used by many universities to select for graduate school.

GUIDANCE AND COUNSELLING

Test scores have long been used in clinical psychology and school guidance to help improve decisions. Results from intelligence, personality, interest, aptitude, and achievement tests can be used by a guidance counsellor to help students make the best decisions about their future schooling, career, and work. In medical school, test data can help counselling for the selection of a medical specialty.

Test and assessment information can also help psychologists and psychiatrists to provide the best possible care for their clients and patients. Test scores alone, however, should never be used to make guidance and counselling decisions. Rather these should be used by the professional to assist in making the best possible decision.

CERTIFICATION AND LICENSING

Nearly all professional organizations (physicians, lawyers, accountants, optometrists, nurses, etc.) and many other groups as well have formal certification and licensing procedures involving tests. Thus, to be eligible to practice as a physician, lawyer, dentist, and psychologist, to name a few, you must write and pass certification exams. In the health professions, it is also common practice to assess practical clinical skills such as conducting a physical exam, taking a patient history, procedural skills, and so forth using standardized objective structured clinical exams (OSCEs). Many organizations have moved to or are moving toward implementing certification and licensing exams utilizing written, CBT, and OSCEs as a means of determining the competency of their licensees. This is likely to expand and increase in the future.

WORKPLACE-BASED ASSESSMENTS

Many health professionals now undergo assessment in the workplace when they are in professional practice. A common assessment is multisource feedback (MSF), also referred to as "360° evaluation." This has emerged as an important approach for assessing professional competence, behaviors, and attitudes in the workplace. Early attempts to develop MSF questionnaires in medicine focused on the assessment of residents in the late 1970s. Today, MSF tools are being used in the United States, Canada, and Europe (in the Netherlands and the United Kingdom) across a number of physician specialties. Typically, this feedback is collected using surveys or questionnaires designed to collect data from various respondents (e.g., peers, coworkers, patients) including the healthcare professional in corresponding self-assessments of the measurement instrument. MSF has gained widespread acceptance for evaluation of professionals and is seen as a catalyst for the practitioner to reflect on where change may be required.[28]

MSF originated in industry because the reliance on a single supervisor's evaluation was considered an inadequate approach to the assessment of a worker's specific abilities. Similarly, physicians work with a variety of people (e.g., medical colleagues, consultants, therapists, nurses, coworkers) who are able to provide a better assessment and contextually based understanding of physician performance than any single person could. In MSF, physicians may complete a self-assessment instrument and receive feedback from a number of medical colleagues, non-physician coworkers (e.g., nurses, psychologists, pharmacists), as well as their own patients. Different respondents focus on characteristics of the physician that they can assess (e.g., patients are not expected to assess a physician's clinical expertise) and together provide a more comprehensive evaluation than what could be derived by any one source alone.

MSF is gaining acceptance and credibility as a means of providing doctors with relevant information about their practice to help them monitor, develop, maintain, and improve their competence. The assessment focuses on clinical skills, communication, collaboration with other healthcare professionals, professionalism, and patient management. This assessment system is a means of maintaining and improving physician competence through systematic feedback.

TYPES OF TESTS AND EVALUATION PROCEDURES

Tests and evaluation procedures are frequently classified into one or more categories. Following are some of the most commonly used categories of test types.

1. **Individual or group administered**. Some tests, like psychological ones such as IQ, or performance medical skills tests (e.g., phlebotomy), must be individually administered. Many educational tests, however, can be administered to a group ranging from a typical classroom to many hundreds of students simultaneously. Almost all medical or healthcare classroom tests are of the group type.
2. **Teacher-made or standardized tests**. Sometimes these tests are also referred to as informal (teacher-made) or formal (standardized tests). Teacher-made tests are obviously constructed by the teacher to measure some specific aspect of achievement (e.g. pathology, anatomy, biochemistry, pediatrics, obstetrics/gynecology) relevant to that course. This test will likely be administered once only to this group of students. Standardized tests, on the other hand, are constructed by testing experts usually to measure some broad range of aptitude or achievement relevant to many medical or other healthcare students. Unlike teacher-made tests, the standardized test is

not designed for one specific course or indeed healthcare school. They are intended to be used (and re-used) in broader jurisdictions such as state-wide (e.g., board certification exams) or perhaps even used nationally (USMLE step exams) or internationally (e.g., MCAT). Moreover, these tests are administered in formal situations according to standardized conditions. Finally, these formal tests have known statistical properties (frequently referred to as psychometric properties), since they have been administered in advance to a peer group of those who will write the test.

3. **Speed or power tests.** Speeded tests obviously have time constraints on completing them. All test-takers are given a fixed amount of time designed so that many or most writers will not be able to complete the test in the allotted time. Power tests, on the other hand, do not have time as a significant constraint. While of course there is some upper limit on the time available, most test-takers can complete the test in the allotted time. Most course tests are power tests where time should not be a significant factor in performance. Tests should only be speeded, if speed of response is a significant element in the dimension measured by the test. For most courses, the professor is not so much interested in students' speed of response but rather the accuracy and depth of response when adequate time is provided.

4. **Supply or selection tests.** Supply or selection refers to the type of items that make up the test. Selection items are those where students or candidates must select a correct answer from several options (e.g. multiple-choice items). For supply items, the student must provide or supply the answer or responses to a question or instructions (e.g. short-answer items). The selection item provides a much more structured task for the test-taker than does the supply item, especially for essay questions. Since for supply items the student must provide the answer, skills such as organization, writing, fluency, and so forth play a prominent role. Supply items are also called constructed-response items, and selection items are called forced choice-items.

5. **Objective or subjective tests.** This distinction refers to how the test is scored and graded and not to the item types. Objective tests are scored objectively by anyone in possession of the key or answer sheet. Indeed, machines (optical scanners or software programs) can score these tests. For subjective tests, only an expert in the subject matter can score these tests, as expert judgment is required to evaluate the constructed answer. Selection items can be generally scored objectively. The objective-subjective refers to the nature of the scoring process.

6. **Norm-referenced or criterion-referenced tests.** Another important way to classify tests is based on how the results are interpreted on norm group performance or against some criterion. For norm-referenced tests, an individual's performance is evaluated against the performance of a norm (peer) group. A professor may interpret a student's physiology test score with reference to the rest of the class, even perhaps using class rank. It may be below average, above average, or about average. For criterion-referenced tests, however, the norm group performance is irrelevant. Rather, a criterion for "passing" or "mastery" performance is established before the test is written

or the skill is performed. Irrespective of the norm groups' performance, an individuals' score is evaluated against this standard, frequently called a cutoff score.

Some standardized tests used in American and Canadian university and healthcare assessment are norm-referenced. The GRE and the MCAT are two tests of this type. The GRE consists of major sections measuring verbal and quantitative skills. Taking the GRE is required for entry to many, but not all, university graduate school in the United States and Canada.

Criterion-referenced tests are widely used more for licensure testing by boards of professional organizations. The USMLE step tests, the Medical Council of Canada exams, and medical licensing exams in Britain are all examples of criterion-referenced tests. To establish minimum performance levels (MPLs) for these tests (cutoff scores) usually requires a complex series of decisions by subject-matter experts with the help of testing experts. While the idea of criterion-referenced measurement is appealing, its use has remained narrow largely because of the theoretical and practical difficulties of establishing standards. The test for acquiring a driver's license is an example of a common criterion-referenced test.

Another set of terms that are used synonymously with criterion-referenced and norm-referenced are mastery tests in contrast to survey tests. For mastery tests, the candidate must exceed some pre-established standard (criterion) to have achieved mastery. By contrast, for the survey test, there is a survey of the candidates' knowledge, but mastery is not evaluated against some standard.

7. **Achievement, intelligence, and personality tests**. Achievement tests attempt to measure the extent to which a student has "achieved" in some subject matter or on some skill. This achievement is thought to represent the level of learning due to motivation, effort, interest, and work habits. A typical test in a cardiovascular course is an example of an achievement test. Intelligence may play a part in the outcome.

Intelligence or aptitude is thought to be the potential for learning or "achieving." The actualization of this potential is achievement itself. Intelligence or this potential for learning is usually measured by IQ tests such as the Wechsler Adult Intelligence Scale and aptitude for medicine is measured by the MCAT.

A personality test measures that aspect of a person's psychological makeup which is not intellectual. Generally, these tests seek to measure the level of a person's adjustment, attitudes, feelings, or specific traits like introversion, sociability, and anxiety. Sometimes personality tests, like the Minnesota Multiphasic Personality Inventory, are used for clinical diagnoses to assess the degree of neuroses or psychosis of an individual.

Researchers have studied personality on medical student selection and performance. One test that has been used for this purpose is the NEO-PI, which is referred to as the Big Five personality inventory, measuring five broad traits, domains or dimensions that are used to describe human personality. These are neuroticism (N), extraversion (E), openness (O), conscientiousness (C), and agreeableness (A). Conscientiousness has been found to be a predictor of performance in medical school and becomes increasingly significant as students and residents advance through medical training. Other traits concerning sociability (i.e. extraversion, openness, and neuroticism) have also been found to be relevant for performance and adaptation in the medical environment.[29] The traits of neuroticism and conscientiousness are related to stress in medical school: low extroversion, high neuroticism, and high conscientiousness results in highly stressed students (*brooders*), while high extroversion, low neuroticism, and low conscientiousness produce low-stressed students (*hedonists*).[30]

8. **Summative, formative, placement, and diagnostic evaluation.** Each of these types of evaluation refers to the use of the test results.

   Summative. This is a "summing up" of all assessments and measurements in order to determine final performance. Assigning the letter grade (A, B…F) or the final percentage value (e.g., 73.4%) is a form of summative evaluation.

   Formative. This is monitoring the situation. During the course of instruction, the professor wishes to monitor if students are moving toward the final objectives so as to take appropriate action. This usually involves quizzes, mid-term tests, etc.

   Placement. Sometimes, it is necessary to determine wherein the educational sequence the student (e.g., advanced, remedial, etc.) should be placed. Professors and administrators may be uncertain, for example, in where to place a student who has failed a clinical rotation or clerkship. Should the student continue on to the next year while remediation is undertaken or should the student be held back until the clinical rotation is redone and passed? Placement evaluation might be conducted using previous records, test data, and interviews to make this decision.

   Diagnostic. When students have persistent learning problems, it may be necessary to diagnose the problem. Psychological, medical, and educational data are frequently necessary to make a diagnostic evaluation. Does the student have visual or hearing impairments? Does the student have any learning disabilities?

THE ORGANIZATION OF THIS TEXTBOOK

This is a comprehensive textbook on how to assess competence in medicine, medical education, and healthcare throughout the clinicians' career. This textbook is organized into three main sections: (1) Foundations, (2) Validity and reliability, and (3) Test construction and evaluation, consisting of a total of 16 chapters.

Foundations

The Foundations section consists of four chapters. Chapter 1, of course, is the introduction that introduces the need for testing and assessment, deals with questions of "what are testing, assessment, measurement, and evaluation?", provides a brief history of testing, describes the common types of tests and assessments, and summarizes the uses of tests.

In Chapter 2, the somewhat controversial topic of competence in medicine is discussed. This chapter deals with the definition of competence, controversies surrounding it, and its multiple forms. In this chapter, there is a discussion of the various methods of assessing competence over the career span.

Chapter 3 deals with somewhat more technical content, the basic statistics in testing. These include descriptive statistics, standard scores, and graphical analyses. Correlational techniques—indispensable methods in testing—are presented, detailed, and discussed in Chapter 4. The following major correlational techniques are presented: Pearson product-moment, Spearman rank-order, biserial, point biserial, regression, multiple regression (linear, logistic), factor analysis (exploratory factor analyses [EFA], confirmatory factor analyses [CFA], structural equation modelling, and hierarchical linear modelling.

Validity and reliability

The section on Validity and reliability contains a discussion on the multiple forms of validity (face, content, criterion-related, construct, advanced methods, unified view of validity) and a rational for the three chapters on validity and two on reliability for a total of five chapters.

Chapter 5—Validity I—deals with logical and content validity and describes the uses of tables of specifications (blueprint) to enhance these types of validity. Chapter 6—Validity II—contains correlational based and between group differences aspects of validity such as criterion-related (concurrent and predictive) and construct (between group differences, factorial validity, experimental, and data structure—regression, discriminant, and cluster analyses). Chapter 7—Validity III—advanced methods, is about advanced techniques of validity such as multi-trait multi-method (MTMM), confirmatory factor analyses, structural equation modelling, systematic reviews and meta-analyses, hierarchical linear modelling, and a unified view of validity.

Reliability is discussed in two chapters. Chapter 8—Reliability I—deals with the multiple forms of reliability (test–retest, internal consistency, parallel forms, inter-rater, intra-rater, Ep^2, S_e, etc.). The technical and mathematical theories of CTT are developed and detailed in this chapter. Chapter 9—Reliability II—contains the technical and mathematical theories of IRT and Ep^2 which are developed and detailed in this chapter.

Test construction and evaluation

In Chapter 10, the various formats of testing for cognition, affect, and psychomotor skills are summarized. These include selection type items (MCQs, constructed response, checklists, and other item formats). There is a discussion of Bloom's taxonomies of cognitive, affective, and psychomotor skills; Miller's Pyramid; and further work on the use of tables of specifications.

Chapter 11 deals specifically with multiple-choice items especially on how to write items, types of MCQs, number of options, how to construct MCQs, and appropriate levels of measurement. In Chapter 12, constructed response items are detailed. These include essays, short answer, matching, and hybrid items such as the script concordance tests. Measuring clinical skills with the OSCE is discussed in Chapter 13. The focus is on describing the OSCE and its use in measuring communications, patient management, clinical reasoning, diagnoses, physical examination, case history, etc. Additional issues of case development and scripts, training assessors, and training standardized patients are detailed.

Chapter 14 deals with checklists, questionnaires, rating scales, and direct observations. The following commonly used assessments are discussed: in-training evaluation reports (ITERs), mini-CEX, multisource feedback, chart audits, and semi-structured interviews. Chapter 15 is about evaluating tests and assessments using item analyses: conducting classical item analyses with MCQs (item difficulty, item discrimination, and distractor effectiveness), conducting item analyses with OSCEs, conducting item analyses with constructed response items, and computing the reliability coefficient and errors of measurement.

Grading, reporting, and methods of setting cutoff scores (pass/fail) are discussed in Chapter 16. The focus is on norm-referenced versus criterion-referenced approaches, setting a MPL utilizing the Angoff method, Ebel method, Nedelsky method, as well as empirical methods (borderline regression, cluster analyses, etc.)

The book also will contain a Glossary (of testing and statistical terms—e.g., reliability, validity, standard error of measurement, biserial correlation, etc.), problems and data (fundamental problems will be presented—e.g., calculating reliability, conducting item analyses, running confirmatory factor analyses; here appropriate software (e.g., SPSS, Iteman, EQS, etc.) and example of its use will be demonstrated. There will be comprehensive references and several Appendices.

SUMMARY

The assessment and evaluation of learning has its origins in antiquity but is only now beginning to emerge as a unified field. This is due to developments in statistical and mathematical theory, test theory, and advances in computer hardware and software, and also the developing internet. Testing and assessment are the acts of quantifying an educational or psychological dimension or assigning a numerical value to it. Evaluation requires a value judgment to be made based on the measurement. While the history of testing dates back two millennia, it has emerged on a large scale only in the 20th century, coincidental with mass education.

The current status of testing is paradoxical: it is on the increase and receives overwhelming public support and yet most teachers, instructors, and professors (who construct, administer, and interpret the vast majority of tests) have little or no formal education in testing. Tests can be used to motivate students, enhance learning, provide feedback, evaluate educational programs, and for research. Other functions include curriculum revisions, selection and screening, certification, and guidance and counselling. Tests can be used in a variety of ways and for several evaluation functions. Testing is likely to expand in modern society. The improvement of healthcare professional competence depends, in part, on the improvement of testing and assessment of medical competence. The alarming rate of medical errors that currently result in death or negative outcomes may be reduced.

REFLECTIONS

1. How can assessment and evaluation reduce medical errors? (500 words maximum)
2. Distinguish between testing, assessment, quantification, and evaluation. (500 words maximum)
3. Briefly summarize the history of testing from antiquity to modern times. (500 words maximum)
4. Describe the various functions of testing as used in medical education. (500 words maximum)
5. Compare and contrast formative, summative, and placement evaluation. (500 words maximum)
6. Describe the various types of tests and evaluation procedures. (500 words maximum)
7. What roles have statistics and computers had in the development of testing? (500 words maximum)

REFERENCES

1. Kohn KT, Corrigan JM, Donaldson MS (1999). *To Err Is Human: Building a Safer Health System*. Washington, DC: National Academy Press.
2. Makary MA, Daniel M (2016). Medical error—The third leading cause of death in the US. *British Medical Journal* 353:i2139. doi:10.1136/bmj.i2139.
3. Schoen C, Osborn R, Doty M, Bishop M, Peugh J, Murukutia N (2007). Toward higher performance health systems: Adults' healthcare experiences in seven countries. *Health Affairs* 26(6):717–734.
4. Brand C, Ibrahim J, Bain C, Jones C, King B (2007). Engineering a safe landing: Engaging medical practitioners in a systems approach to patient safety. *Internal Medicine Journal* 37:295–302.
5. Newman-Toker DE, Pronovost PJ (2009). Diagnostic errors—the next frontier for patient safety. *Journal of the American Medical Association* 301:1060–1062.
6. Sibinga EM (2010). Clinician mindfulness and patient safety. *Journal of the American Medical Association* 304:2532–2533.
7. Magner LN (2005). *A History of Medicine* (2nd edition). New York: Taylor & Francis, pp. 154–155.
8. Debre P (2000). *Louis Pasteur*. Baltimore, MD: Johns Hopkins University Press.

9. Eamon W (2010). *The Professor of Secrets*. Washington, DC: National Geographic Publishing.

10. Hodges B, Lingard L (eds) (2013). *The Question of Competence: Reconsidering Medical Education in the Twenty-First Century*. Ithaca, NY: Cornell University Press.

11. Violato C (2016). A brief history of the regulation of medical practice: From Hammurabi to the national board of medical examiners. *Wake Forest Journal of Science and Medicine* 2:122–129.

12. American New Standard Bible, *Book of Judges*, 12: 6.

13. Dubois PH (1970). *A History of Psychological Testing*. Boston, MA: Allyn Bacon.

14. Miyazaki I (1981). *China's Examination Hell: The Civil Service Examinations of Imperial China*. New Haven, CT: Yale University Press.

15. Wang R (2013). *The Chinese Imperial Examination System*. Plymouth, UK: Scarecrow Press.

16. Johns CH (2000). *The Oldest Code of Laws in the World: The Code of Laws Promulgated by Hammurabi, King of Babylon*. Union, NJ: Lawbook Exchange, Ltd.

17. Sigerist HE (1961). *History of Medicine, Volume II: Early Greek, Hindu, and Persian Medicine*. New York: Oxford University Press.

18. Flexner A (1910). *Medical Education in the United States and Canada: A Report to the Carnegie Foundation for the Advancement of Teaching, Bulletin No. 4*. New York City, NY: The Carnegie Foundation for the Advancement of Teaching.

19. McArthur DL (1983). *Educational Testing and Measurement: A Brief History*, (Report #216). Los Angeles, CA: Center for the Study of Evaluation, University of California.

20. Cronbach LJ, Nageswari R, Gleser GC (1963). Theory of generalizability: A liberation of reliability theory. *The British Journal of Statistical Psychology* 16:137–163; Cronbach LJ, Gleser GC, Nanda H, Rajaratnam N (1972). *The Dependability of Behavioral Measurements: Theory of Generalizability for Scores and Profiles*. New York: John Wiley.

21. Rose LC, Gallup AM (2007). The 39th annual Phi Delta Kappa/Gallup poll of the public's attitudes toward the public schools. *Phi Delta Kappa* 89(1):33–48.

22. Holmboe ES, Ward DS, Reznick RK, Katsufrakis PJ, Leslie KM, Patel VL, Ray DD, Nelson EA (2011). Faculty development in assessment: The missing link in competency-based medical education. *Academic Medicine* 86(4):460–467.

23. Donnon T, Violato C, DesCôteaux JG (2006). Engagement with online curriculum materials and the course test performance of medical students. *International Journal of Interactive Technology and Smart Education* 10:150–156.

24. Foos PW, Fisher RP (1988). Using tests as learning opportunities. *Journal of Educational Psychology* 80:179–183.

25. Pastotter B, Bauml KH (2014). Retrieval practice enhances new learning: The forward effect of testing. *Frontier in Psychology* 5. doi:10.3389/fpsyg.2014.00286.

26. Schmidt HG, Rotgans JI, Yew EH (2011). The process of problem-based learning: What works and why. *Medical Education* 45:792–806.

27. Donnon T, Violato C (2006). Medical students' clinical reasoning skills as a function of basic science achievement and clinical competency measures: A structural equation model. *Academic Medicine* 81(10 Suppl):S120–S123.

28. Donnon T, Al Ansari A, Al Alawi S, Violato C (2014). The reliability, validity, and feasibility of multisource feedback physician assessment: A systematic review. *Academic Medicine* 89(3):511–516.

29. Doherty EM, Nugent E (2011). Personality factors and medical training: A review of the literature. *Medical Education* 45(2):132–140.

30. Tyssen R, Dolatowski FC, Røvik JO, Thorkildsen RF, Ekeberg O, Hem E, Gude T, Grønvold NT, Vaglum P (2007). Personality traits and types predict medical school stress: A six-year longitudinal and nationwide study. *Medical Education* 41(8):781–787.

2

Competence and professionalism in medicine and the health professions

ADVANCED ORGANIZERS

- Competence and professionalism are complex, interrelated, multidimensional constructs commonly based on three primary components: knowledge, skills, and attitudes. Miller described a four-tier pyramid of clinical ability, identifying the base of the pyramid as knowledge (measuring what someone knows), followed by competence (measuring how they know), performance (shows how they know), and last at the summit, action (behavior).
- Entrustable professional activities (EPAs) are clinical activities that require the use and integration of several competencies and milestones critical to safe and effective clinical performance. Each EPA is based on a number of competencies and milestones where EPAs are units of work and competencies are abilities of persons. To assess the competence of physicians for EPAs requires complex and comprehensive assessments.
- In the English-speaking world, the present views define medical competence and professionalism as the ability to meet the relationship-centered expectations required to practice medicine competently.
- A variety of professional organizations have recently weighed in on the constructs of competence and professionalism: the American Board of Internal Medicine (ABIM) in the early 1990s, the Association of American Medical Colleges (AAMC), the Accreditation Council for Graduate Medical Education (ACGME), and the National Board of Medical Examiners (NBME) focused on professionalism. In addition, the ABIM in partnership with the American College of Physicians, American Society of Internal Medicine, and the European Federation of Internal Medicine developed a Physician Charter.

- Another model of medical competence is the Canadian Medical Education Directions for Specialists (CanMEDS) Framework. The CanMEDS consists of seven roles: manager, communicator, professional, scholar, expert, health advocate, collaborator and have been used as theoretical underpinnings of physician competencies.
- British and American views of medical professionalism are quite similar. For Asian countries, however, professionalism is a Western concept without a precise equivalent in Asian cultures.
- Instruments and procedures that are designed to measure competence and professionalism are challenged on validity, reliability, and practicality.
- Assessing competence: objective structured clinical examinations, assessment of language and communication, in-training evaluation reports, workplace assessment and multisource feedback, direct observations and competence.
- Teaching and physician competence—does teaching medicine make you a better doctor?
- The overall results provide evidence of effectiveness of the present direct observation and assessment in a clinical environment. The repeated measures analyses showed that students improved substantially on clinical skills, communications, and professionalism.
- Reflection, particularly self-reflection, is thought to be an important part of competence and professionalism. Unfortunately, reflection has been used with nearly as many meanings as has competence, but in the health science professions, it is viewed as an important part of lifelong personal and professional learning and competence.

INTRODUCTION

Competence and professionalism are complex, interrelated, multidimensional constructs. They are commonly based on four primary components: knowledge, skills, attitudes, and behavior. Miller has described a four-tier pyramid (Table 10.2) of clinical ability, identifying the base of the pyramid as knowledge (measuring what someone knows), followed by competence (measuring how they know), performance (shows how they know), and last at the summit, action (behavior).[1] Clinical competence involves a complex interplay between attributes displayed within the physician–patient encounter, which enables physicians to effectively deliver care. These attributes share an intimate relationship with one another and include the ability to take a proper history, complete a physical examination, communicate effectively, manage a patient's health, interpret clinical results, synthesize information, collaborate with other health professionals, advocate for population health, and so forth. These attributes are seen as integral to almost all medical practice and practice in other health professions.

Competence is composed of many different measurable variables, latent variables, and factors relating behavior to environment. Medical competence is a reciprocal link and interaction of a person's medical knowledge, skills, attitudes, and behavior. Clinical competence is determined and standardized as it relates to the practice of medicine in treating patients. Competence and performance are frequently distinguished from one another. Performance in the practice of medicine is the appropriate application of clinical competence to a clinical situation.

Clinical competence is a construct that is not easy to measure directly. Professionalism as it relates to practice of medicine is another construct which has not been adequately defined and is difficult to measure. Epstein's and Hundert's definition of professional competence is that it is the "habitual and judicious use of communication, knowledge, technical skills, clinical reasoning, emotions, values and reflection in daily practice for the benefit of the individual and community being served."[2]

Hodges and Lingard have pointed out that in the past decade competence has grown to the status of a "god term" in medicine and other healthcare professions.[3] Together with professionalism, it has become a principle notion of what medical education should be striving for in the 21st century. They express concern that the concept of competence and competency-based medical education (CBME) have become ubiquitous but only vaguely defined and poorly understood. Although CBME has promise (commitment to outcomes, focus on learner-centeredness, move away from time-based education), there are perils (reductionism, emphasis on minimum performance levels, utilitarianism focus, logistical challenges for individually paced progress). According to Hodges and Lingard, competence is so widely used, in so many different ways, that it risks having no meaning at all. They concluded that the question, "what is competence?" remains to be satisfactorily answered.

MEDICAL COMPETENCE

Competence refers to an area of performance that can be described, operationalized, and measured.[4] These are performance areas in patient care, medical knowledge, professionalism, practice-based learning and improvement, systems-based practice, and interpersonal and communication skills. Although multi-faceted, medical competence can be determined through testing and assessments. There has been a great deal of activity in testing and assessment in the past 100 years, and these are likely to play an even larger role in the determination of competence for licensure and regulation of medical practice in the future.[5] The future focus will be on competency-based testing of, among other things, entrustable professional activities (EPAs).

ENTRUSTABLE PROFESSIONAL ACTIVITIES

An EPA is a clinical activity that requires the use and integration of several competencies and milestones critical to safe and effective clinical performance.[6] Each EPA—for example, #8: "Give or receive a patient handover to transition care responsibility"—is based on a number of competencies and milestones where EPAs are units of work and competencies are traits of persons. To assess the competence of physicians for this, EPA requires complex and comprehensive assessments.

Although EPA-based assessment is gaining momentum, challenges of feasibility of implementation remain. This assessment strategy also provides an opportunity to improve training and assessment by increasing focus on appropriate supervision and regulation of students, residents, and physicians to assess competence. Entrustability is achieved when the learner can perform the professional activity safely and effectively without supervision.

HEALING, COMPETENCE, AND PROFESSIONALISM

There have been healers in society since time immemorial. The tradition of *physician* healer in Western society dates back to Hippocrates and is known and cherished by medical practitioners everywhere. The healer offers advice and support in matters of health and ministers to and treats the sick. For centuries, the Hippocratic Oath and its modern derivatives have served as the foundation of competence in medicine.

There are two important major elements of medicine as a profession: a specialized body of knowledge and a commitment to service. But, according to Swick,[7] modern medical professionals have become more closely connected to the application of expert knowledge at the expense of functions central to the good of the public they serve. He warns that medical professionals have become distracted from their public and social purposes and thus lost a distinctive voice. Strengthening medical professionalism becomes one way to the distinctive voice.

DEFINITION OF MEDICAL PROFESSIONALISM

In the English-speaking world, the service of the physician–healer has been organized around the concept of the professional. The present views define medical competence and professionalism as the ability to meet the relationship-centered expectations required to practice medicine competently.

The concept of professionalism has evolved over the past several decades. There are three stages in the evolution of medical professionalism: the first (1980s–early 1990s) was dominated by the debates of professionalism and commercialism; a second (1990s) was dominated by calls to define medical professionalism as a concept and as a competency; the third (late 1990s–current) called for definitions by highlighting the need to develop measures and metrics.[8]

A review in 2002 reported that half of the medical schools in the United States had identified between four and nine elements of professionalism and had developed written criteria and specific methods for their assessment. Northeastern Ohio Universities College of Medicine described professionalism by eight elements: (1) reliability and responsibility, (2) honesty and integrity, (3) maturity, (4) respect for others, (5) critique, (6) altruism, (7) interpersonal skills, and (8) absence of impairment. The University of New Mexico School of Medicine contained similar elements, but it included communication skills and respect for patients while omitting altruism. The University of California, San

Francisco School of Medicine, just focused on four aspects of professionalism: (1) professional responsibility, (2) self-improvement and adaptability, (3) relationships with patients and families, and (4) relationships with members of the healthcare team.[9] Professional values common to the undergraduate medical curricula are altruism, respect for others, and additional humanistic qualities such as honor, integrity, ethical and moral standards, accountability, excellence, and duty/advocacy.

A variety of professional organizations have recently weighed in on the constructs of competence and professionalism. The ABIM began its humanism project that led to project professionalism in the early 1990s. Similarly, the AAMC, the ACGME, and the NBME focused on professionalism. In addition, the ABIM in partnership with the American College of Physicians, American Society of Internal Medicine, and the European Federation of Internal Medicine developed a Physician Charter.[10]

According to the ABIM, professionalism in medicine requires the physician to serve the interests of the patient above self-interest. Professionalism aspires to altruism, accountability, excellence, duty, service, honor, integrity, and respect for others. The elements of professionalism required of candidates seeking certification and recertification from the ABIM encompass: a commitment to the highest standards of excellence in the practice of medicine and in the generation and dissemination of knowledge; a commitment to sustain the interests and welfare of patients; and a commitment to be responsive to the health needs of society.[11] Altruism is the essence of professionalism and fundamental to this definition. It demands that the best interests of patients, not self-interest, guide physicians. Respect for others (ranging from patients to medical students) is the essence of humanism.

A second large organization defining professionalism is the ACGME: professionalism is manifested through a commitment to carrying out professional responsibilities, adherence to ethical principles, and sensitivity to a diverse patient population. Moreover, it lists the positive aspects of professionalism: respect, regard, integrity, and responsiveness to patient and society that supersede self-interest. The 2015 joint initiative of the ACGME and the ABIM has resulted in The *Internal Medicine Milestone Project*, a definition of medical competence and professionalism.[12]

The NBME has identified 60 behaviors of professionalism and has created an intriguing pictorial representation of professionalism composed of a circular core of knowledge and skills surrounded by seven supporting qualities: altruism; responsibility and accountability; leadership; caring; compassion and communication; excellence and scholarship; respect, and honor and integrity.

The ABIM, the ACGME, the NBME, AAMC, the Society of Academic Emergency Medicine and European Federation of Internal Medicine mostly concur with elements such as altruism, accountability, excellence, duty/advocacy, humanistic qualities, ethical and moral standards, service, honor, integrity, and respect for others. In 1995, the ACGME and the Royal College of Physicians and Surgeons of Canada (RCPSC) endorsed "professionalism" as one of the six general competencies for physicians.

CanMEDS and competence

Another model of medical competence has been developed by the RCPSC: the Canadian Medical Education Directions for Specialists (CanMEDS) Framework (Figure 2.1). The CanMEDS consists of seven roles: manager, communicator, professional, scholar, expert, health advocate, collaborator and have been used as theoretical underpinnings of physician competencies.

The CanMEDS roles are thought to be dynamic and interrelated, but they are also distinct and cohesive. The CanMEDS diagram is designed to illustrate how these roles fit together and describe the competent physician. Competence in this model goes well beyond medical expert (although central) to the six other competencies.

Cross-cultural concepts of medical professionalism

The British approach to medical professionalism is grounded in patient-centered professionalism in the structural and normative context of medicine in the United Kingdom. The professional physician requires medical knowledge, skills, modernity, empathy, honesty, listening, and communication skills to be an

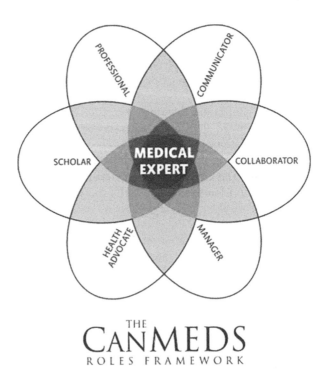

Figure 2.1 Adapted from the CanMEDS Physician Competency Framework with permission of the Royal College of Physicians and Surgeons of Canada. Copyright © 2005.

effective team player. Professionalism is composed of expert knowledge and skill, ethicality, and service to patients.

There are some differences between the American and British views on professionalism. British definitions of professionalism are more patient-centered than in the United States. Additionally, the British emphasize service but not altruism as a core element of professionalism as in the United States. In general, however, British and American views of medical professionalism are quite similar.

For Asian countries, professionalism is a Western concept without a precise equivalent in Asian cultures. The term does not easily translate into any Asian language or ways of thinking regarding autonomy, service, and justice which are understood quite differently in the East, with the 2,000-year-old Confucian tradition gives priority to collectivist, authoritarian, and hierarchical cultural standards. (In Hong Kong, the ideal of medical professionalism has been adhered to due to the British rule.)

Despite this, Keio University School of Medicine in Tokyo has successfully introduced a professionalism curriculum that both supports Japan's cultural traditions and affirms the school's academic mission by using a sequential, overlapping, and small group discussion approach. The success of this initiative demonstrates that even in a culture unfamiliar with the concept of medical professionalism, it can be taught in a way that is appreciated by students and faculty.[13] In China, medical professional bodies have also been formed and professional ethical standards are acknowledged, and the focus is on individual patients rather than the community. The concepts of patient–physician relationship and primacy of patient interest are in concordance with Western views and has been widely accepted by Chinese society and healthcare workers.[14]

In Taiwan, Tsuen-Chiuan et al.[15] employed the ABIM medical professionalism definitions. They explored the factors of commitment to care, righteous and rule-abiding, pursuing quality patient care, habit of professional practice, interpersonal relationship, patient-oriented issues, physician's self-development, and respect for others and found that "commitment to care" was perceived least important by Taiwanese medical graduates. Culture sensitivity was perceived as pursuing quality patient care rather than respect as in the ABIM definition.

In Vietnam, there has been no clear definition of medical professionalism. The most popular concept which guides physicians' practice is medical ethics. Nhan et al.[16] found that the perceptions of medical professionalism of Vietnamese medical students and physicians were fairly similar to the ABIM definitions: integrity, social responsibility, professional practice habits, ensuring quality care, altruism, and self-awareness. Social responsibility was perceived least important, and self-awareness was perceived most important by Vietnamese medical students. These constructs of medical professionalism were relatively similar with those found in the ABIM definitions but with some Vietnamese cultural differences, focusing on sentimentality. The positive focus on aspects of sentimental culture is humanity and respect of others, but the negative effects are lack of principles, too accommodating, and unreasonableness.

Assessing competence and professionalism

Assessing these two constructs, especially with the multiple definitions, is challenging. Instruments and procedures that are designed to measure competence and professionalism are challenged on:

- Validity—does the instrument measure competence as it is intended to measure?
- Reliability—is the assessment objective and are the results consistent and reproducible?
- Practicality—can it be assessed practically with students, residents, and physicians with available assessors?

MILLER'S PYRAMID OF CLINICAL COMPETENCE

Miller proposed a framework for assessing levels of clinical competence as a pyramid: the lowest two levels test cognition, followed by competence, performance, and at the pinnacle, action. Novice learners may know something about a neurological examination, for example, or they may know how to do a neurological examination. The upper two levels test behavior to determine if learners can apply what they know into practice. They can show how to do a neurological examination; can they actually do a neurological examination in practice?

Structured assessment: Objective structured clinical examinations

The OSCE is a performance-based assessment with some objectivity and concentrates mainly on skills and to a lesser degree on knowledge (see Chapter 13). Even though Barrows and Abrahamson had described the technique of using standardized patients in 1964, the OSCE did not come into general use until the 1970s. The use of oral exams for assessing clinical competence continued for a long time despite its limitations of reliability and validity. Harden et al. combined the use of multi-stations and standardized patients and identified three ideal criteria for assessing clinical competence in an OSCE.[17]

In an OSCE format, the candidates rotate through a series of stations (mostly with an SP; the ones without SPs are referred to as "static stations"), where they are required to perform a clinical task. During this rotation, all the candidates receive the same medical encounter and are assessed by an examiner (physician judges or SPs) who provides a score based on the preset criteria on a checklist.

Some of the attributes measured through OSCEs include the ability to take a proper and adequate history, complete a physical examination, communicate effectively, manage patient's health, interpret clinical results, and synthesize information. The OSCE has been used for assessing competence of health professionals, including physicians, nurses, optometrists, dentists, and others. Their utility, however, is poor for assessing attitudinal and behavioral performance that is better assessed *in situ* during clerkship and residency, for example.

In-training evaluation reports

In-training evaluation is the process of observing and documenting the performance of students, residents, or other trainees in a naturalistic clinical setting. Typically, the attending physician observes the trainee in a particular department, ward, or discipline, one or more times during an assessment period. Then in-training evaluation reports (ITERs) are completed by the preceptor or assessor at the end (or any other point of training), usually on a standardized form assessing clinical knowledge, skills, and attitudes. ITERs are used by most disciplines to assess the clinical competence of residents during the 2–5 year supervised training period. ITERs are also used for giving formative feedback to the trainees on their competence. The construct measured through ITERs can be based on professional roles such as the CanMEDS roles (e.g., communicator, medical expert, collaborator) or those set by professional bodies such as the ABIM (e.g., professionalism, etc.). ITERs have been in use for many years for assessing the clinical competence of residents. ITERs have been improved substantially (reliability and validity) over the last several decades and have been made discipline specific.

Assessment of language and communication

Medical language represents the wide array of terms associated with medical knowledge with the professional language that is needed for communicating effectively with patients and colleagues in the practice of medicine. Professional communication in medicine is also related to the ability to demonstrate clinical skills.

One of the most significant advancement in the assessment of language for professional purposes has been the move toward authentic assessment: language proficiency in situations and tasks that are specific to the professional practice (i.e., situations with ecological validity). The goal of authentic assessment is to simulate the conditions of professional interaction. The conditions need to accurately sample the range of experiences which are most likely to be representative of professional practice. Although not necessarily identical to genuine experiences (the use of SPs in OSCEs), the interaction requires candidates to engage strategically in solving unpredictable problems by communicating in real time.

Analytic criteria can be employed on rating scales to assess fluency, pronunciation, comprehensibility, vocabulary, grammar, etc. Overall or holistic assessment allows the assessor to provide an overall impression of professional language proficiency. The OSCE is useful for the authentic assessment of professional language proficiency as it can employ multiple cases and examiners, authentic tasks, real-time communication, and psychometrically based rating scales. An example of such a scale is the Canadian Language Benchmark Assessment (CLBA) that has been adapted to reflect medical contexts (cultural-communication, legal, ethical, and organizational aspects of the practice of medicine). For more naturalistic assessment, both spoken and written language samples, *in situ* can be collected and analyzed for authentic assessment of language and communication proficiency.

Workplace assessment and multisource feedback

The Physician Achievement Review (PAR) in Alberta is probably the best case of medical workplace assessment employing multisource feedback (MSF). This MSF was developed specifically for assessing performance of practicing physicians. The instruments of PAR were developed in the late 1990s in response to The College of Physicians and Surgeons of Alberta's initiative to improve the quality of medical practice.[18] The approach consists of four types of data: self, medical colleagues (physicians), coworkers (non-physicians), and the patients, all completing standardized questionnaires. The competencies assessed by the four instruments vary and include clinical competence for self and peer physician questionnaires only: humanistic attributes, patient communication professionalism, collegiality, etc. are in all the instruments. The PAR instruments have been used for assessing surgical, pediatrics, and other specialties.[19]

Violato et al.[19] factor-analyzed PAR instruments and identified a number of factors of physician performance such as communication skills, patient management, clinical assessment, psychosocial and humanism, and professional development. The instruments were found to have evidence of adequate reliability ($\alpha > 0.90$ for most scales; $Ep^2 > 0.65$ for most assessments) and had substantial evidence for validity (face, content, factorial, convergent, and discriminant).

A comparative factor analytic study was conducted by Violato and Lockyer, comprising 2,306 peer surveys for 304 participating physicians from internal medicine, pediatrics, and psychiatry; a four factor solutions was reported (patient management, clinical assessment, professional development, communication).[20] They reported adequate reliability ($\alpha = 0.98$ and $Ep^2 = 0.83$) and nearly 70% of the variance was accounted for by the four factors. These studies provide empirical evidence for the reliability and validity of the PAR instruments. A recent MSF 5-year longitudinal study employing family physicians shows considerable stability and evidence of construct validity of the PAR instruments.[21] This workplace-based approach employing MSF has been employed in the Netherlands, Britain, United State, Bahrain, and elsewhere.

TEACHING AND PHYSICIAN COMPETENCE

Teaching has been regarded as part of medical competence and professionalism since antiquity.[22] Over the millennia, physicians, from Hippocrates, Galen, and Osler to current professors, have taught patients, medical students, and other health professionals, either through direct instruction, modelling, or by publications.

An interesting question that has arisen is, "Does teaching medicine make you a better doctor?" Perhaps, teaching requires the physician to have a more complex and subtle understanding of the subject matter than do non-teachers. Moreover, perhaps the teachers have an understanding of how to convey this subject matter to novices and learners thus developing meta-cognitive awareness of the knowledge, skills, attitudes, and professionalism of medical competence. Additionally, the need to role model medical competence and professionalism for learners may improve these qualities in the teacher. Physicians themselves identify teaching as a factor that enhances performance although existing data to support this relationship has been limited.

Researchers in Alberta[23] recently studied more 3,500 physicians some of whom had academic teaching appointments at university medical schools and some who didn't to determine whether there were differences in clinical performance scores as assessed through MSF data based on clinical teaching.

MSF data for 1,831 family physicians, 1,510 medical specialists, and 542 surgeons were collected from physicians' medical colleagues, co-workers (e.g., nurses and pharmacists), and patients. Typically, an average of around eight colleagues, eight co-workers, and 25 patients anonymously rated the doctors on standardized instruments. These data were analyzed in relation to information about physician teaching activities including percentage of time spent teaching during patient care and academic appointments.

The results indicated that higher clinical performance scores were associated with holding any academic appointment and generally with any time teaching versus no teaching during patient care. This was most evident for data from medical colleagues, where these differences existed across all specialty groups. Patient data results were mixed as were the data for co-workers. For ratings by colleagues (i.e., other physicians), the results were clear: teachers in family medicine, medical specialists and surgeons were rated as more competent, better clinicians and more professional than were non-teachers.

In this study, higher involvement in teaching was associated with higher clinical performance ratings from medical colleagues and co-workers for all physicians. These results suggest teaching as a method to enhance and maintain high-quality clinical performance and promote maintenance of competence and improving professionalism. They also support the idea that teaching medicine is integral to competence and professionalism.

DIRECT OBSERVATIONS AND COMPETENCE

The evaluation of the clinical competence of medical students and residents can be done through the use of direct observation. There has been inconsistency in how best to measure and compare performance on clinical skill domains, however. In response to this problem, the ABIM proposed the use of the mini-clinical evaluation exercise (mini-CEX) to evaluate learners' in the completion of a patient history and physical examination that results in the demonstration of organized clinical judgments and efficient counseling skills.

In its standard form, the mini-CEX is a seven-item, global rating scale that is designed to evaluate medical students' and residents' patient encounters in about 15–20 min. The mini-CEX is specifically designed to assess the skills that learners require in actual patient encounters and also to reflect the educational requirements that are expected of those learners. As described by Norcini et al.,[24] the multiple uses of the mini-CEX with trainees allows for a greater variability across different patient encounters that results in improved reliability and validity as a measure of clinical skill practice and development. It is a performance-based evaluation method that is used to assess selected clinical competencies (e.g., patient interview and physical examination, communication, and interpersonal skills) within a clinical training context.

The mini-CEX can be used widely in a broad range of clinical settings. There is mounting psychometric evidence of it for direct observation of single-patient encounters. Kogan et al.[25] in a systematic review identified the mini-CEX as having the strongest validity evidence of instruments for direct observation and assessment of clinical skills of medical trainees. In a recent meta-analysis, Alansari et al.[26] supported this finding with evidence of construct and criterion-related validity of the mini-CEX as an important instrument for the direct observation of trainees' clinical performance and competence.

The mini-CEX assesses seven dimensions: (1) medical interviewing, (2) physical examination, (3) humanistic qualities/professionalism, (4) clinical judgment, (5) counseling skills, (6) organization/efficiency, and (7) overall competence. According to Norcini et al.,[24] the mini-CEX assesses candidates at the top of Miller's Pyramid (i.e. "shows how" and "does").

Growth of competence

Objective performance in medical competence domains (e.g., professionalism, patient management) can be measured by collecting and analyzing activities *in situ*, but collecting the necessary amount of data can be difficult. Nonetheless, this can be done through repeated measures designs where the student, resident, or physician can be repeatedly observed in structured situations by trained observers, and their performance can be assessed objectively on standardized instruments (e.g., mini-CEX).

This growth or the rate of learning can be usefully represented by learning curves. They allow assessment in real time and may allow us to determine how much practice or learning is required to achieve a particular level of competence. According to the Thurstone classical learning curve,[27] learning increases with time or practice according to a negative exponential function (improvement decreases over time as learning occurs), the rate of learning can be determined (slope of the curve), maximal performance can be determined for the practice or time period (the upper asymptote). Learning curves have not been used very much in medical education generally.

In a recent study,[28] faculty members were trained how to assess students and provide formative feedback during a clinical encounter with the adapted mini-CEX utilizing principles of CBME and direct observation of third-year clerkship students (Table 2.1). There were 27 assessors, 108 students for a total of 1,001 assessments during required clerkships from May–February. The mean number of assessments per student was 8.97 (SD = 2.57) with range 1–15. The mean time for assessment was 25.31 min and for feedback 19.69 min. Students were rated on a five-point scale based on their degree of entrustability on that competency (1 = not close to meeting criterion; 2 = not yet meets criterion; 3 = meets criterion; 4 = just exceeds criterion; 5 = well exceeds criterion). The data used for the analyses were primarily of direct observations of student–patient encounters in naturalistic situations in the clinical environment during the clerkships.

Table 2.1 Means, standard deviations and range of direct observation of patient encounters with the mini-CEX in structured clinical settings

Mini-CEX competency		Time (mean days in clerkship)						
		27	65	108	154	213	271	Total
1. Communication	Mean	3.08	3.44	3.40	3.48	3.60	3.67	3.44
Range: 1–5	SD	0.68	0.87	0.73	0.67	0.63	0.68	0.73
2. Medical interview	Mean	2.81	3.18	3.15	3.30	3.30	3.39	3.18
Range: 1–5	SD	0.79	0.91	0.71	0.72	0.67	0.68	0.77
3. Physical exam	Mean	2.63	3.09	3.01	3.16	3.19	3.22	3.03
Range: 1–5	SD	0.72	0.66	0.46	0.67	0.56	0.64	0.66
4. Professionalism	Mean	3.31	3.58	3.47	3.63	3.68	3.70	3.56
Range: 2–5	SD	0.72	0.79	0.69	0.64	0.68	0.71	0.72
5. Clinical reasoning	Mean	2.74	3.01	3.17	3.22	3.33	3.44	3.15
Range: 1–5	SD	0.70	0.83	0.64	0.65	0.65	0.67	0.73
6. Management planning	Mean	2.65	3.05	3.04	3.11	3.20	3.31	3.06
Range: 1–5	SD	0.70	0.78	0.62	0.65	0.59	0.57	0.68
7. Organizational efficacy	Mean	2.77	3.03	3.15	3.24	3.20	3.34	3.12
Range: 1–5	SD	0.73	0.84	0.61	0.62	0.60	0.66	0.70
8. Oral presentation	Mean	2.81	3.04	3.08	3.20	3.14	3.29	3.09
Range: 1–5	SD	0.74	0.77	0.59	0.57	0.49	0.51	0.64
9. Overall assessment	Mean	2.86	3.19	3.22	3.30	3.33	3.39	3.21
Range: 1–5	SD	0.61	0.75	0.57	0.56	0.57	0.58	0.63
Observation & feedback		**Range**	**Mean**	**SD**	—	—	—	—
Observing time (min)		10–90	25.31	11.05	—	—	—	—
Coach feedback (min)		5–45	19.69	7.45	—	—	—	—

The descriptive statistics for the variables in the analyses are presented in Table 2.1. As can be seen from these data, the smallest total means for the mini-CEX items is 3.03 (Physical Exam) while the largest is 3.56 (Professionalism). The SDs are in the two-thirds to three-quarters of a scale point range (mean SD = 0.73). Items all range from 1 to 5 with the exception of professionalism (2–5). The mean time for assessment was 25.31 min (range: 10–90 min). The mean time for feedback to the students by the assessor was 19.69 min (range: 5–45 min).

Growth and learning curves

Figures 2.2 and 2.3 contain a longitudinal analysis for six time periods (sextiles) during the assessments (10 months; May 2016–February, 2017). There were approximately 165 observations for each of the six time periods.

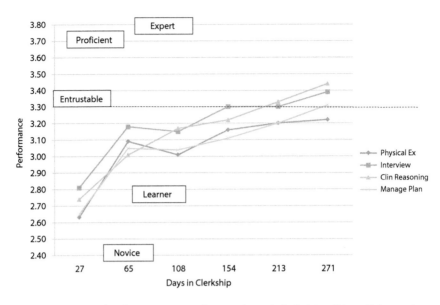

Figure 2.2 Growth of competence during clinical clerkships (May–February).

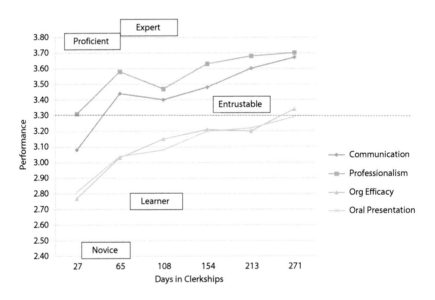

Figure 2.3 Growth of competence during clinical clerkships (May–February).

Each of the eight competencies from the mini-CEX is depicted on the graphs. A close inspection of Figure 2.2 reveals that there was an increase in the means of four competencies over time ($p < 0.01$) as theoretically expected; student competence grows over this time period (also Table 2.1). Figure 2.3 shows that there was an increase in the means of the other four competencies over time ($p < 0.01$) as student competence grows. Figures 2.2 and 2.3 depict Thurstone's classical learning curves where learning increase with time according to a negative exponential function.

The results from the eight competencies indicate that most of the rapid learning occurs within the first 100 days (about 3 months) of the clerkship ranging from 1.95 (Management Planning) to 9.5 (Physical Exam). The mean increase in the Overall Assessment was 0.627 standard deviation which results in a large effect size (Cohen's $d = 0.86$); the ratio of the two time periods for Overall Assessment was 3.27.

Entrustability, as well as other student performance levels (novice, learner, proficient, expert) are set as criteria in Figures 2.2 and 2.3. The scale score 3 is defined and used by the assessors as "meets expectation" for entrustability. The standard error of measurement around the scale score of 3 is 0.15, so we set the cutoff score for entrustability at the upper level of the 95% confidence interval = $3 + (2 \times 0.15) = 3.30$.

Employing this rigorous cutoff for entrustability, it can be seen from Figures 2.2 and 2.3 that average performance on various competencies reach entrustability at different times: professionalism (27 days), communication (65 days), medical interview (154 days), clinical reasoning (213 days), management planning (271 days), organizational efficacy (271 days), and oral presentation (271 days). Entrustability (≥ 3.30) is achieved at 154 days (about 5 months) for Overall Assessment. Interestingly, on Physical Exam most students had not yet achieved entrustability at 271 days.

The repeated measures analysis showed that students improved substantially on clinical skills, communications, and professionalism. These results show that the assessment system is feasible and works effectively for assessing competence, professionalism, and clinical skills.

SELF-ASSESSMENTS, PORTFOLIOS, AND REFLECTIONS

Reflection, particularly self-reflection is thought to be an important part of competence and professionalism. Unfortunately, reflection has been used with nearly as many meanings as has competence. In the health science professions, it is viewed as an important part of lifelong personal and professional learning and competence.

Self-reflection that can be achieved in the development of a portfolio may also facilitate behavioral change. The process of producing a portfolio usually involves synthesis of past experiences and future planning and therefore may be a useful method of improving the impact of feedback. In a recent review and analysis, Nguyen, Fernandez, Karsenti, and Charlin[29] identified five core components of reflection, and two extrinsic elements were identified as characteristics of reflective thinking. Reflection is defined as the process of engaging the self in attentive, critical, exploratory, and iterative interactions with one's thoughts and actions and their underlying conceptual frame, with a view to changing them and a view on the change itself.

Reflective portfolios are one tool that can incorporate the results of peer and self-assessment and their relationships. Electronic portfolios (ePortfolios), web-based in format, have the capacity to enhance student responsibility for their learning, and shape their understanding of their growth. In reflective portfolios, students articulate the value and meaning of their work and how it has contributed to their growth.

Reflection can be defined as "critical self-assessment." The self-reflection process requires the learner to analyze and synthesize their learning in the context of thought and action. Both as product and process, reflective ePortfolios have the potential to promote learning and transfer of knowledge by fostering the ability to make connections between professional behaviors and learning experiences.

A number of factors are relevant to the efficacy of feedback; the impact of the perceived value of the feedback is related to the likelihood of behavioral change. Factors include the characteristics of the assessment system, such as facilitators to encourage reflection, credibility of the source, the value of the information and receptivity to the feedback. There continues to be a lack of clarity whether peers or professors are more effective facilitators of feedback. Also ePortfolios can be used for reflection of feedback of self- and peer assessments of professional behavior leading to possible behavioral changes. Accordingly, self-assessment feedback and the use of an ePortfolio can improve professional competence.

SUMMARY AND CONCLUSIONS

Competence and professionalism are complex, interrelated, multidimensional constructs commonly based on three primary components: knowledge, skills, and attitudes. Entrustable professional activities are clinical actions that require the use and integration of several competencies and milestones critical to safe and effective clinical performance. To assess the competence of physicians for this, EPA requires complex and comprehensive assessments.

In the English-speaking world, the present views define medical competence and professionalism as the ability to meet the relationship-centered expectations required to practice medicine competently. British and American views of medical professionalism are quite similar. For Asian countries, however, professionalism is a Western concept without a precise equivalent in Asian cultures. Instruments and procedures that are designed to measure competence and professionalism are challenged on validity, reliability, and practicality.

A variety of professional organizations have recently weighed in on the constructs of competence and professionalism. The Canadian Medical Education Directions for Specialists (CanMEDS) framework consists of seven roles: manager, communicator, professional, scholar, expert, health advocate, collaborator and have been used as theoretical underpinnings of physician competencies.

Studies of the direct observation of learners provide evidence of effectiveness of direct observation and assessment in the clinical environment. The repeated measures analyses showed that students improved substantially on clinical skills, communications, and professionalism.

Reflection, particularly self-reflection is thought to be an important part of competence and professionalism. Unfortunately, reflection has been used with nearly as many meanings as has competence, but in the health science professions, it is viewed as an important part of lifelong personal and professional learning and competence.

REFLECTIONS

Reflection 2.1

Compare and contrast the meaning of the terms *competence* and *performance*. Write a brief essay (1,000 words) that discusses how the two terms are similar or different and how confusion may arise due lack of clarity. Ensure that you cite relevant empirical evidence for your arguments.

Reflection 2.2

How is Miller's Pyramid useful in assessing competence? Your response should not exceed 1,000 words. Ensure that you cite relevant empirical evidence for your answer.

Reflection 2.3

Describe how direct observation can be employed to assess *performance*. Write a brief essay (1,000 words) discussing the techniques and issues surrounding direct observation methods.

Reflection 2.4

Describe how multisource feedback in workplace-based assessment can be employed to assess *competence*. Write a brief essay (1,000 words) discussing the techniques and issues surrounding multisource feedback.

Reflection 2.5

Compare and contrast the meaning of the terms *professionalism* and *competence*. Write a brief essay of about 1,000 words. Cite relevant empirical evidence for your arguments.

REFERENCES

1. Miller GE. The assessment of clinical skills/competence/performance. *Academic Medicine*, 1990; 65:s63–s67.
2. Epstein RM, Hundert EM. Defining and assessing professional competence. *JAMA*, 2002; 287(2):226–235. p 226.
3. Hodges B, Lingard L (eds). *The Question of Competence: Reconsidering Medical Education in the Twenty-First Century*. Cornell University Press: Ithaca, NY, 2013.

4. Hawkins RE, Welcher CM, Holmboe E, Kirk LM, Norcini JJ, Simons KB, Skochelak SE. Implementation of competency-based medical education: Are we addressing the concerns and challenges? *Medical Education*, 2015; 49:1086–1102; ten Cate O, Snell L, Carraccio C. Medical competence: The interplay between individual ability and the health care environment. *Medical Teacher*, 2016; 32:669–675.

5. Violato C. A brief history of the regulation of medical practice: From Hammurabi to the National Board of Medical Examiners. *Wake Forest Journal of Science Medicine*, 2016; 2:122–129.

6. Carraccio C, Englander R, Gilhooly J, Mink R, Hofkosh D, Barone MA, Holmboe ES. Building a framework of entrustable professional activities, supported by competencies and milestones, to bridge the educational continuum. *Academic Medicine*, 2017; 92(3):324–330.

7. Swick HM. Toward a normative definition of medical professionalism. *Academic Medicine*, 2000; 75(6):612–616.

8. Hafferty FW. Definitions of professionalism. *Clinical Orthopaedics and Related Research*, 2006; 449:193–204.

9. Arnold L. Assessing professional behavior: Yesterday, today, and tomorrow. *Academic Medicine*, 2002; 77(6):502–515.

10. van Mook W, de Grave W, Wass V, O'Sullivan H, Zwaveling JH, Schuwirth LW, van der Vleuten CP. Professionalism: Evolution of the concept. *European Journal of Internal Medicine*, 2009; 20:e81–e84.

11. ABIM. Project Professionalism, 2006. Available at: www.abim.org/pdf/profess.pdf.

12. The internal medicine milestone project, 2015. Available at: www.acgme.org/Portals/0/PDFs/Milestones/InternalMedicineMilestones.pdf.

13. Plotnikoff GA, Amano T. A culturally appropriate, student-centered curriculum on medical professionalism. *Minnesota Medicine*, 2007; 90(8):42–43.

14. Hui E. The physician as a professional and the moral implications of medical professionalism. *Hong Kong Medical Journal*, 2005; 11(1):67–69.

15. Tsai TC, Lin CH, Harasym PH, Violato C. Students' perception on medical professionalism: The psychometric perspective. *Medical Teacher*, 2007; 29(2):128–134.

16. Nhan VT, Violato C, Le An P, Beran TN. Cross-cultural construct validity study of professionalism of Vietnamese medical students. *Teaching and Learning in Medicine*, 2014; 26(1):72–80.

17. Harden R, Stevenson M, Wilson Downie W, Wilson G. Assessment of clinical competence using objective structure examination. *British Medical Journal*, 1975; 1:447–451.

18. Hall W, Violato C, Lewkonia R, Lockyer J, Fidler H, Toews J, Jennett P, Donoff M, Moores D. Assessment of physician performance in Alberta: The Physician Achievement Review Project. *Canadian Medical Association Journal*, 1999; 161:52–57.

19. Violato C, Lockyer JM, Fidler H. Multi source feedback: A method of assessing surgical practice. *British Medical Journal*, 2003; 326:546–548.

20. Violato C, Lockyer J. Self and peer assessments of paediatricians, psychiatrists and medicine specialists: Implications for self-directed learning. *Advances in Health Sciences Education*, 2006; 11(3):235–244.

21. Violato C, Lockyer J, Fidler H. Changes in performance: A 5-year longitudinal study of participants in a multi-source feedback. *Medical Education*, 2008; 42(10):1007–1013.

22. Nuland SB. *Doctors: The Biography of Medicine*. Random House: New York, 1988.

23. Lockyer JM, Hodgson CS, Lee T, Faremo S, Fisher B, Dafoe W, Yiu V, Violato C. Clinical teaching as part of continuing professional development: Does teaching enhance clinical performance? *Medical Teacher*, 2016; 38(8):815–822.

24. Norcini JJ, Blank LL, Duffy FD, Fortna GS. The mini-CEX: A method for assessing clinical skills. *Annals of Internal Medicine*, 2003; 138:476–481.

25. Kogan JR, Holmboe ES, Hauer KE. Tools for direct observation and assessment of clinical skills of medical trainees: A systematic review. *JAMA*, 2009; 302(12):1316–1326.

26. Al AnsariA, Ali SK, Donnon T. The construct and criterion validity of the mini-CEX: A meta-analysis of the published research. *Academic Medicine*, 2013; 88(3):413–420.

27. Thurstone LL. The learning curve equation. *Psychological Review*, 1919; 34:278–286.

28. Violato C, Askew K, Ellis L. *Growth of Medical Competence: Direct Observation of Students during Third Year Clinical Clerkships*. Association of Medical Education of Europe: Helsinki, Finland, 2017.

29. Nguyen QD, Fernandez N, Karsenti T, Charlin B. What is reflection? A conceptual analysis of major definitions and a proposal of a five-component model. *Medical Education*, 2014; 48:1176–1189.

3

Statistics and test score interpretation

- Descriptive statistics are essential for teaching. Anyone who works in a professional capacity with people should learn about statistics—as is almost an article of faith in education and the health professions—each person is unique and an individual. Statistics allows you to go beyond the declaration of this truism and to quantify the uniqueness and similarity of people.
- Important graphs and frequency distributions for statistics include histograms and frequency polygons. There are four important types of frequency polygons in test data analysis. These include the following distributions: normal, skewed, bimodal, and rectangular.
- Measures of central tendency summarize the tendency of test scores to cluster around the center of the distribution and produce an "average" score. There are three measures of central tendency, or average, which shall be discussed in turn: the mode, median, and mean.
- There are two basic measures of dispersion, the range and standard deviation. A full description of a distribution must include an indication of its dispersion or variability. The range conveys some indication of the dispersion of a dataset, but it is very crude and unstable since it is based on only two scores, the maximum and the minimum.
- A preferred, much more stable and better measure of variability is the SD which includes every score in the distribution.
- The SD is a direct measure of a group's variability or the dispersion of scores. A small SD indicates that the group is quite homogeneous, while a large SD indicates that the group is heterogeneous.
- Norms provide information about the performance of a particular group on a specified measure. Any individual's score can thus be compared to that reference group, usually employing standard scores including z-scores, T-scores, stanines, and percentiles.

INTRODUCTION: WHY STATISTICS?

Why should prospective instructors, teachers, and professors learn about statistics? The answer to this question is very simple. Anyone who works in a professional capacity with people should learn about statistics—as is almost an article of faith in education and the health professions—each person is unique and an individual. Statistics allows you to go beyond the declaration of this truism and to quantify the uniqueness and similarity of people. This allows the instructor to make precise inferences and evaluations of learners on the basis of numerical information and statistics. Teachers should know enough statistics to analyze and describe the results of their own tests, understand and interpret statistics in test manuals and research reports, and comprehend and discuss standard scores used in reporting learner performance as commonly found in the health professions. Such common tests, for example, include the MCAT, NBME board exams, National Council Licensure Examination for Registered Nurses (NCLEX-RN), and the National Council Licensure Examination for Practical Nurses (NCLEX-PN).

Before the advent of computers, computations involved in statistics were tedious and prone to errors. Nowadays, however, the widespread availability of computers and customized software has made the computations of statistics as simple as striking a key on a keyboard or a click of the mouse. If you have entered the data correctly, you can also be sure that the results of the computations will be error free. There are a number of user-friendly computer programs, which will allow you to do all of the computations necessary in your assessment course and in your eventual course and teaching practice. Once you learn to use a program, statistical calculations will become routine and very simple.

This chapter is devoted to descriptive statistics, which are essential for classroom practice. You will learn about graphs and frequency distributions, measures of central tendency, measures of dispersion and variability, and norms and standard scores.

HISTOGRAMS AND FREQUENCY POLYGONS

Histograms

A histogram is a method of graphing and displaying data to indicate the shape of a distribution. It is particularly useful when there are a large number of observations. We begin with an example consisting of the scores of 169 medical students in a first-year Neuroscience Test. The test consists of 250 items, each graded as "correct" or "incorrect" and the percent value of each student was computed. The students' scores ranged from 64.8% to 93.7%. The first step is to create a frequency table but a simple frequency table would be too big, containing over 100 rows. To simplify the table, we group scores together in intervals of two as shown in Table 3.1.

Frequency polygon

A frequency polygon is very similar to a histogram, except that frequency polygons can be used to compare sets of data or to display a cumulative frequency

Table 3.1 Frequency table for neurosciences exam

Score range	Frequency	Percent	Cumulative percent
63–65	1	0.6	0.6
66–68	1	0.6	1.2
69–71	1	0.6	1.8
73–75	2	1.2	3.0
76–78	7	4.1	7.1
79–81	19	11.2	18.3
82–83	18	10.7	29.0
84–85	17	10.1	39.1
86–87	14	8.3	47.3
88–89	14	8.3	55.6
90–91	17	10.1	65.7
92–93	18	10.7	76.3
94–95	17	10.1	86.4
96–97	17	10.1	96.4
98–99	6	3.6	100.0
Total	169	100.0	

distribution. In addition, histograms tend to be rectangles, while a frequency polygon resembles a line graph. Figure 3.1 contains a frequency polygon of 163 first-year medical students in the **Essentials of Clinical Medicine Course**. The mean was 93.8%.

IMPORTANT DISTRIBUTIONS

There are four important types of frequency polygons in test data analysis. These include the following distributions: normal, skewed, bimodal, and rectangular.

The normal distribution

This distribution is depicted in Figure 3.2. Notice that it is a frequency polygon that has a smooth shape and is symmetrical. The normal curve was developed mathematically in 1733 by DeMoivre and re-discovered 1924 by Karl Pearson.[1] Subsequently, Gauss used the normal curve to analyze astronomical data in 1809; this curve is often called the Gaussian distribution. A common everyday term for it is the bell-shaped curve.

If you were to find the center of the distribution and draw a line through it, you could see that the left half of the curve is a mirror image of the right half. This property of symmetry is very important for statistical use of this curve. From the mid-point of the curve, it drops sharply as you move both to the left and right of center, but the "tails" never actually touch the x-axis. This is the asymptotic property of the distribution. Theoretically, the tails are thought to extend to infinity. This is expressed in equation 3.1:

$$f(x) = \frac{1}{\sqrt{2\pi}} e^{\frac{-x^2}{2}}$$

(3.1)

Three examples of the normal distribution are depicted in Figure 3.2.

The first variable (Figure 3.2a) is the MCAT scores. Notice that most of the heights from this group cluster around the center and become very infrequent at the extremes of high and low scores. This is hardly surprising as most medical students are around an "average" performance and very few score either extremely high or extremely low.

Like the MCAT scores of medical students, the distribution of the birth weight of neonates depicted in Figure 3.2b is also normally distributed. Again you can see that the ounces have a central tendency and become very rare at the extremes of the distribution, very heavy or very light. The same is true of the Total Optimism scores of adult Americans (Figure 3.2c).

Clearly, there is some general principle underlying the properties of the variables depicted in Figure 3.2. Indeed, this pattern (normal distribution) is widespread and does represent a general principle of variability. It is thought that variability among living things exist in this pattern and that is how things normally are. Hence, *the normal distribution*.

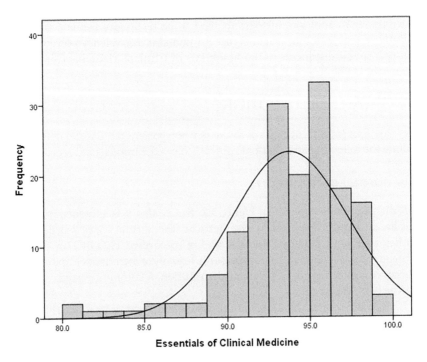

Figure 3.1 A frequency polygon overlaid on a histogram.

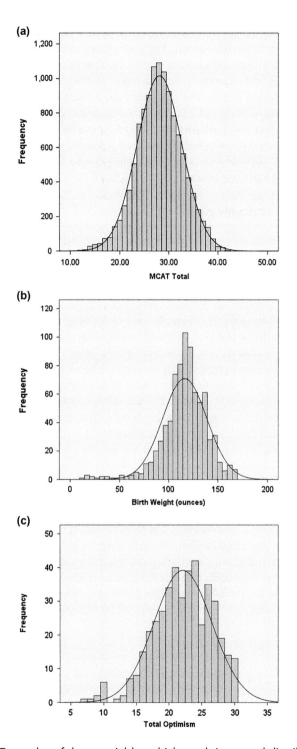

Figure 3.2 Examples of three variables which result in normal distributions.

What is the reason for this? The explanation has to do with a principle of probability: when differences among the objects measured are due to random or chance factors, a normal distribution results. In all of the examples in Figure 3.2, the differences *between* measurements are due to chance factors and therefore a normal distribution results. For our purposes, in dealing with most physical, psychological, and educational variables, you can assume an underlying normal distribution. As you may have already noticed, in practice when you get a set of scores from a class, it usually doesn't resemble a normal distribution at all. Why is this? To answer this question, it is necessary to digress briefly into a distinction between samples and populations.

Populations and samples

A population is defined as *all* of the objects (people, fish, rats, trees, rocks, test scores, or anything else that is measured) in the set that is of interest. You may define all American medical students as a set, for example, and call that a population. Then at least one or all but one of the medical students constitutes a subset or sample of the population. Populations are usually very large and samples are usually small by comparison. A single class of medical students would constitute a sample, while the population would be all medical students. An instructor, teacher, or tutor is usually dealing with a sample (class), which may range from small (e.g., less than ten in small group sessions) to somewhat larger for the whole medical class (e.g., 150 in basic courses such as Anatomy and Embryology) and perhaps idiosyncratic. Thus, data from one class may not appear much like a normal distribution. The assumption, however, is that this class is a sample from a population which itself is normally distributed.

A further complication arises because sometimes professors treat their class as a sample and sometimes as a population. When the teacher is interested only in their particular class and not in any larger group, then that class is the whole set or population. This is the case, for example, when an instructor is deriving final grades for a class—there is no interest in comparing to other classes. Alternatively, when an instructor is interpreting scores from standardized tests (e.g., the NBME Subject Matter Exams), the reference group is a much larger one than only the teacher's own class, which, in this case, is a subset or a sample. In any case, for most purposes, these distinctions are obvious in actual practice. Using idiosyncratic or small samples like particular classes can produce skewed distributions.

Skewed distributions

Like a hat that has gone askew, skewed distributions are off-center. There are two types of skew: one where the scores bunch up to the right and one where they bunch up to the left. When the scores pile up to the left, the distribution is referred to as a positive skew and a negative skew when the scores are at the other end (see Figure 3.3a). While this may seem counter intuitive, it is the direction of the "tail" of the distribution that indicates positive or negative.

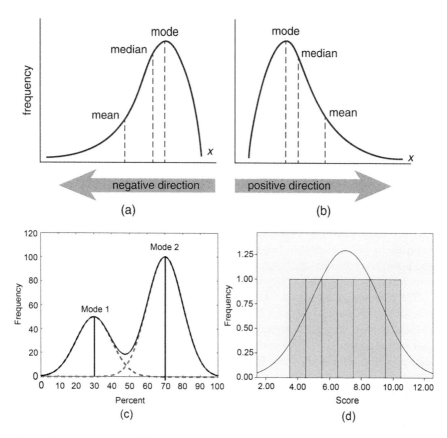

Figure 3.3 Examples of skewed, bimodal, and rectangular distributions (a) and (b) Skewed distributions. (c) Bimodal distribution. (d) Rectangular distribution.

What causes a skewed distribution? If we assume that the underlying population distribution is normal, then there are two possible reasons for a skewed distribution: (1) the sample on which the data are based is biased or (2) the test you have given is either too difficult or too easy. In most circumstances, the first possibility in not tenable. By statistical definition, 19 classes out of 20 are not biased or unusual but are "normal." That is, they represent the underlying normal distribution. When a skewed distribution occurs, then, the instructor must ask herself whether or not the class is unrepresentative such as a group of very high performers or conversely, low achievers. If this is not true, then the second possibility is probably tenable.

When the distribution is negatively skewed, the test used was too easy for these learners. Notice (Figure 3.3a) that the scores are piled up toward the high end of the distribution and very few learners achieved low scores. This is called a "ceiling" effect, as the scores are piled against the ceiling. For a positive skew (Figure 3.3b), this is called a "floor" effect as the scores bunch up on the low end, or the floor. A positive skew indicates that the test was too difficult and learners with considerable knowledge of the subject were classified with those with only superficial knowledge (i.e., on the floor). In any case, whenever there is a skewed distribution, this signals the instructor that something is amiss. A bimodal distribution is also a signal that something is unusual about the class.

Bimodal distributions

A bimodal distribution is shown in Figure 3.3c. Notice that the distribution has two "humps" with a dip between them. The dotted lines indicate the probable underlying populations that have been combined to give this bimodal distribution. If you follow the solid line and then the dotted line at the dip, you can see that two normal distributions have been "jammed" together. A simple example of such a bimodal distribution is a frequency polygon of the heights of adult men and women together (say 1,000 of each). Of course you really have two underlying populations (with respect to height) such that when you mix them together, you end up with a bimodal distribution. Anytime that you have a bimodal distribution, it suggests that there really are two underlying populations mixed together.

The example in Figure 3.3c is of the results of a biostatistics test in an undergraduate class (Medical Sciences 407). Many of the class score on the right "hump" of the distribution, while a separate group scored on the left "hump." Upon further investigation, the higher scoring group were biological science majors who were required to take the class for their majors, while the lower scoring group were humanities majors fulfilling a science requirement. Another common distribution in testing is the rectangular distribution.

Rectangular distributions

A rectangular distribution looks like a rectangle (Figure 3.3d). This distribution may occur with very small classes (say less than 15). If you gave a class of ten learners, for example, a test out 50, no two learners might achieve the same score. Thus, each score would occur only once (a frequency of 10%). When these data are plotted on a frequency polygon, a rectangular distribution results. The data in Figure 3.3d are from a PhD seminar with only seven students in it. Each scored a unique score on a quiz that resulted in a rectangular distribution. This merely results because of the very small group involved.

To summarize then, a number of distributions can arise in practice even though the underlying population may be normally distributed. A knowledgeable teacher can usually make good inferences about the test or underlying composition of the samples based on the nature of the distribution whether it is skewed, bimodal, or rectangular. Further insights into the data, however, require statistical analysis beginning with central tendency.

CENTRAL TENDENCY

As has already been alluded to several times in this chapter, test scores have a central tendency or tend to cluster around the center of the distribution and produce an "average" score. In fact there are three measures of central tendency or average, which shall be discussed in turn: the mode, median, and mean.

The mode

The mode (Mo) is the most popular or the modal score. To determine the mode in a distribution, you must inspect the data and find the most frequently occurring score. An example of some data that depicts central tendency is given in Table 3.2. The Mo on Quiz 1 is 14, while the Mo on Quiz 2 is 12 as they are the most frequently occurring scores on the two distributions.

It is possible of course to have more than one score occurring with equally high frequency. In that case, you may have a bimodal or even a trimodal distribution. Recall that above the juxtaposition of male and female heights produced a bimodal distribution. That is, two modes (or most frequent scores) were evident; one for the height of males and one for the height of females.

The median

The median (Md) is the score that divides the distribution into half (as the median on a boulevard divides the road in half). It is also called the counting average because in order to determine the Md, you must arrange a set or scores in rank order and then count to the point where that score divides the distribution

Table 3.2 Measures of central tendency

Scores on quiz 1	Scores on quiz 2
10	6
14	7
14 Mo = 14	8
14	8
15	9
16 Md = 16	10 Md = 10.5
17	11
18	12
19	12 Mo = 12
21	12
<u>24</u>	13
$\Sigma X = 182$	<u>14</u>
	$\Sigma X = 122$

$$\text{Mean} = \sum_{i=1}^{n} \frac{X}{n-1}$$

Mean for quiz 1	Mean for quiz 2
$182/n - 1 = 182/10$	$122/n - 1 = 122/11$
18.2	11.1

in half. The data in Table 3.2 have been arranged in rank order, and for Quiz 1, the Md has been determined to be 16. That is because there are 11 scores on Quiz 1 such that the mid-point score turns out to be 16. Half of the scores are above this point (5 scores) and half are below it (5 scores).

The matter becomes a little more complicated with the scores on Quiz 2. Here there are 12 scores so that no real occurring score constitutes the mid-point. Rather, the Md falls between two scores and is a hypothetical point. Since there are 12 scores, the mid-point occurs between score 6 and 7 (thus 6 scores are below and 6 above). The Md then is halfway between the sixth and seventh scores (11 and 10), which is 10.5 (see Table 3.2).

A formula to compute the score, which is the Md once the scores have been rank ordered is given as

$$\text{Mdn} = n \times \frac{1}{2} \tag{3.2}$$

where
$\quad$ n is the number of scores
$\quad$ Mdn is the number of the score, which is the median.

If there are 25 scores in the rank-ordered distribution, Mdn $= 25 \times 1/2 = 13$th. The 13th score of this distribution is the median. When n is an odd number, then the median will always be an actual score. If $n = 26$, for example, Mdn $= 26+1/2 = 13.5$. Thus, the score that is the median will fall between the 13th and 14th scores. When n is an even number, the median will always be a hypothetical number.

The mean

The mean (M or $\bar{X}$) is the most widely used measure of central tendency and is also known as the arithmetic average. The mean is calculated in the following manner:

$$\text{Mean} = \frac{\text{Sum of all scores}}{\text{Number of scores}},$$

For a population, the mean is computed and represented using Greek letters and symbols in equation 3.3:

$$\mu = \sum_{i=1}^{n} \frac{X}{N} \tag{3.3}$$

where
$\quad$ $\mu = \text{mean}$
$\quad$ $\Sigma = $ summation operator (i.e., "add them up") from the 1st to the nth score
$\quad$ N is the number of scores in a population

For a sample, the mean is computed and represented using Roman letters (same as English alphabet) and symbols in equation 3.4:

$$\text{Mean} = \sum_{i=1}^{n} \frac{X}{n-1} \qquad (3.4)$$

where

Σ = summation operator (i.e., "add them up") from the 1st to the nth score
X is any score
n is the number of scores in a sample

Examples of how to calculate the mean is given in Table 3.2.

Comparing the mean, mode, and median

For any dataset, the values of the three measures of central tendency can give you an indication of the nature of the underlying distribution. If all three values are identical or very similar, for example, this indicates that the underlying distribution is normal (see Figure 3.2). If, on the other hand, the mean is greater than the median, which in turn is greater than the mode, this indicates a positively skewed distribution. For a situation where the mode is largest with the median next and the mean smallest, the underlying distribution is negatively skewed (Figure 3.3a and b). When there are two modes with the mean and median having the same values both intermediate between the modes, a bimodal distribution is indicated (Figure 3.3c). Finally, the measures of central tendency have little meaning in a rectangular distribution (Figure 3.3d).

Without actually plotting a frequency polygon, you can make a good estimate about the nature of the underlying distribution just by comparing the values of the mean, mode, and median in any given data set. If these measures are identical or within a point or two of each other, a normal distribution is indicated. Skewed distributions can be inferred by noticing the relative values of the three measures as in a bimodal distribution. While the inferences based on the central tendency are not definitive indicators of the underlying distribution, they are useful albeit rough guidelines for classroom practice.

Which of the three measures is best? This turns out to be a nonsensical question because each measure of central tendency conveys meaning in relation to the others. It is true, however, that the mean is probably the most widely used measure of central tendency and indeed is synonymous with the term "average." Nevertheless, each measure can have quite a different numerical value (as in skewed distributions) but still be a "correct" measure of central tendency.

Astute users of statistics can convey different meaning with the same data by using different measures of central tendency. Consider a salary dispute between a health district and its nurses who are mostly young and novice (the salary distribution will be positively skewed). When the nurses go out on strike, the board, in an attempt to turn public opinion against them, reports in the local newspaper that the average (mean) nurse salary is $64,500 per annum. In the same newspaper, the nurses report that the average (mode) salary is $44,343 per annum. Readers of this newspaper will undoubtedly become confused, skeptical, and conclude that someone is prevaricating. Both parties of course are telling the truth but in a way that supports their point of view. Newspaper readers encountering such data probably conclude that statistics are meaningless and are used for propaganda purposes. Knowledgeable persons, of course, are not likely to be taken in by these simple statistical tricks.

In addition to central tendency, accurate description of any dataset must also include a description of dispersion or variability.

DISPERSION AND VARIABILITY

Two basic measures of dispersion, the range and standard deviation, will be discussed here. A full description of a distribution must include an indication of its dispersion or variability.

The range

Consider two distributions; both are normally distributed with the exact same central tendencies. If all you were told was that the values of the central tendencies were identical, you might conclude that the distributions are the same. If you saw the distributions, and A had a greater dispersion or more variability in the scores than distribution B, it would be obvious that they are not the same distributions. This further piece of information, therefore, is required to distinguish the distributions. It is as though you had two names, both Jordan, in front of you. You might conclude that they represent the same person until you discovered that one had the surname Winthrop; the other, Petrovic. Similarly, for a distribution, a "surname" or measure of dispersion is required to describe it fully. If, for distribution A, you knew that the Range (maximum score − minimum score) is 50 (80 − 30) and for B it is 30 (70 − 40), you could conclude that they are different distributions. While the range does convey some indication of the dispersion of a dataset, it is very crude and unstable since it is based on only two scores, the maximum and the minimum. A preferred, much more stable and better measure of variability is the SD which includes every score in the distribution.

The standard deviation

For a population, this is defined by equation 3.5:

$$\sigma = \sqrt{\frac{\sum_{i=1}^{n}(\mu - X_i)^2}{N}} \tag{3.5}$$

where σ is the symbol for standard deviation
   X is any score
   μ is the mean
   N is the number of test scores in a population

For a sample, this is defined by equation 3.6:

$$SD = \sqrt{\sum_{i=1}^{n} \frac{(M - X_i)^2}{n-1}} \qquad (3.6)$$

where
SD is the symbol for standard deviation
X is any score
M is the mean
n is the number of test scores

The SD, as the name implies, is a standardized deviation score. Notice from the formulas (equation 3.5) that the mean is subtracted from each score producing a deviation score. That is, each score is deviated around the mean. These are then squared, summed, and averaged (i.e., divided by N or $n - 1$; see equations 3.4 and 3.5). In short, the deviation scores are standardized and the resulting figure (the standard deviation) is directly interpretable as a measure of dispersion. The larger SD is the greater the dispersion of the distribution.

The meaning of the standard deviation

Computing SD is a relatively simple matter but it is much more important to understand what it means. The SD is a direct measure of the group's variability or the dispersion of scores. A small SD indicates that the group is quite homogeneous, while a large SD indicates that the group is heterogeneous.

Suppose that you gave a physiology test to three sections of first-year medical students for a total of 60 learners, you could calculate the mode, median, mean, and standard deviation of this group. Now suppose you gave the same test to a group made up of first, second, and third-year classes for a total of 60 learners. Again compute the measures of central tendency as well as the SD. How do you think the values will compare across the two groups? Probably, the measures of central tendency will be the same (or very similar) across the two groups, while the SDs will be quite different. The SD will be greater for the second group than the first group since the former is much more heterogeneous than the latter, because it is made up of first, second, and third-year learners rather than just first-year learners. Even though the measures of central tendency might be similar, comparing SD gives a clear indication of the differences in homogeneity.

The SD is also widely used in interpreting test scores in SD units (standard scores) as we shall see later in this chapter. Finally, SD is used by test publishers as well as by researchers to make inferences about individual and group performance on tests and other measures. Which do you think is larger—the SD of all those who wrote the MCAT in 2014 or the SD of those that were admitted to medical school for that cohort?

NORMS AND STANDARD SCORES

Norms provide information about the performance of a particular group on a specified measure. Any individual's score can thus be compared to that reference group, usually employing standard scores including z-scores, T-scores, stanines, and percentiles. In this section, we will discuss each of these standard scores and norms.

What are Norms? Norms are statistics such as the mean and SD on a norm group that give precise numerical values on some measure such as an IQ test or height measurement. Norm group is probably closest in meaning to "peer" group, and its purpose is to establish a reference for comparison of a particular person.

In many educational and other kinds of performance, there are no absolute standards by which you can evaluate or judge performance. Even in athletic performance such as sprinting, for example, determination of a person's achievement must be necessarily based on a comparison to some norm or peer group values. How good a sprinter is a high-school student who runs the 100 m in 14.2 s? If judged in relation to the world record of under 10 s held by Olympic athletes, the high school student's time seems poor. This is the wrong norm or peer group for interpreting the student's time, however. A more appropriate group for comparison is the performance of other high school students. Even more precisely, you would need to know if the student is a male or female. The main point is that the sprinter's time only makes sense in relation to some group norms, particularly a relevant group or a peer group.

Performance on standardized tests is usually interpreted on the basis of the performance of a peer or norm group. Norms, however, are not standards but only statistics that are useful for comparison. A standard is some absolute criterion against which all are judged. IQ, for example, is a norm-referenced type test since each examinee is judged against the performance of their peer group. IQ makes no sense as an absolute measure.

It is imperative that the norm group be based on a representative sample, which is relevant. Judging the performance of a freshman student on a basic skills test against the performance of a graduate student, for example, would violate the first requirement of representativeness. It is crucial that the norms that are established for the measure be based on a representative sample. The norms against which the sprinting achievement of the high school student is to be judged should be based on other high school students and not Olympic athletes.

Norm groups should also be relevant. It is common in Canada, for example, to use American norms for interpreting Canadian examinee's scores. This is common practice on IQ tests such as the Wechsler Intelligence Scale for Children—Revised (WISC-R) even though the test and norms are clearly biased toward American examinees. Here the relevancy of the norms are in question as you may very well wonder how the performance of, say, rural Hispanic children in the southern states is relevant to urban, white children living in Calgary. This norm group may be quite irrelevant for Canadian children taking the WISC-R.

Another way that norms can become irrelevant is when they become dated. The original norm group for the Wechsler Adult Intelligence Scale (WAIS) was selected in the 1950s such that examinees in 1980 were judged according to those dated norms. It wasn't until 1981 that revised norms were published for the

WAIS-R (revised). The earlier norms had probably become inappropriate given the social, economic, and political changes that have occurred since the 1950s. Another version of the test, the WAIS-III, was released in 1997; by then the 1981 norms had become obsolete. The next version is scheduled to be released in 2019. In making norms relevant, it is important to take into account the geographical region of the sample, its socioeconomic status, educational level, ethnic composition, gender composition, as well as other characteristics. Norms then should adhere to the three "Rs." They must be recent, representative, and relevant.

An individual's performance on a standardized test is usually interpreted on the basis of standard scores based on the normal distribution.

Standard scores and the normal distribution

The basis for deriving standard scores is the normal distribution. This curve, as you have seen, is symmetrical and bell-shaped and has many useful mathematical properties, which underlie a great deal of statistical theory. For test interpretation, one of the most useful properties is the fact that the curve can be divided into SD units, which define a fixed and known percentage of the area under the curve.

The normal distribution is depicted in Figure 3.4 together with the SD units and the percentage of area under each unit. Notice that the curve is divided into six pieces. Imagine that the curve was rectangular. Then each of the SD units would contain an equal amount of area. Since the curve is bell-shaped, however, as you move away from the center, the amount of area bounded by an SD unit falls sharply. The first SD unit on either side of the mean, therefore, contains most area (~34% each). The next two units contain approximately 13.5% of the area each, while the two most extreme units have about 2.5% each. The tails of the curve theoretically extend to infinity—are asymptotic—but for all practical purposes, nearly all of the area under the curve is bounded by three SD units on either side of the mean.

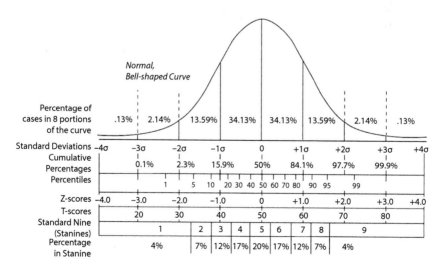

Figure 3.4 The standard normal curve.

The curve depicted in Figure 3.4 is called the *standard normal curve* because it has been transformed into SD units. The mean of this curve is 0 (the mean is 0 SD units from itself), while the first value to the right of the means is +1 (i.e., one SD above the mean). The first value to the left is −1 because it is 1 SD below the mean. The remaining values indicate how many SDs they are above (positive) or below (negative) the mean. Any normally distributed variable can be translated into the standard normal curve.

The standard normal curve is the common metric of comparing across different tests as well as comparing to a norm group. We may use world currencies as an analogy. Each country has its own peculiar currency, which are not directly comparable to one another. Which is more, 10 dollars or 100 yen? To the naive observer, 100 yen might seem more because it is numerically greater. Such comparisons are inappropriate, however, as these currencies are not directly comparable. Rather both must be translated into a common metric, the gold standard, which is the standard for all world currencies. If we translate 10 dollars into the gold standard and then to yen, it turns out to be worth about 112 yen, a higher value.

The standard normal curve is the gold standard for test scores. Suppose that Felicia received a score of 30 on Test A and 35 on Test B. On which test did she do better? While you may be tempted to answer Test B, you have inadequate information. Test A has 40 questions, while Test B has 50 questions so that Felicia received 75% on Test A but only 70% on Test B. You might be forgiven for concluding that Felicia did better on Test A but your conclusions would still be wrong. This is like directly comparing dollars to yen. You must go to the standard metric, the standard normal curve. Suppose that you now knew that the mean on Test A was 25 and the SD was 5. Therefore, Felicia scored 5 points above the mean (30–25), which is exactly 1 SD unit above the mean. On Test B, the mean was 37 and the SD was 2. Felicia, therefore, scored 1 SD below the mean (35–37/2) on Test B. Clearly, Felicia did better on Test A than she did on Test B (see Figure 3.4). By thus standardizing a score on any test, you can compare across tests for any person, as well as across people on any test. The type of standard score (i.e. SD units) that has been described here is called a *z*-score. Figure 3.4 summarizes a number of standard scores under the normal distribution, which will be discussed in turn.

z-Scores

The simplest standard score and the one that the others are based on is the *z*-score. Formalizing the computations above, the following formula defines this standard score:

$$z = \frac{X - M}{SD} \tag{3.7}$$

where
    z is the *z*-score
    M is the mean on the test

X is the raw score
SD is the standard deviation on the test

If you transformed any normally distributed raw scores into *z*-scores, you would produce the standard normal curve with a mean of 0 and an SD of 1. Thus, if you were to take IQ data and transform all the scores into *z*-scores by subtracting the IQ mean from each (100) and dividing the result by the SD (15; in short, applying equation 3.7), you would produce the standard normal curve (see Figure 3.4).

The *z*-scores, which come from raw scores less than the mean, are always negative, while those coming from raw scores above the mean are always positive. This, of course, is intuitively obvious since the mean produces a *z*-score of 0. If the difference between the mean and a raw score is a fraction of an SD, then the resulting *z*-score will have a decimal value. This is illustrated by the example of a raw score of 52 on a test with a mean of 50 and an SD of 8 ($z = 52 - 50/8 = 0.25$). Locate this value in Figure 3.4.

While *z*-scores are well understood and readily utilized by testing experts, they can be confusing and distressing to learners and some instructors. This is because *z*-scores have the properties of having negative values (and 0) as well as decimal or fractional values. Most non-experts are accustomed to test scores as whole, positive numbers. An instructor may encounter difficulty trying to explain to a student that he has a *z*-score of 0 (perhaps suggesting 0 knowledge), or worse yet, a *z*-score of −1.3 (find this value in Figure 3.4). In order to overcome these difficulties with negative and decimal values, *T*-scores have been developed.

T-Scores

This standard score is a linear transformation of *z*-scores. The decimal values are eliminated by multiplying each *z*-score by 10 (this has the effect of moving the decimal place one to the right) and adding 50 to each result (thus, setting the mean at 50 since it was previously 0) as follows:

$$T = 10(z) + 50 \tag{3.8}$$

Notice now that there are no negative scores (if $z = -0.5$ then $T = 10(-0.5) + 50 = 45$) or decimal values (always round *T*-scores to the nearest whole number). *T*-scores, then, have more intuitive appeal and are less likely to be misunderstood than *z*-scores by non-experts (see Figure 3.4). Nevertheless, *T*-scores have shortcomings of their own.

A *T*-score of 50 indicates "average" performance since it is the mean of the distribution. Most people would interpret a test score of 50 as a marginal passing score since they have been exposed to years of school use where this number magically indicates a "pass." Moreover, a *T*-score of 60, which would indicate to these same people a passing but lackluster performance, in reality indicates quite superior performance since it is 1 SD above the mean. The problem is that most people interpret *T*-scores as though they are percentage test scores and thus misunderstand them. In a continuing attempt to develop simple standard scores that are not misinterpreted by the lay person, testing experts have invented the stanine.

Stanines

This standard score (from the two words *standard nines*) is an attempt to divide the standard normal curve into nine intervals rather than points so as to classify scores by categories rather than points. Notice that all *T*-scores between 47 and 53 receive a stanine 5 (see Figure 3.4) so that now a single-digit index of performance is used. To derive stanines, you need to have either a *z*-score or a *T*-score and then read the stanine equivalent from Figure 3.4.

The main advantage of stanines is that a single-digit reporting system is used that ranges from 1 to 9. On the surface of it, this is apparently very easy to understand. There are two main disadvantages to this system, however.

First, differences between learners in performance are obscured. While you may be able to justify the grouping together of two learners whose IQs are 97 and 104 into stanine 5, you would have greater difficulty justifying putting both IQ scores of 127 and 150 into stanine 9. Similarly, IQs 72 and 43 are classified together in stanine 1. In the extreme stanines then, real differences between people are obscured. Here then, two-digit reporting, such as *T*-scores or *z*-scores, is required.

Second, like *T*-scores and *z*-scores, stanines are subject to misinterpretation because of people's preconceived notions. A stanine 5, for example, indicates "average" performance as does a *T*-score 50 since both are means, but for many people, this is marginal passing. A stanine 7 is 2 SDs above the mean and thus indicates very good performance but might mean just an adequate performance for many people. In a continuing attempt to devise a simple, non-misleading, and easy-to-understand reporting system, testing and measurement experts have devised the percentile.

Percentiles

This ranking system can be computed directly from *z*-scores. Look back momentarily at Figure 3.4. It becomes clear that if you were to score at the mean on any standard scoring system (e.g., *z*-score or *T*-score), you have scored higher than half (50%) of the norm group and thus you are at the 50th percentile (also termed %ile). Similarly, if you score 1 SD above the mean ($z = +1.0$), you have scored higher than 84% of the norm group (add up all the area to the left of the *z*-score) and are thus in the 84th %ile. You can see then, that like *z*-scores, *T*-scores, stanines, and percentiles are just another way of reporting standard scores. It becomes a little trickier to compute the percentile rank of decimal values of *z*-scores.

The mathematics in computing the area under the normal curve to the left of any *z*-score are quite complex and require some calculus. Fortunately, erstwhile mathematicians have already done this for a great number of *z*-scores, and the results are summarized in Table 3.3. You need to only look-up the *z*-score and its associated area in this table and thus avoid complex calculations.

Table 3.3 has two sets of columns, *z*-scores (column A) and the area beyond *z* (the remaining columns). The area in columns is given as a proportion rather than a percentage. In order to translate this into a percentage, merely move the decimal place 2 to the right and round to the nearest whole number. Thus, for $z = 0.30$, the percentage equivalent is 62 since the proportion is .6179 (see Figure 3.4). Thus, a

Table 3.3 Percent of area under the standard normal curve for z-scores

z	0.00	0.01	0.02	0.03	0.04	0.05	0.06	0.07	0.08	0.09
0.0	0.5000	0.5040	0.5080	0.5120	0.5160	0.5199	0.5239	0.5279	0.5319	0.5359
0.1	0.5398	0.5438	0.5478	0.5517	0.5557	0.5596	0.5636	0.5675	0.5714	0.5753
0.2	0.5793	0.5832	0.5871	0.5910	0.5948	0.5987	0.6026	0.6064	0.6103	0.6141
0.3	0.6179	0.6217	0.6255	0.6293	0.6331	0.6368	0.6406	0.6443	0.6480	0.6517
0.4	0.6554	0.6591	0.6628	0.6664	0.6700	0.6736	0.6772	0.6808	0.6844	0.6879
0.5	0.6915	0.6950	0.6985	0.7019	0.7054	0.7088	0.7123	0.7157	0.7190	0.7224
0.6	0.7257	0.7291	0.7324	0.7357	0.7389	0.7422	0.7454	0.7486	0.7517	0.7549
0.7	0.7580	0.7611	0.7642	0.7673	0.7704	0.7734	0.7764	0.7794	0.7823	0.7852
0.8	0.7881	0.7910	0.7939	0.7967	0.7995	0.8023	0.8051	0.8078	0.8106	0.8133
0.9	0.8159	0.8186	0.8212	0.8238	0.8264	0.8289	0.8315	0.8340	0.8365	0.8389
1.0	0.8413	0.8438	0.8461	0.8485	0.8508	0.8531	0.8554	0.8577	0.8599	0.8621
1.1	0.8643	0.8665	0.8686	0.8708	0.8729	0.8749	0.8770	0.8790	0.8810	0.8830
1.2	0.8849	0.8869	0.8888	0.8907	0.8925	0.8944	0.8962	0.8980	0.8997	0.9015
1.3	0.9032	0.9049	0.9066	0.9082	0.9099	0.9115	0.9131	0.9147	0.9162	0.9177

(Continued)

Table 3.3 (Continued) Percent of area under the standard normal curve for z-scores

z	0.00	0.01	0.02	0.03	0.04	0.05	0.06	0.07	0.08	0.09
1.4	0.9192	0.9207	0.9222	0.9236	0.9251	0.9265	0.9279	0.9292	0.9306	0.9319
1.5	0.9332	0.9345	0.9357	0.9370	0.9382	0.9394	0.9406	0.9418	0.9429	0.9441
1.6	0.9452	0.9463	0.9474	0.9484	0.9495	0.9505	0.9515	0.9525	0.9535	0.9545
1.7	0.9554	0.9564	0.9573	0.9582	0.9591	0.9599	0.9608	0.9616	0.9625	0.9633
1.8	0.9641	0.9649	0.9656	0.9664	0.9671	0.9678	0.9686	0.9693	0.9699	0.9706
1.9	0.9713	0.9719	0.9726	0.9732	0.9738	0.9744	0.9750	0.9756	0.9761	0.9767
2.0	0.9772	0.9778	0.9783	0.9788	0.9793	0.9798	0.9803	0.9808	0.9812	0.9817
2.1	0.9821	0.9826	0.9830	0.9834	0.9838	0.9842	0.9846	0.9850	0.9854	0.9857
2.2	0.9861	0.9864	0.9868	0.9871	0.9875	0.9878	0.9881	0.9884	0.9887	0.9890
2.3	0.9893	0.9896	0.9898	0.9901	0.9904	0.9906	0.9909	0.9911	0.9913	0.9916
2.4	0.9918	0.9920	0.9922	0.9925	0.9927	0.9929	0.9931	0.9932	0.9934	0.9936
2.5	0.9938	0.9940	0.9941	0.9943	0.9945	0.9946	0.9948	0.9949	0.9951	0.9952
2.6	0.9953	0.9955	0.9956	0.9957	0.9959	0.9960	0.9961	0.9962	0.9963	0.9964
2.7	0.9965	0.9966	0.9967	0.9968	0.9969	0.9970	0.9971	0.9972	0.9973	0.9974
2.8	0.9974	0.9975	0.9976	0.9977	0.9977	0.9978	0.9979	0.9979	0.9980	0.9981
2.9	0.9981	0.9982	0.9982	0.9983	0.9984	0.9984	0.9985	0.9985	0.9986	0.9986
3.0	0.9987	0.9987	0.9987	0.9988	0.9988	0.9989	0.9989	0.9989	0.9990	0.9990
3.1	0.9990	0.9991	0.9991	0.9991	0.9992	0.9992	0.9992	0.9992	0.9993	0.9993
3.2	0.9993	0.9993	0.9994	0.9994	0.9994	0.9994	0.9994	0.9995	0.9995	0.9995
3.3	0.9995	0.9995	0.9995	0.9996	0.9996	0.9996	0.9996	0.9996	0.9996	0.9997
−3.4	0.0003	0.0003	0.0003	0.0003	0.0003	0.0003	0.0003	0.0003	0.0003	0.0002
−3.3	0.0005	0.0005	0.0005	0.0004	0.0004	0.0004	0.0004	0.0004	0.0004	0.0003

(Continued)

Table 3.3 (Continued) Percent of area under the standard normal curve for z-scores

z	0.00	0.01	0.02	0.03	0.04	0.05	0.06	0.07	0.08	0.09
-3.2	0.0007	0.0007	0.0006	0.0006	0.0006	0.0006	0.0006	0.0005	0.0005	0.0005
-3.1	0.0010	0.0009	0.0009	0.0009	0.0008	0.0008	0.0008	0.0008	0.0007	0.0007
-3.0	0.0013	0.0013	0.0013	0.0012	0.0012	0.0011	0.0011	0.0011	0.0010	0.0010
-2.9	0.0019	0.0018	0.0018	0.0017	0.0016	0.0016	0.0015	0.0015	0.0014	0.0014
-2.8	0.0026	0.0025	0.0024	0.0023	0.0023	0.0022	0.0021	0.0021	0.0020	0.0019
-2.7	0.0035	0.0034	0.0033	0.0032	0.0031	0.0030	0.0029	0.0028	0.0027	0.0026
-2.6	0.0047	0.0045	0.0044	0.0043	0.0041	0.0040	0.0039	0.0038	0.0037	0.0036
-2.5	0.0062	0.0060	0.0059	0.0057	0.0055	0.0054	0.0052	0.0051	0.0049	0.0048
-2.4	0.0082	0.0080	0.0078	0.0075	0.0073	0.0071	0.0069	0.0068	0.0066	0.0064
-2.3	0.0107	0.0104	0.0102	0.0099	0.0096	0.0094	0.0091	0.0089	0.0087	0.0084
-2.2	0.0139	0.0136	0.0132	0.0129	0.0125	0.0122	0.0119	0.0116	0.0113	0.0110
-2.1	0.0179	0.0174	0.0170	0.0166	0.0162	0.0158	0.0154	0.0150	0.0146	0.0143
-2.0	0.0228	0.0222	0.0217	0.0212	0.0207	0.0202	0.0197	0.0192	0.0188	0.0183
-1.9	0.0287	0.0281	0.0274	0.0268	0.0262	0.0256	0.0250	0.0244	0.0239	0.0233
-1.8	0.0359	0.0351	0.0344	0.0336	0.0329	0.0322	0.0314	0.0307	0.0301	0.0294
-1.7	0.0446	0.0436	0.0427	0.0418	0.0409	0.0401	0.0392	0.0384	0.0375	0.0367
-1.6	0.0548	0.0537	0.0526	0.0516	0.0505	0.0495	0.0485	0.0475	0.0465	0.0455
-1.5	0.0668	0.0655	0.0643	0.0630	0.0618	0.0606	0.0594	0.0582	0.0571	0.0559
-1.4	0.0808	0.0793	0.0778	0.0764	0.0749	0.0735	0.0721	0.0708	0.0694	0.0681
-1.3	0.0968	0.0951	0.0934	0.0918	0.0901	0.0885	0.0869	0.0853	0.0838	0.0823
-1.2	0.1151	0.1131	0.1112	0.1093	0.1075	0.1056	0.1038	0.1020	0.1003	0.0985
-1.1	0.1357	0.1335	0.1314	0.1292	0.1271	0.1251	0.1230	0.1210	0.1190	0.1170

(Continued)

Table 3.3 (Continued) Percent of area under the standard normal curve for z-scores

z	0.00	0.01	0.02	0.03	0.04	0.05	0.06	0.07	0.08	0.09
−1.0	0.1587	0.1562	0.1539	0.1515	0.1492	0.1469	0.1446	0.1423	0.1401	0.1379
−0.9	0.1841	0.1814	0.1788	0.1762	0.1736	0.1711	0.1685	0.1660	0.1635	0.1611
−0.8	0.2119	0.2090	0.2061	0.2033	0.2005	0.1977	0.1949	0.1922	0.1894	0.1867
−0.7	0.2420	0.2389	0.2358	0.2327	0.2296	0.2266	0.2236	0.2206	0.2177	0.2148
−0.6	0.2743	0.2709	0.2676	0.2643	0.2611	0.2578	0.2546	0.2514	0.2483	0.2451
−0.5	0.3085	0.3050	0.3015	0.2981	0.2946	0.2912	0.2877	0.2843	0.2810	0.2776
−0.4	0.3446	0.3409	0.3372	0.3336	0.3300	0.3264	0.3228	0.3192	0.3156	0.3121
−0.3	0.3821	0.3783	0.3745	0.3707	0.3669	0.3632	0.3594	0.3557	0.3520	0.3483
−0.2	0.4207	0.4168	0.4129	0.4090	0.4052	0.4013	0.3974	0.3936	0.3897	0.3859
−0.1	0.4602	0.4562	0.4522	0.4483	0.4443	0.4404	0.4364	0.4325	0.4286	0.4247

Table entry for z is the area under the standard normal curve to the left of z.

z-score of 0.30 results in a percentile of 62. A z-score of 1.10 has an associated area of .8643 (Figure 3.4), which is the 86th %ile (0.8643×100 and rounded to the nearest whole number). Calculate the percentile of a z-score of 2.15 (it is the 98th %ile).

What if the z-score is negative? This will of course result in a percentile equivalent of less than 50 since negative z-scores fall below the mean. Remember that the standard normal curve is symmetric and thus the area beyond z for scores greater than the mean (positive) is the same as the area to the left of z for z-scores less than the mean (negative). A negative z-score therefore results in a percentile equivalent as listed in the bottom half of Table 3.3. Find the percentile equivalent for $z = -0.55$ (Column A). The corresponding value is 0.2912, which is 29th %ile. This is the percentile equivalent because it is the area to the left of a negative z-score.

The main advantage of percentiles is that they are accurate and easy to understand even by non-experts. There are two main disadvantages with percentiles, however. First, they are somewhat more difficult to derive than other standard scores though Table 3.3 can simplify matters. Second, not all intervals are equal on the percentile scale. A difference of 3 %ile point between 61 and 64, for example, represents a trivial difference, while the same three points between the 96th and 99th %ile represents a huge difference in performance. Like the stanine scale, at the extreme ends of the distribution, the percentile scale distorts and obscures differences in performance.

Standard scores have strengths and weaknesses. There is no scoring and reporting system that is free of problems. Perhaps the best strategy is to use several standard scores to report such as T-scores in combination with percentiles. For further clarification, the actual raw score and the total percentage correct on the test should also be reported. In any case, there is no single reporting system that is devoid of problems.

SUMMARY AND MAIN POINTS

Some understanding of statistics and data analysis is a requirement for virtually all professionals that work with people, especially teachers. This allows for a greater appreciation of the differences and similarities between learners and also helps the teacher better organize and interpret test scores and other educational measures. The normal curve is a particularly important distribution as are skewed, bimodal, and rectangular distributions. A notable characteristic of many frequency distributions is their central tendency—the scores tend to cluster around the center. There are three measures of central tendency or average: the mode, median, and mean. A full description of distributions also requires measures of dispersion, the range, and SD. Relationships between scores, as summarized statistically by the correlation coefficient, play a large role in data analysis and understanding of test scores. Norms and standard scores are an important aspect of test score interpretation and reporting. There are four types of standard scores: z-scores, T-scores, stanines, and percentiles.

- Descriptive statistics are essential for classroom practice. Anyone who works in a professional capacity with people should learn about statistics—as is almost an article of faith in education and the health professions—each person is unique and an individual. Statistics allows you to go beyond the declaration of this truism and to quantify the uniqueness and similarity of people.

- Important graphs and frequency distributions for statistics include histograms and frequency polygons. There at four important types of frequency polygons in test data analysis. These include the following distributions: normal, skewed, bimodal, and rectangular.
- Measures of central tendency summarize the tendency of test scores to cluster around the center of the distribution and produce an "average" score. There are three measures of central tendency or average, which shall be discussed in turn: the mode, median, and mean.
- There are two basic measures of dispersion, the range and standard deviation. A full description of a distribution must include an indication of its dispersion or variability. The range conveys some indication of the dispersion of a dataset, but it is very crude and unstable since it is based on only two scores, the maximum and the minimum.
- A preferred, much more stable and better measure of variability is the SD which includes every score in the distribution.
- The SD is a direct measure of a group's variability or the dispersion of scores. A small SD indicates that the group is quite homogeneous, while a large SD indicates that the group is heterogeneous.
- Norms provide information about the performance of a particular group on a specified measure. Any individual's score can thus be compared to that reference group, usually employing standard scores including z-scores, T-scores, stanines, and percentiles.

REFLECTIONS AND EXERCISES

Descriptive statistics and standard scores

30 marks

Purpose: to compute descriptive statistics for actual data from 25 students in a university level health sciences course.

Directions

1. Use the dataset for 25 students from this assignment. Create an electronic file of the data in SPSS. **(10 marks)**
2. **Descriptive Statistics:** use SPSS to compute the mean, mode, median, range, variance, and standard deviations for Quiz 1, Quiz 2, Quiz 3, Essay, and Final. Record this information in a table. (see example below) **(10 marks)**
3. Write three paragraphs commenting on the nature of the distributions. Speculate on what the measures of central tendency and dispersion of the five assignments tell about the achievement in this class. Your response should address issues of magnitude, skewness, and heterogeneity. **(10 marks)**

TO SUBMIT TO THE INSTRUCTOR

1. A Table of Descriptive Statistics for the five assessments.
2. Three paragraphs describing your inferences about distributions.

Performance data for 25 students in health sciences

Person	Quiz 1(20)	Quiz 2(15)	Quiz 3(10)	Essay(25)	Final(75)
1	19	14	10	19	70
2	11	7	6	17	35
3	11	11	6	14	51
4	18	13	8	20	68
5	10	9	6	23	40
6	16	12	8	16	62
7	18	14	10	21	61
8	7	10	4	21	40
9	4	6	6	11	37
10	8	7	5	20	35
11	16	9	8	19	66
12	15	11	7	16	69
13	7	9	5	18	41
14	18	14	9	24	64
15	10	10	5	21	31
16	7	10	6	20	50
17	8	8	6	17	50
18	5	7	3	22	30
19	19	15	9	23	66
20	11	8	5	19	34
21	19	14	8	14	62
22	10	7	6	20	37
23	19	13	9	20	68
24	20	15	10	18	66
25	5	15	4	13	41

Norms and standard scores

4. Using all the learners from the Health Sciences data, compute each one's z-score, T-score, stanine, and percentile rank on Quiz 1 and the Final.
5. Below is a table of various standard scores and raw scores for a test with a mean of 65 and SD = 12. Convert each one that is given into the other scores.
6. If a cutoff score of 125 on the Wechsler IQ tests was used to admit children into a program for the gifted, how many children would qualify in a school district with 75,000 children (assume a normal distribution)?

Raw score	z-Score	T-Score	Stanine	Percentile
	1.00			
		40		
71				
	0.50			
			7	
				70
		65		
69				
				93
			3	
	0.75			
43				

7. If all children who scored in the 10th%ile or less on a basic skills test were admitted into a remedial educational program, how many children would qualify in a school of 250 (assume a normal distribution)?

When you first open SPSS, you will get the following screen.
1. Click on Close. You will get the following screen.

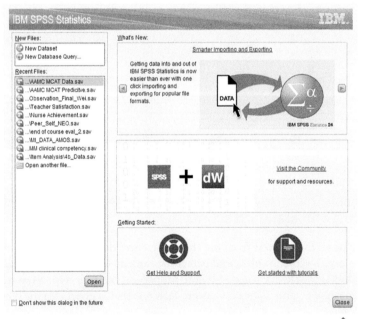

2. Click on Variable View. The following screen will appear.

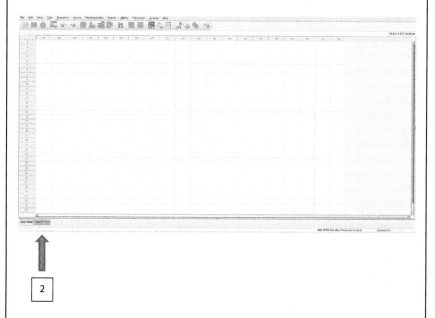

2

3. Name the first variable, "Person," etc.

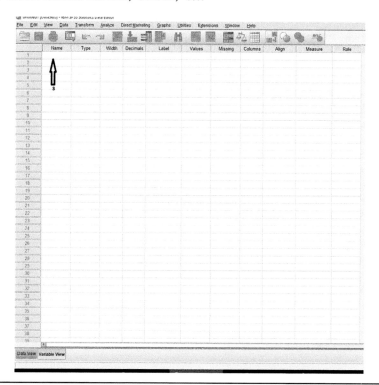

REFERENCES

1. Le Cam L, Lo Yang G (2000). *Asymptotics in Statistics: Some Basic Concepts* (2nd ed.). New York: Springer.

4

Correlational-based methods

- The correlation coefficient, r, must always take on values between +1.0 and −1.0 since it has been standardized to fit into this range. The sign indicates the direction of the relationship (i.e., either positive or negative), the magnitude indicates the strength of the relationship (weak as r approaches 0; strong as r increases and approaches +1.0 or −1.0), and the coefficient of determination (r^2) which is an indicator of the variance accounted for in y by x.
- Cause and effect cannot be interpreted from correlation which only indicates a relationship
- Other correlations that are important in assessment and measurement: Spearman's rho coefficient, the Biserial (r_b), and Point-Biserial (r_{pb}) correlation coefficients. When both x and y are continuous, Pearson's r is the appropriate coefficient. If both x and y are ordinal, then Spearman's rho is the correct correlation. When x is continuous and y is an artificial dichotomy, r_b is the correct coefficient. Finally, when x is continuous and y is a natural dichotomy, the r_{pb} is correct.
- We employ several independent variables to improve the predicted outcome on a dependent variable. The multiple regression equation is:
  $Y' = \beta_1 X_1 + \beta_2 X_2 + \cdots \beta_k X_k + c$
- Factor analysis is a collection of methods used for exploring the correlations between a number of variables seeking the underlying clusters or subsets called factors or latent variables. It addresses the following:
  - Number of factors are needed to summarize the pattern of correlations in the correlation matrix
  - The amount of variance in a dataset is accounted by the factors
  - Factors that account for the most variance
  - Meaning and how are the factors to be interpreted
- Discriminant analysis can evaluate whether, based on a discriminant function calculated, participants can be correctly categorized into pass/fail groups based on prior test scores

- Cluster analysis categorizes data into homogenous groups. It has been useful in several applications in medical education such as exploring the validity of standard setting for cutoff scores.

CORRELATION

The correlation is a statistical technique that is based on the work of the 19th century mathematicians and statisticians, Francis Galton and Karl Pearson and bears the latter's name, the *Pearson product–moment correlation coefficient*.[1] Fortunately, it is common practice to refer to it by the much shorter term "correlation" or by its symbol, *r*.

This statistic is very easy to understand as it simply indicates the relationship between two variables. As the name implies, it is a "co-relation" between two variables. Some examples of related variables that are intuitively obvious are height and weight, effort and achievement, ages of husband and wife, and heights of fathers and sons. The correlation coefficient summarizes both the magnitude and direction of the relationship between two variables. The coefficient is given by the following:

$$ r = \frac{\sum_{i=1}^{n}\left(X_i - \bar{X}\right)\left(Y_i - \bar{Y}\right)}{\sqrt{\sum_{i=1}^{n}\left((X_i - \bar{X})\right)^2 \sum_{i=1}^{n}\left(Y_i - \bar{Y}\right)^2}} \tag{4.1}$$

where
  r is the correlation coefficient
  Σ is the summation sign
  X is any variable
  Y is any other variable
  n is the number of students measured

The coefficient, *r*, must always take on values between +1.0 and −1.0 since it has been standardized to fit into this range (the denominator on the formula— Equation 4.1—is the product of the standard deviations of the two variables). The coefficient can also take on the value 0 which indicates that there is no relationship whatsoever between the two variables.

Equation 4.1 looks quite complex and intimidating but really only involves adding, subtracting, multiplying, dividing, and taking square roots, all of which are elementary arithmetic operations. Even so, it is rare nowadays to calculate a correlation coefficient by hand since it is quite tedious and subject to arithmetic error. With the wide availability of computers, it is very easy to compute the correlation coefficient. This allows you to focus on the meaning of the coefficient rather than on the tedious and unrewarding exercise of computing it.

There are four elements of *r* to attend to in interpreting it: the sign, the magnitude, the statistical significance, and the coefficient of determination (r^2). The sign indicates the direction of the relationship (i.e., either positive or negative), the magnitude indicates the strength of the relationship (weak as r approaches 0; strong as r increases and approaches +1.0 or −1.0), the significance which indicates the probability that the r value is truly different from 0, and the coefficient of determination which is an indicator of the variance accounted for in x by y.

To run a Pearson's r with SPSS, use the following.

Select "Analyze" then "Bivariate Correlations." The following dialogue window should be open.

1. Select "Step 1_Total [step1] and Step 2_Total [step2]" from the left pane and click over to the right ("Variables:") pane.
2. Leave the pre-selected "Pearson"
3. Select "OK"

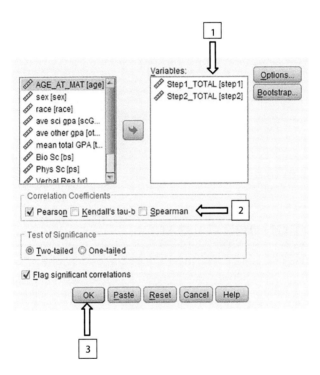

The results are tabulated as follows.

Correlations		Step 2_Total
Step 1_Total	Pearson's r	0.775[a]
	Sig. (two-tailed)	0.000
	n	1,771

[a] Correlation is significant at the 0.01 level (two-tailed).

The Pearson's $r = 0.775$ based on 1,771 medical students who wrote both Steps 1 and 2. The coefficient is statistically significant at the $p < 0.01$ for a two-tailed test. Computing the coefficient of determination (r^2) by squaring the correlation coefficient ($0.775 \times 0.775 = 0.60$) results in 60% ($0.60 \times 100$) of the variance in performance in Step 2 is accounted for by the performance in Step 1. The Venn diagram below illustrates r and the coefficient of determination (r^2) visually.

Coefficient of determination (shared variance)

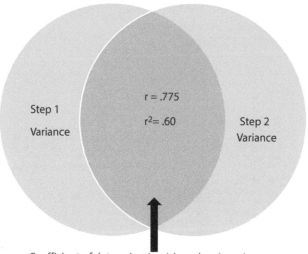

Coefficient of determination (shared variance)

CORRELATION AND CAUSATION

Cause and effect cannot be interpreted from correlation which only indicates a relationship. It is sometimes tempting to conclude that one variable causes changes in the other variable, but such inferences cannot be justified on the basis of correlation. Frequently, to make causal inferences on this basis is nonsensical. Achievement and IQ, for example, are known to be correlated, but it is nonsensical to state that IQ "causes" achievement. The height of father and sons is also correlated but it doesn't make sense to say that father's height causes son's height. Both are controlled by underlying laws of genetic inheritance and thus the two variables are correlated. Experimental evidence in addition to correlational data is required to make inferences about cause and effect of two variables.

In addition to the Pearson product–moment correlation coefficient, there are several other correlations that are important in assessment and measurement: Spearman's rho coefficient, the Biserial (r_b), and Point-Biserial (r_{pb}) correlation coefficients. As with Pearson's r, these coefficients are measures of association but depend on the scales of measurement. When both x and y are continuous, Pearson's r is the appropriate coefficient. If both x and y are ordinal, then

Table 4.1 Various correlation coefficients depending on scales of measurement

Variables X and Y	X is continuous	X is ordinal	X is nominal
Y is continuous	Pearson's r	Biserial r_b	Point-Biserial r_{pb}
Y is ordinal	Biserial r_b	Spearman's rho	
Y is nominal	Point-Biserial r_{pb}		

Spearman's rho is the correct correlation. When x is continuous and y is artificially nominal, the r_b is the correct coefficient. Finally, when x is continuous and y is naturally nominal, the r_{pb} is correct (Table 4.1).

Interval and ratio scales are generally categorized together as continuous for the purposes of calculation of the correlation. Nominal variables are dichotomous (two categories such as male and female), while ordinal variables refer to rank-order (e.g., class rank).

Spearman rank-order correlation

Spearman's rank correlation coefficient (rho; ρ) is a nonparametric measure of rank correlation. It assesses how well the relationship between two ordinal variables that increase or decrease together. A perfect Spearman correlation of +1 or −1 occurs when each of the variables is a perfect rank-order of the other. The Spearman correlation between two variables will be high when observations have a similar rank between the two variables and low when observations have different ranks between the two variables. Spearman's rho is appropriate for ordinal variables. When all ranks are integers, Spearman's rank-order correlation is:

$$r_s = 1 - \frac{6 \sum d^2}{n(n^2 - 1)}$$

where
  r_s = Spearman's rho
  $\sum$ = summation sign
  d^2 = difference between the ranks squared
  n = the number of observations

To run a Spearman's rho with SPSS, use the following.

Select "Analyze" then "Bivariate Correlations." The following dialogue window should be open.

1. Select "Bio Sc [bs] and Phys Sc [ps]" from the left pane and click over to the right ("Variables:") pane.
2. Select "Spearman" and de-select "Pearson"
3. Select "OK"

The result is tabulated as follows.

Correlations

		Phys Sc
Bio Sc	Spearman's rho	0.649[a]
	Sig. (two-tailed)	0.000
	N	1,782

[a] Correlation is significant at the 0.01 level (two-tailed).

The Spearman's rho = 0.649 based on 1,782 medical students who wrote both Bio Sc and Phys Sc. The coefficient is statistically significant at the $p < 0.01$ for a two-tailed test. Computing the coefficient of determination ($r^2 = 0.649 \times 0.649 = 0.42$) results in 42% of the variance in performance in Phys Sc is accounted for by the performance in Bio Sc.

Point-biserial correlation

Suppose in the dataset that we have been working with, we wished to know if sex is correlated with performance on Step 2. We can run a point-biserial correlation between sex (dichotomous variable) and Step 2 (continuous variable), which is a special case of the Pearson correlation.

To run a Pearson's *r* with SPSS, use the following.

Select "Analyze" then "Bivariate Correlations." The following dialogue window should be open.

1. Select "Sex and Step 2_Total [step2]" from the left pane and click over to the right ("Variables:") pane.
2. Leave the pre-selected "Pearson"
3. Select "OK"

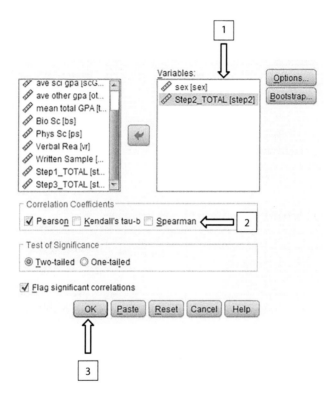

The SPSS results are tabulated as follows:

Correlations		
		Step2_Total
Sex	Point biserial	0.017
	Sig. (two-tailed)	0.462
	n	1,771

The point-biserial = 0.017 based on 1,771 medical students who wrote Step 2. The coefficient is statistically non-significant (denoted p = ns) for a two-tailed test. There is no need for any further interpretation, because there is no correlation between sex and Step 2 performance: men and women perform equally.

The biserial correlation can be computed in precisely the same way as the point-biserial except that one variable is artificially dichotomous (e.g., high scorers vs low scorers), while the other is continuous. In Chapter 15, we will make extensive use of the point-biserial in item analysis of tests by calculating it as the discrimination coefficient.

SIMPLE REGRESSION

Simple regression refers to the situation which we have only a dependent variable (y) and one independent variable (x). The regression equation is depicted:

$$Y' = \beta_1 X_1 + c \tag{4.2}$$

Y': dependent variable to be predicted
β_1: standardized beta weight for the independent variable
X_1: independent variable
c: constant

To run a simple regression with SPSS, use the following.

Select "Graphs" then "Legacy Dialogs" and then "Scatter/Dot." The following dialogue window should be open:

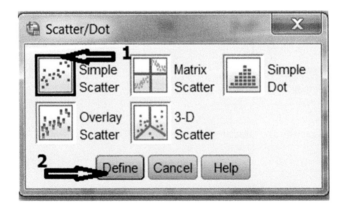

1. Select "Simple Scatter"
2. Select "Define"

The following window should be open:

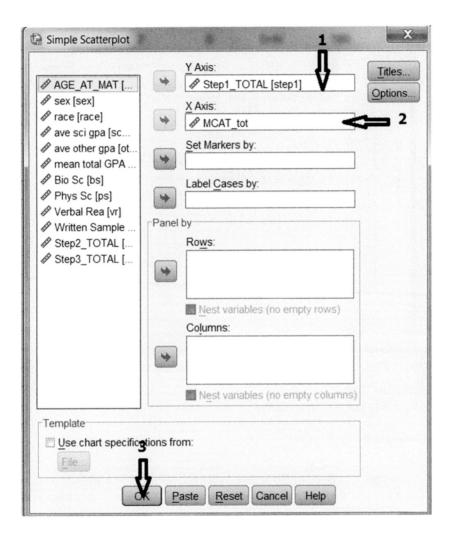

1. Select the dependent variable (*y*)—Step1_Total
2. Select the independent variable (*x*)—MCAT_tot
3. Select OK

Double click on the Graph output to produce the following Chart Editor window.

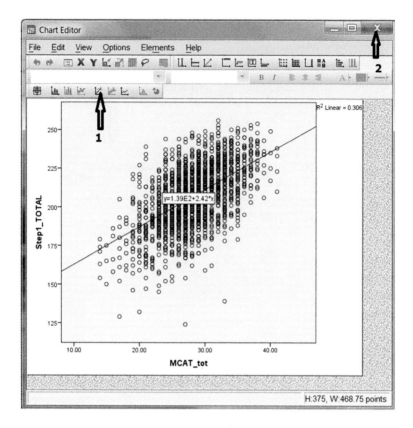

1. Select the "best fit line" icon
2. Select X to exit the Chart Editor

Following is the SPSS result:

Model	R	R^2	Adjusted R^2	SE of estimate	R^2
1	0.553	0.306	0.305	16.514	0.306

Model		Coefficients	
		B	Std. Error
1	Constant	138.638	2.473
	MCAT_tot	2.422	0.086

From equation 4.2, a prediction of Jason's MCAT total score of 30 for performance on Step 1 of the USMLE becomes:

$$Y' = 2.422 \times 30 + 138.638 = 211.298$$

MULTIPLE REGRESSION

It is rare to predict a dependent variable (y) from only one independent variable (x). Frequently, we employ several independent variables so as to improve the predictive validity of the dependent variable. The multiple regression equation is depicted:

$$Y' = \beta_1 X_1 + \beta_2 X_2 + \cdots \beta_k X_k + c \qquad (4.3)$$

Y': dependent variable to be predicted
β_1: standardized beta weight for an independent variable
X_1: an independent variable
β_2: standardized beta weight for another independent variable
X_2: another independent variable
β_k: standardized beta weight for the kth independent variable
X_k: k^{th} independent variable
  c: constant

To run a multiple regression with SPSS, use the following.

Select "Analyze" then "Regression" then "Linear." The following dialogue window should be open.

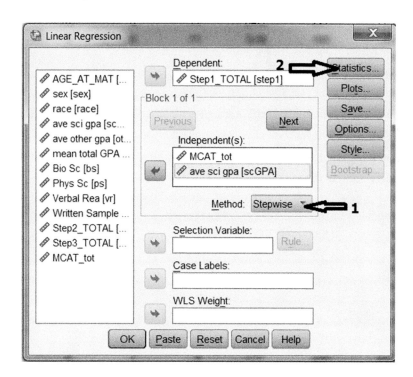

Select "Step 1_Total [step1]" for the "Dependent" and "MCAT_tot" and "ave sci gpa [scGPA] as the Independent(s).

1. Select "Stepwise"
2. Select "Statistics"

The following window will open.

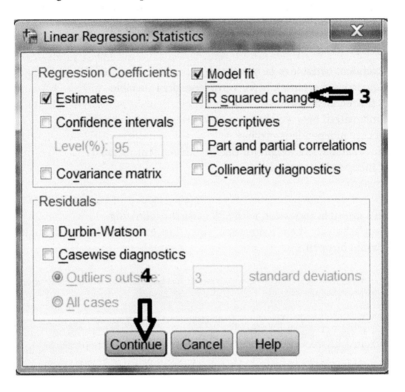

3. Select "*R* squared change"
4. Select "Continue"
5. Select "OK" in the next window.

Model	R	R^2	Adjusted R^2	SE of estimate	R^2
1	0.553	0.306	0.305	16.530	0.306
2	0.588	0.345	0.345	16.055	0.040

Model		Unstandardized coefficients	
		B	Std. error
1	Constant	138.655	2.476
	MCAT total	2.422	0.087
2	Constant	112.972	3.452
	MCAT total	2.232	0.086
	Ave Science GPA	9.171	0.884

FACTOR ANALYSIS

Factor analysis is a collection of methods used for exploring the correlations between a number of variables seeking the underlying clusters or subsets called factors or latent variables. According to the principles of factor analysis, variables correlate because they are determined in part by common underlying influences. Patterns of correlations among individual personality variables, for example, are thought to reflect underlying processes that effect students' behaviors and performance. "Conscientiousness" is thought to be a personality trait characterized by organization, purposeful action, self-discipline, and a drive to achieve. These behaviors, therefore, should be highly correlated.

A particular use of factor analysis in health sciences education can be used in the development of objective tests for the measurement of personality and other noncognitive attributes (e.g., empathy, compassion, communication). Researchers employ factor analysis to reduce a large number of variables to a smaller number of factors, to describe and potentially understand the relationships among observed variables, or to test theory about underlying processes.

Important questions addressed by factor analysis are:

1. How many factors are needed to summarize the pattern of correlations in the correlation matrix?
2. How much variance in a dataset is accounted for by the factors?
3. Which factors account for the most variance?
4. How many reliable and interpretable factors are there in the data?
5. What is the meaning and how are the factors to be interpreted?

We begin with a large number of items reflecting a theoretical "guess" about the items or variables that are most meaningful. The variables are given to candidates and factors are derived. As a result of the first "exploratory" factor analysis, variables are added and deleted, a second test is devised, and that test is given to other participants. The process continues until a test is developed with numerous items forming several factors that represent the area to be measured.

Reducing several variables to a few factors

Mathematically, factor analysis produces several linear combinations of observed variables, each linear combination a factor. The factors summarize the patterns of correlations in the observed correlation matrix.

Steps in factor analysis include:

1. Collecting, editing, and preparing a dataset for analysis
2. Extracting a set of factors from the correlation matrix

3. Rotating the factors to increase interpretability
4. Determining the number of factors
5. Interpreting the results

Although there are relevant statistical considerations to most of the steps listed above, an important test of the analysis is its interpretability. Does the result make sense? Is the number of factors the correct one? Are they cohesive? Can they be meaningfully interpreted? The interpretation and naming of factors depend on the meaning of the particular combination of observed variables that correlate highly with each factor. A factor is more easily interpreted when several observed variables correlate highly with it and do not correlate with other factors.

How many factors?

A very widely used extraction method is the principal components analysis (PCA). This is a mathematical method of identifying the underlying components of the correlations. Important criteria computed during PCA are eigenvalues. These are indices that tell how good a component (factor) is as a summary of the data. An eigenvalue = 1.0 means that the factor contains the same amount of information as a single variable. Eigenvalues > +1.0 account for more information or variance than a single variable and should be retained as a factor.

The *Kaiser Rule* is the most commonly used approach to selecting the number of components (factors): retain all components with eigenvalues ≥ 1.0. In other words, eigenvalues equal to or greater than the information accounted for by an average single item should be retained.

Rotation of factors

A primary goal of factor analysis employing extraction is to discover the optimum number of factors in the solution that (1) accounts for the maximum variance, but (2) remains parsimonious. This is usually the first step in factor analysis that results in an "unrotated" matrix. It is a compromise between a large number of factors to account for maximal variance and the fewest factors to maintain parsimony or simplicity.

A second major goal is to rotate the factors so as to maximize their interpretability with a "rotated" matrix producing a simple structure. This is a pattern of loadings where each item loads strongly (i.e., >0.70) on only one of the factors but weakly on the other factors (i.e., <0.30). The factor solution must be rotated to be interpretable. If the factors are orthogonal (i.e., not correlated with each other), the factor axes are all at right angles to one another. Factor loadings (correlations of the items to the factor) are interpreted directly (Table 4.2).

Rotations are of two types: orthogonal or oblique.

Table 4.2 Guidelines for interpreting loadings

Loading on the item	Overlapping variance (%)	Evaluation
>0.71	>50	Excellent
0.63–0.70	40–49	Very Good
0.55–0.62	30–39	Good
0.45–0.54	20–29	Fair
0.32–0.44	10–19	Poor

Methods of rotation

Varimax, the most common rotation option, is an orthogonal rotation of the factors to maximize the variance extracted that is accounted by that factor. A varimax solution yields results which make it as easy as possible to identify each variable with a single factor.

Direct oblimin rotation is the method for a non-orthogonal (oblique) solution: that is, the factors are allowed to be correlated with each other. While there are other rotation methods, they are not widely applicable in medical education.

Interpretation of factors

Factors are usually interpretable when some observed variables load highly on them and the rest do not. Ideally, each variable would load on one and only one factor. The greater is the item loading, the more the variable is considered to be a clean measure of the factor. Sometimes there are "split" loadings when a variable loads on two factors (e.g., 0.65 on one factor and 0.52 on another). This means that the variable measures elements of both factors. The cutoff size of loading to be interpreted is somewhat subjective but a good rule of thumb is that only variables with loadings of 0.40 and above are interpreted.

A final aspect of the interpretation is to characterize a factor by assigning it a name, a process that is just as much an art as it is a science. Interpretation of factors can be based on the variable names with the largest loadings, and the types of variables are grouped by their correlations with factors (e.g., several reading, writing, and speaking tests may group together so we call the factor "Language").

The usefulness, replicability, and complexity of factors are also considered in interpretation. Is the solution replicable with different samples? Are some factors trivial or outliers or do they fit in the hierarchy of theoretical explanations about a phenomenon?

The most critical element of a factor analysis is the identification of the number of factors, even more important than extraction and rotation techniques.

Extraction effectiveness is tied to the number of factors. The more factors extracted, the better the fit and the greater the percent of variance in the data "accounted for" by the factor solution. The more factors extracted, however, the less parsimonious the solution. Extracting as many factors as variables would account for 100% of the variance, but this is a trivial solution. The main goal is to extract as few factors as possible while accounting for as much variance as possible. The goal of parsimony (as few factors as necessary) is an important goal and should not be lost.

In confirmatory factor analysis (Chapter 7), the number of factors is a selection of the number of theoretical processes underlying a research area. A hypothesized factor structure can be confirmed by asking if the theoretical number of factors adequately fits the data. Construct validity evidence of the factors requires that scores on the latent variables (factors) correlate with scores on other variables or that scores on latent variables change with experimental conditions as predicted by theory.

Running factor analysis

The following example illustrates the use of factor analysis. Direct observations have been widely accepted as a good way to evaluate the clinical competence of medical students and residents. It has been proposed to use mini-clinical evaluation exercise (mini-CEX) to assess a set of clinical competencies (e.g., medical interview, physical examination, professionalism, and communications) in the completion of a patient history within a medical training context. The mini-CEX is designed to reflect educational requirements during the teaching round and to assess skills that residents require in the actual patient encounters. Some good characteristics including direct observations, instant use in day-to-day practice, and immediate feedback to the learner after the physical examination make the mini-CEX an excellent educational tool that helps learners to be aware of their strengths and opportunities for improvement.

The following study illustrates the use of the mini-CEX with third-year medical students participating in mandatory clerkship rotations (surgery, pediatrics, obstetrics/gynecology, internal medicine, psychiatry, emergency medicine, family medicine, neurology, radiology). There were 108 students (57 men; 52.8% and 51 women; 47.2%) in the study. Students were observed by faculty members in real patient encounters *in situ*. An adapted version of the mini-CEX to directly assess clerkship students' medical competence (Table 4.3) was employed. Students were rated on a five-point scale based on their degree of entrustability on that competency (1 = not close to meeting criterion; 2 = not yet meets criterion; 3 = meets criterion; 4 = just exceeds criterion; 5 = well exceeds criterion).

The data were entered into SPSS.

To run a factor analysis with SPSS, use the following.

Select "Dimension Reduction" then select "Factor." The following dialogue window should be open.

Table 4.3 Adapted version of the mini-CEX to directly assess clerkship students' medical competence

Mini-CEX Assessment Form

Assessor_____Student_____Date_____

Patient Problem/Dx(s)_____ Patient Age___ Patient Sex: M/F

Setting (I/O)_____ **ENCOUNTER COMPLEXITY: Low/Moderate/High**

Mini-CEX time: Observing____min Assessor providing feedback to student____min

Variables	Mean (SD)	Median	Min	Max	Skewness
1. Communication skills	3.47 (0.71)	3.00	1.00	5.00	0.06
2. Medical interviewing skills	3.22 (0.76)	3.00	1.00	5.00	0.13
3. Physical examination skills	3.09 (0.64)	3.00	1.00	5.00	0.20
4. Professional /humanistic qualities	3.57(0.69)	3.00	2.00	5.00	0.44
5. Clinical reasoning	3.23 (0.73)	3.00	1.00	5.00	0.21
6. Management planning	3.13 (0.70)	3.00	1.00	5.00	0.31
7. Organization/efficacy of encounter	3.16 (0.71)	3.00	1.00	5.00	0.31
8. Oral presentation	3.25 (0.64)	3.00	1.00	5.00	0.36
Observing time (min)	25.94 (11.0)	25.00	10.00	100.00	3.01
Feedback time (min)	20.19 (7.0)	20.00	5.00	45.00	0.63
Encounter complexity	2.06 (0.57)	2.00	1.00	3.00	0.01

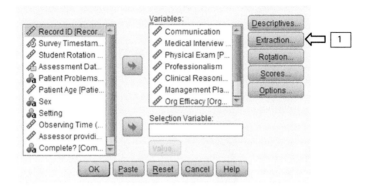

Select the mini-CEX items click over to the "Variables:" pane as above.

1. Select "Extraction." The following dialogue window should open.
2. The default "Method" should be "Principal components." If not select it.
3. "Extract" should be "Based on eigenvalue." Eigenvalue greater than 1 should be the default. If not select it. (You could use any number of factors by selecting "Fixed number of factors" if you had a good reason—theoretical or practical—to extract a particular number of factors which may not correspond to Eigenvalue greater than 1).
4. The maximum number of iterations for this iterative process is 25. Leave this as the default unless you have a very good reason to change it.
5. Click on "Continue."

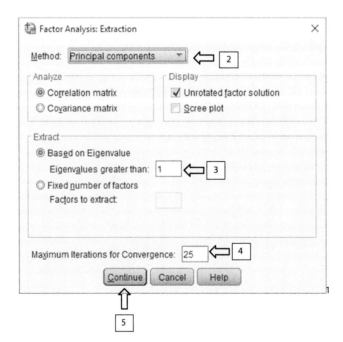

Select "Rotation" button in the dialogue box.

6. Under "Method," select "Varimax."
7. In "Display," "Rotated Solution" should be selected. If not, select it.
8. The maximum number of iterations for this iterative process is 25. Leave this as the default unless you have a very good reason to change it.
9. Click on "Continue."

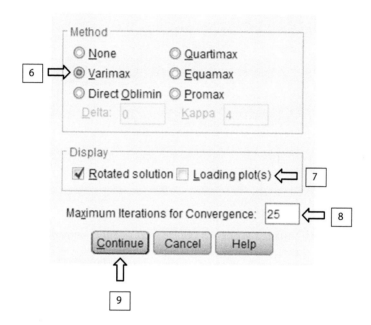

Click on "Options" in the Dialogue box.

10. For "Missing Values," "Excluded cases listwise" should be selected.
11. Under "Coefficient Display Format" the "Absolute value below:" should be set at 0.40.
12. Click on "Continue."

Now you should be back at the main dialogue box and the factor analysis is ready to run. Click on "OK" and the procedure should execute.

Output from SPSS

A large amount of output will ensue from the analysis. The key is to identify and interpret the output relevant for the present analysis and problem.

We begin with Table 4.4 which contains the initial eigenvalues and the variance accounted for. The eigenvalues are listed hierarchically from largest to smallest

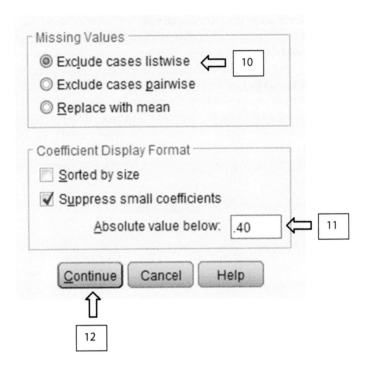

Table 4.4 Total variance explained principal component extraction

Component		Initial eigenvalues	
	Total	Variance (%)	Cumulative %
1. Communication	5.774	64.151	64.151
2. Medical interview	1.225	8.051	72.202
3. Physical exam	0.586	6.514	78.716
4. Professionalism	0.451	5.009	83.726
5. Clinical reasoning	0.390	4.330	88.056
6. Management planning	0.323	3.584	91.640
7. Organizational efficacy	0.287	3.191	94.831
8. Oral presentation	0.264	2.930	97.761
9. Overall	0.202	2.239	100.000

for the nine variables. Notice that Component 1 has a corresponding eigenvalue of 5.774 which accounts for 64.151% of the variance in the data. The magnitude of the next several eigenvalues decreases markedly accounting small amounts of the variance. A close inspection of Table 4.4 reveals that there are two eigenvalues greater than 1 and that accounts for 72.202% of the variance. Additionally, the table contains how much of the variance in this solution is accounted for by each component; e.g., Component 2 accounts for 8.051% of the common variance as determined by the rotation sums of squared loadings. Therefore, two factors are selected in this analysis.

Interpreting the factors

Table 4.5 contains the varimax (orthogonally) rotated factors; convergence occurred in three iterations. Based on the factor loadings, theoretical meaning and coherence, the next task is to name the factors. Factor 1 is *Clinical Competence* because the main large loadings (0.680–0.814) are from the following variables all reflecting clinical competence:

1. Physical exam
2. Clinical reasoning
3. Management planning
4. Organizational efficacy
5. Oral presentation

Factor 2 (*Professionalism & Communication*) is named based on the factor loadings, theoretical meaning, and coherence as it has large primary loadings from communication, medical interview, and professionalism ranging from 0.649 to 0.841. There are several "split-loadings" (variables load on more than one factor) in Table 4.5: medical interview, management planning, organizational efficacy, oral presentation, and overall. Variable #2 (Medical Interview), for example, loads both on factor 1 (*Clinical Competence*) at 0.518 and factor 2 (*Professionalism & Communication*) at 0.649. This split makes theoretical sense as medical interviewing skills is part of both clinical competence and communication skills and

Table 4.5 Varimax-rotated component matrix[a]

	Factors	
	1	**2**
Variables	**Clinical competence**	**Professionalism and communication**
1. Communication		0.813
2. Medical interview	0.518	0.649
3. Physical exam	0.704	
4. Professionalism		0.841
5. Clinical reasoning	0.814	
6. Management planning	0.808	
7. Organizational efficacy	0.680	0.510
8. Oral presentation	0.710	0.468
9. Overall	0.733	0.531

[a] Convergence in three iterations.

professional demeanor. The other split-loading also make theoretical sense since they are part of more than one factor.

The results of this factor analysis allow us to identify the underlying theoretical structure of the various distinct but interrelated variables of the mini-CEX. The following conclusions can be drawn from the results.

1. A number of items (9) are reducible to a few basic underlying elements, latent variables, or factors.
2. Based on the eigenvalues > 1.0 rule, there are two clear factors.
3. The two factors account for nearly three-fourths (72.20%) of the total variance, a good result.
4. The magnitude of the variance accounted for by the factors themselves provide theoretical support for construct validity. *Clinical Competence* accounts for the largest proportion of the variance—64.15% while professionalism & communication accounts for a smaller proportion, 8.051%. This is a theoretically meaningful result.
5. The factors overall provide theoretical support and are meaningful and cohesive. The split-loadings also provide supporting evidence since it is expected that some items are part of more than one factor.

The overall factor analysis then helps us reduce the complexity of understanding the patient encounter of medical students into fundamental underlying factors.

DISCRIMINANT ANALYSIS

Sometimes we wish to investigate factors that result in group differences (e.g., passing or failing an assessment). Candidates can be grouped based on prior performance on related assessments. We can investigate, for example, if performance on institutionally based tests (e.g., physiology, cellular biology, etc.) is related to passing the USMLE Step 1 board examination by employing discriminant analysis. This procedure can evaluate whether, based on a discriminant function calculated, participants can be correctly categorized into pass/fail groups such as based on prior test scores. Can our discriminant analysis correctly classify pass/fail students based on the prior test scores? If so, this may allow the school to provide early detection of students who may be at risk for failing Step exams.

For the purposes of discriminant analyses, a grouping (dependent) variable can be identified (e.g., pass/fail). The independent variables are the tests scores from the Year 1 institutional exams. During the analysis, a central mean score is calculated for the dependent variable and Wilks, Lambda statistic indicates whether there is a statistically significant difference between the two group means. A canonical correlation is calculated to indicate the strength of the relationship between the test scores. A canonical discriminant function coefficient is calculated for each test; the larger the absolute value of the variable (test), the greater its contribution to the discrimination between the two groups. Finally, a classification table is created that compares the actual classification of candidates based on their test scores with the statistical classification of group membership based on a classification function created by the statistical analysis of the test data. Even more precisely, how well can we classify students based on our discriminant function into pass/fail in Step 1? Effective classification based on this known group differences analysis may allow early detection of student academically at risk.

CLUSTER ANALYSIS

Cluster analysis categorizes data into homogenous groups. It has been useful in several applications in medical education such as exploring the validity of standard setting for cutoff scores. Cluster analysis can be used to identify groups of similar performances in a cohort using mathematical concepts of distance and similarity among performances. Cluster analysis is considered more objective than is human judgments in setting cutoff score for passing an exam. Thus, it is has been used for validating standard setting methods requiring expert judgments setting pass/fail percentages, for example. Can a group of experts set authentic cutoff scores to make pass/fail decisions about students?

To explore the validity of expert judgment for this purpose, cluster analysis can be used to identify the natural number of distinct groups (pass versus fail) of students based on their performance. Similarly, we can identify three groups such as pass, fail, and borderline. Based on performance patterns of the three clusters on an assessment (e.g., clinical skills), we can identify them as pass, borderline, and fail. The valid cutoff score may lie at some point between borderline and fail scorers.

SUMMARY AND MAIN POINTS

The correlation is a statistical technique to study the relationship between and among variables. Several other statistical techniques have evolved based on the original Pearson's r: rank-order correlation, biserial correlation, regression analyses, factor analysis, discriminant analysis, and cluster analysis.

- The correlation coefficient, r, must always take on values between +1.0 and −1.0 since it has been standardized to fit into this range. The sign indicates the direction of the relationship (i.e., either positive or negative), the magnitude indicates the strength of the relationship (weak as r approaches 0; strong as r increases and approaches +1.0 or −1.0), and the coefficient of determination (r^2) which is an indicator of the variance accounted for in x by y.
- Cause and effect cannot be interpreted from correlation which only indicates a relationship
- Other correlations that are important in assessment and measurement: Spearman's rho coefficient, the Biserial (r_b), and Point-Biserial (r_{pb}) correlation coefficients. When both x and y are continuous, Pearson's r is the appropriate coefficient. If both x and y are ordinal, then Spearman's rho is

the correct correlation. When x is continuous and y is artificially nominal, the r_b is the correct coefficient. Finally, when x is continuous and y is naturally nominal, the r_{pb} is correct.

- We employ several independent variables to improve the predict outcome on a dependent variable. The multiple regression equation is
  $Y' = \beta_1 X_1 + \beta_2 X_2 + \cdots \beta_k X_k + c$
- Factor analysis is a collection of methods used for exploring the correlations between a number of variables seeking the underlying clusters or subsets called factors or latent variables. It addresses the following:
  - Number of factors are needed to summarize the pattern of correlations in the correlation matrix
  - The amount of variance in a dataset is accounted for by the factor
  - Factors that account for the most variance
  - Meaning and how are the factors to be interpreted
- Discriminant analysis can evaluate whether, based on a discriminant function calculated, participants can be correctly categorized into pass/fail groups based on prior test scores
- Cluster analysis categorizes data into homogenous groups. It has been useful in several applications in medical education such as exploring the validity of standard setting for cutoff scores

REFLECTION AND EXERCISES

Reflections 4.1: Write brief response (250 words maximum) for each item below

1. Describe the use of correlation in health sciences education.
2. Compare and contrast r, rho, regression, and biserial correlation.
3. What is multiple regression and how is it used?
4. Summarize the theory underlying factor analysis.
5. Compare and contrast discriminant and cluster analysis.

Exercise 4.1: Clerkship clinical scores

Dataset from clerkships clinical scores (pediatrics, surgery, internal medicine), grade point average (GPA), and a knowledge MCQ test.
Enter the above data into an SPSS file.

1. Compute descriptive statistics of all five variables. Describe the nature of the distributions (i.e., heterogeneity—variance/SD, skewness, central tendencies)—**250 words maximum**
2. Compute Pearson's r among all five variables. Interpret the results (i.e., magnitude, direction, and coefficient of determination)—**250 words maximum**

ID	Peds	Surgery	IM	GPA	MCQ
1	70	35	31	3.0	112
2	80	40	33	2.0	93
3	65	27	38	2.2	98
4	64	32	32	3.1	114
5	55	26	29	2.0	95
6	62	34	28	2.5	106
7	58	34	24	2.5	107
8	73	43	30	3.3	132
9	67	35	32	3.5	123
10	62	36	26	3.3	127
11	68	34	34	3.9	136
12	60	31	29	2.6	102
13	64	36	28	2.1	92
14	59	28	31	2.5	98
15	52	27	25	1.8	87
16	63	35	28	2.0	90
17	69	35	34	3.8	134
18	58	24	34	1.7	83
19	47	22	25	3.4	133
20	65	33	32	3.4	124
21	56	29	27	2.5	104
22	53	33	20	2.4	110
23	59	30	29	2.7	109
24	52	22	30	2.3	104
25	60	33	27	3.0	111
26	62	31	31	3.2	109
27	49	28	21	2.4	100
28	52	31	21	2.1	97
29	52	23	29	2.6	103
30	75	42	33	3.1	110
31	53	24	29	2.9	103
32	59	29	30	2.4	96
33	57	26	31	2.3	95
34	54	31	23	3.4	117
35	51	33	18	2.9	100
36	66	37	29	2.4	101
37	69	40	29	2.5	96
38	59	25	34	2.0	88
39	71	37	34	1.8	85
40	56	27	29	2.0	90

Exercise 4.2: Factor analysis

Using the above data, run a factor analysis (i.e., determine the number of factors, the rotation method, etc.). Interpret the results (e.g., how much variance was accounted for, name the factors, specify if the factors are cohesive)—**500 words maximum**

Exercise 4.3: Multiple regression

Using the above data, run a multiple regression with GPA as the dependent variable and the remaining variables as independent. Use a stepwise regression method. Interpret the results (e.g., how much variance was accounted for, which is the optimal model)—**500 words maximum**

REFERENCES

1. Pearson K. (1895) Notes on regression and inheritance in the case of two parents. *Proceedings of the Royal Society of London*, 58: 240–242.

SECTION II

Validity and reliability

IMPORTANT CHARACTERISTICS OF MEASUREMENT INSTRUMENTS

There are three critical elements of any assessment procedure or measurement instrument: validity, reliability, and usability or feasibility. Reliability has to do with the consistency of measurement; usability deals with the practicality of using an assessment procedure, while validity has to do with the extent to which the instrument measures, whatever it is supposed to measure. That is, validity focuses on the question of how well an assessment carries out its intended function. The question is about the extent to which an assessment or test measures, whatever it is supposed to measure.

Face validity, the most superficial of the four types, focuses on the test's appearance: does it appear to fit its intended purpose? Content validity deals with the issue of the adequacy of the sampling of the test: does it contain the correct content? Both of these types of validity can be considered logical validity.

Criterion-related validity, an empirically based concept, pertains to the correlations between a test and current performance on other relevant criteria (concurrent validity) and a test's ability to predict future performance on a relevant criterion (predictive validity). Finally, construct validity subsumes all of the other forms of validity in establishing the extent to which the test measures the hypothesized entity, process, or trait.

There has been a fifth form of validity proposed recently, consequential validity*. This refers the consequences of the use of a particular assessment instrument or

* Messick S. Validity. In RL Linn (Ed.), Educational measurement (3rd ed., pp. 13–103). New York: Macmillan, 1989.

test. There may be positive and negative outcomes for the test-takers, educational institutions, and society as a whole. Consequential validity may also be referred to as utility, in that it refers to a measure's application. The use of and social consequences of assessment as a whole has received little empirical examination in comparison to statistical validity (criterion-related and construct). A measure cannot be used appropriately—and therefore lacks validity—if it does not measure what it purports to measure. Conversely, a measure will not be valid—quantify what it is intended to measure—if it is not used appropriately for its intended purpose. Each purpose affects the other (empirical evidence and consequences of use), so both purposes have been referred to as a type of validity.

While there are three critical elements of any measurement instrument, including educational tests—validity, reliability, and usability—reliability is a precondition to validity. A test must be reliable to be valid. A test which is reliable, however, is not necessarily valid. Reliability, therefore, is a necessary but not sufficient condition for validity. (For a further discussion of reliability see Chapters 8 and 9.) Finally, neither validity nor reliability can guarantee usability or practicality. The polygraph illustrates an instrument with low practicality under some conditions. This device measures physiological arousal on various modalities such as the electroencephalograph, Galvanic skin response, heart rate, and so on. It is highly reliable and valid for measuring fear responses in the laboratory. The polygraph is not very practical or usable for the same measurement under naturalistic conditions, because a person must be strapped into electrodes and other equipment. This limitation greatly reduces the use value of the polygraph.

Before we begin a detailed examination of validity, let us further illustrate the interrelations between validity, reliability, and usability. If your wristwatch is five minutes fast and you always keep it that way, it is highly reliable but lacks validity (since it produces the wrong time). Alternatively, if your watch is both consistent and tells the correct time, then it has both high reliability and validity. Finally, your watch may sometimes run fast and sometimes run slow in unpredictable ways so that it is neither reliable nor valid.

In all of the above cases, however, the watch has high usability as you can strap it onto your wrist and go about your daily affairs. By contrast, a grandfather clock or an atomic clock may be far more reliable and valid than your watch, but both lack practicality and usability. Similarly, the balance arm weight scales that are common in physicians' offices are probably more reliable and valid than your bathroom weight scale, but they are not as usable or practical (due to cost and size). Ultimately, the value of a measuring instrument (including educational tests) must involve a carefully balanced consideration of reliability, validity, and usability.

THE NATURE OF VALIDITY

Does a ruler measure length? Does a clock measure time? Does a thermometer measure temperature or a speedometer measure velocity? These questions may appear trite and the answers self-evident, but they are the essence of validity.

Does the Stanford–Binet (an IQ test) really measure intelligence, or the Law School Admission Test (LSAT) measure a predilection for legal knowledge? Does the Medical School Admission Test (MCAT) measure an ability to acquire medical knowledge? Did the final exam in history that you wrote in college really measure your knowledge of history? These questions are less trite than the first set and the answers are less evident. Indeed, these are essential questions about test validity. These questions have to do with the nature of validity.

In daily life, we are surrounded by a myriad of measurements that you rarely question. We accept automatically the information imparted by the thermometer, the wristwatch, weight scale, ruler, or many other instruments. We may not be so quick to accept without question the results of an anatomy test, however. Perhaps we felt the test was unfairly difficult or didn't ask central questions about the subject matter. These are concerns about the test's validity.

Validity, however, is not an all or none phenomenon—it is not discrete. It is a matter of degree. An atomic clock is more valid than an inexpensive wristwatch but both validly measure time. Your physician's weight scale is more valid than your bathroom scale though both measure weight. Another point about validity is that it is situation specific. The validity of an instrument is clearly restricted to particular conditions. A speedometer is clearly valid for measuring velocity but not temperature. Similarly, the Stanford–Binet is valid for predicting academic achievement (to some extent) but not for predicting eventual happiness in life, economic success, or leadership qualities. The central questions for the validity of a test is "What is it valid for?"

To answer this question adequately, there are four levels of analysis:

1. Face Validity
2. Content Validity
3. Criterion-related Validity
   a. predictive
   b. concurrent
4. Construct Validity

In some conventional discussions, three forms of validity are generally recognized (content, criterion related, and construct). Face validity is not regarded as a form of validity per se. A joint committee of the American Psychological Association, National Council on Measurement in Education, and the American Educational Research Association has prepared a document, *Standards for Educational and Psychological Testing* (Washington, D C: American Psychological Association, 2014), which describes validity and sets standards for test use. In this treatment, face validity is not regarded as a form of validity. Some textbook writers also do not discuss this form as a separate kind of validity. Nevertheless, in the present discussion and in Chapter 5, it is discussed as a separate type of validity because it influences classroom climate and many aspects of assessment in the health professions. Therefore, for present purposes, face validity is considered a form of validity. It also has become particularly important recently because of the emphasis on "performance" assessment such as assessing clinical competency where face validity is critical.

The levels of validity are generally regarded as hierarchical so that a higher level includes those below it. It is not always necessary to analyze every level of validity for every situation or use of an assessment. Indeed, there are some useful rules of thumb for classifying the validities and procedures for establishing them. These are summarized in Table 1.

The first two levels of validity, face and content, are not fully empirical in nature. The other two levels, criterion-related and construct are empirical in nature. In short, face and content validity can be established without recourse empirical evidence, while criterion-related and construct validity requires data for their demonstration.

THE NATURE OF RELIABILITY

Reliability has to do with the consistency of measurement. It is a necessary condition for validity. While reliability is a precondition for validity, it does not

Table 1 Four types of validity

Type	Definition	Evidence	How to establish
Face Validity	The appearance of the instrument	Non-empirical	Make the instrument appear appropriate
Content Validity	The adequacy with which an instrument samples the domain of measurement	Non-empirical	Construct a table of specifications (blueprint)
Criterion-related Validity	The extent to which the instrument relates to some criterion of importance	Empirical (correlation, regression, exploratory factor analysis, discriminant analysis, etc.)	Study the relationship of the scores with some criterion of importance
Construct Validity	The psychological processes that underlie measurement on the assessment device	Empirical (multiple correlation, confirmatory factor analysis, structural equation modelling, experimental)	Manipulate the test scores through experimental procedures and observe results. Study relationships among the latent variables or constructs

guarantee it. That is, a measurement instrument which is reliable is not necessarily valid. As we have seen, a clock which always runs ten minutes fast is reliable since it is consistent but it is not valid since it gives the incorrect time. It is evident then, that *reliability is a necessary but not sufficient condition* for validity. Alternatively, an instrument which is valid must be reliable.

What is meant by the consistency of measurement? What factors can lead to the inconsistency of measurement? How can you tell if some measurement is consistent or not? These questions are at the heart of the concept of reliability. A simple example can help to clarify the nature of reliability.

Suppose that you measured the length of your kitchen table with a ruler and it turned out to be 50 inches long. Later that day, you began to doubt this measurement so next morning you measured the table again. This time it turned out to be 46 inches long. Which is correct? To settle the matter, you measured the table a third time and this time it was 53 inches long. Still unsure you measured the table several more times with a different result each time. What is the problem here? There are two possibilities: (1) the table keeps changing length every time it is measured or (2) something is wrong with your measurement instrument.

Under normal conditions, of course, tables do not change length, so in this case the problem must be the measurement instrument. Upon closer examination you discover that your ruler is made of rubber and the differential results are due to the inconsistency of the measurement. This is why of course, rulers are made from wood, plastic, or metal so that they don't stretch and shrink from time to time.

This example is not merely unlikely or trite, though, as many tests and assessments in health professions education do behave like rubber rulers, as they produce inconsistent results or unreliable measurements. The concern with reliability in educational, psychological, and health professions education measurement is paramount because of the difficulty of producing consistent measures of achievement and psychological constructs. In measuring physical properties of the universe, reliability is usually not a big problem (For example, think of measuring height, velocity, temperature, weight, and so on.), while it is a central problem for educational and performance characteristics of health professionals and other people.

Reliability is a multifaceted concept rather than a singular idea. Indeed, there are several ways of thinking about and discussing reliability. Four methods of establishing reliability are usually recognized.

The four methods or techniques for determining the reliability of a measurement instrument are summarized in Table 2 and listed below.

1. Test–Retest
2. Parallel Forms
    a. given at the same time
    b. given at different times
3. Split-Half
4. Internal Consistency

Table 2 Various methods of estimating reliability

Method	Reliability measure	Procedure
Test–retest	Stability over time	Give the same tests to the same group of subjects at different times (hours, days, weeks, months, etc.)
Parallel Forms (same time)	Form Equivalence	Give two forms of the same test to the same group at the same time
Parallel Forms (different time)	Form Equivalence and stability over time	Give two forms of the same test with a time interval between the two forms
Split-half, Cronbach's α, KR20, Ep^2	Internal consistency	Give the test once and apply the Kuder–Richardson formula, Cronbach's alpha coefficient formula, generalizability analysis. Apply analysis of variance methods to get variance components.

These techniques are not only different methods for establishing reliability but each type produces a somewhat different type of reliability as well. While all forms of reliability focus on consistency, there are different aspects of the testing to which the consistency is relevant. These various methods of understanding and determining reliability are discussed in detail in Chapters 8 and 9.

5

Validity I: Logical/Face and content

ADVANCED ORGANIZERS

- This chapter deals with two forms of validity, logical and content, commonly referred to as face and content validity.
- Face validity has to do with appearance: does the test appear to measure whatever it is supposed to measure? Face validity provides an initial impression of what a test measures but can be crucial in establishing rapport, motivation, and setting classroom climate.
- An issue with face validity is that many educators, psychologists, and others judge assessments only on the basis of face validity. When judgments are made under uncertainty, a number of cognitive biases and heuristics involving superficial aspects of the assessments result in an overreliance on face validity.
- Content validity involves sampling or selecting. The domain of measurement must be clearly defined and detail the cognitive processes involved employing levels of Bloom's taxonomy (knows, comprehends, applies, analyzes, synthesizes, evaluates/creates).
- Enhancing content validity may be achieved most directly through the use of a table of specifications (TOS). A well-designed and carefully developed TOS will provide a sound plan for a test. The closer is the match between the test's accuracy in sampling of the content and learning outcomes, the higher is the content validity.
- Prior to developing a TOS, we must know what the instructional objectives of the program or course are. Instructional objectives are goals of instruction that specify student or learner behavior as an outcome of instruction.
- The Delphi procedure, a method employing a systematic procedure to achieve consensus of group judgments, may be used to further enhance the content validity of a test or other assessment. Evidence for content validity therefore is supported from consultations with experts in the relevant field and a high degree of agreement among experts on the relevancy of the contents to measure the domain of interest.

LOGICAL AND CONTENT

This chapter deals with the first two forms of logical validity that are most commonly referred to as face and content validity (see Table 1 in section 2).

FACE VALIDITY

Although it is sometimes considered to be only a superficial type, face validity can play a crucial role in many assessment situations. Face validity has to do with appearance: does the test appear to measure whatever it is supposed to measure? From the candidate's perspective, does the instrument *seem* to measure the relevant domain?

Besides providing an initial impression of an assessment, face validity can be crucial in establishing rapport, motivation, and determining how seriously it will be taken. There is little that can undermine a respondent's motivation and seriousness than an assessment that is perceived to be inappropriate or unfair. Face validity thus plays a pivotal role in assessment as we shall see in this chapter.

While some testing authorities understate the importance of face validity and even regard it as a misnomer, it can play a crucial role in many testing situations. In addition to the question, "Does the test appear to measure whatever it is supposed to measure?" another relevant question is, "Does the test look right and fair?" Why is this so important?

Besides providing an initial impression of what a test measures, face validity can be crucial in establishing rapport, motivation, and setting classroom climate. There is little that makes a group of students hostile as quickly as a test that is perceived to be inappropriate or unfair.

Here are typical medical student-written comments on a gastrointestinal exam they perceived as unfair:

- "This was not adequately covered in lecture and certainly wasn't a learning objective"
- "We DID NOT do histology"
- "These questions are unfair"
- Another student offered a divine invocation: "DIOS MIO!"

Students may react with dismay and anger toward the exam, instructor, and course, resulting in poor motivation and a negative learning environment. Classroom climate may become generally negative. Face validity thus plays an important role in testing.

The Wechsler tests of intelligence also provide examples of the importance of face validity. These tests were developed by David Wechsler at Bellevue Hospital in New York to be used with Americans. Two main tests, the *Wechsler Intelligence Scale for Children* now in its fifth edition (WISC-V) and the *Wechsler Adult Intelligence Scale* currently in its fourth edition (WAIS-IV), have been widely used historically throughout the world to measure IQ. The *Information* subtest of these IQ tests contained some questions which are clearly intended for Americans. Such questions as, "Name two men who have been president of the United States since 1950", and "What are the colors of the American flag?", have clear American cultural reference.

People in Canada, England, Australia, New Zealand, and elsewhere are going to be taken aback by these and other items that are supposed to measure the respondents' general knowledge about their culture. Such items can make the respondent hostile, unmotivated, and negative toward the test and the psychologist administering the test.

Psychologists in many countries have made the tests more culturally relevant by substituting questions that are pertinent to the culture of the test-taker but sometimes with surprising results. In a Canadian study,[1] for example, changing the American-biased question about presidents to naming prime ministers of Canada actually made the question more difficult for Canadians. Nearly all Canadians (98%) tested answered the American president question correctly, while only about half (55%) answered the Canadian prime minister question correctly ($p < 0.001$). This surprising finding is likely due to the larger number of American presidents during that time period than Canadian prime ministers (since the latter can serve an indefinite number of terms while presidents are limited to two terms). Moreover, American presidents enjoy much more publicity (even in Canada) than do prime ministers. So while face validity was improved in this case, the properties of the test were altered in an unexpected way. Face validity does play a crucial but complex role in such testing situations.

Another useful example of the face validity problem is the *Rorschach Inkblot Test*, probably the most famous psychological test of all. This test consists of 10 inkblot figures on cards that provide ambiguous forms. The test-taker is required to describe what the inkblots represent and the responses are analyzed for content and structure that have been "projected" onto the inkblots. This test is now so well-known and has been lampooned in films, television programs, as well as novels and stories that anyone taking this test is likely not to take it seriously. Rapport, motivation, and effort may thus be seriously compromised.

In classroom and standardized educational testing, multiple-choice tests also suffer from face validity problems. Many people believe that multiple-choice items only measure rote knowledge, even though the items can be constructed to measure higher level cognitive processes. This general belief about multiple-choice items can influence reaction and orientation toward these types of items and undermine rapport, credibility, and general classroom climate. It is common to hear students say that, "I just can't take multiple-choice tests." When using these tests, you should be aware that they have validity limitations.

Alternatively, the general public probably overestimates the ability of essay tests to measure higher level cognitive outcomes such as synthesis and evaluation. While the open-ended question of the essay test provides a format for measuring outcomes requiring organization and creation of ideas, there is no guarantee that such responses will necessarily be forthcoming. Indeed, the essay test format probably overestimates the importance of saying something but underestimates the importance of having something to say.

Another exam format, the objective structured clinical exam (OSCE), is very widely used in the health professions to assess a variety of skills, procedures, and cognitive processes. These include taking a case history, conducting a physical exam, interpreting X-rays, blood pressure, etc., providing a diagnosis, and prescribing treatments. Although the OSCE has been used extensively for more than 40 years, there continues to be issues with its empirical validity (discussed in detail in Chapter 13). As it involves clinical situations frequently including actors portraying patients, the OSCE has high face validity.

An issue with face validity is that many educators, psychologists, and others judge assessments only on the basis of face validity. Nearly every medical school employs the personal interview as a major criterion for selection into medical school, for example. In a recent systematic review of 75 studies assessing the use of interviews involving many thousands of medical school applicants, Patterson, Knight, Dowell et al.[2] found that the medical school interview has near zero predictive validity for medical school. Many of these studies have also shown that the interview has nearly zero reliability or agreement between interviewers whether the interviews are done in a panel or individually. In other words, the personal interview is of little or no value in distinguishing between suitable and unsuitable candidates for medical school. The personal interview for law school, dentistry, optometry, and other health professions is equally dismal for selection.

Similar findings pertain to the job interview where prospective candidates for a job are interviewed individually or in a panel. Many decades of research have shown that the job interview lacks both reliability and predictive validity in selecting for a job. The job interview is probably the most widely used criterion for job selection even though it has poor reliability and validity.

The unavoidable conclusion about the personal interview for job selection, admission to medical school or other programs is that they are poor assessment methods lacking in reliability and validity. Nonetheless, the personal interview continues to be widely used at great effort and expense.

Consider the medical school personal interview. A typical mid-sized medical school with a class of 120 will interview around 500 applicants every year. An interview can last for 1–3 h and may involve several interviewers. Accordingly, 500–1,500 h of candidates' time is involved and 1,500–2,000 h of professors' time as more than one professor generally interviews each candidate. Many of the applicants may travel from out of town or out of state at considerable expense. Overall then, the personal interview is a massive undertaking costing thousands of hours of human time and financial costs in professors' salaries and applicants' time and travel. This is repeated in the United States more than 150 times every year and perhaps thousands of times worldwide. How can such massive effort continue with such a useless activity?

One of the explanations is face validity. Most people have a firm belief that they can discern human qualities (whether for a job or medical school suitability) by interviewing or talking with prospective candidates. When people—even experts—are faced with complex judgment without complete information, they typically rely on the intuitive system of judgment versus the analytic cognitive system. Daniel Kahneman—the Noble Laureate psychologist—and his colleague

Amos Tversky concluded that when judgments are made under conditions of uncertainty, a number of cognitive biases and heuristics involving superficial aspects of the assessments result in an overreliance on face validity.[3] In this context, a cognitive *heuristic* is simple procedure that helps find answer to difficult questions. When faced with uncertainty or incomplete information, experts frequently rely on intuition to answer difficult questions.

One of the cognitive heuristics that comes into play under such conditions is the illusion of validity of expert judgment; those who make the judgments express a high degree of confidence even though they are likely to be wrong.[4] This double interplay between the intuitive illusion of validity and a high degree of confidence probably explains the continued persistence of medical school interviews where professors want to "look candidates in the eye" or discern the "cut of their jib." Candidates also favor the interview—thereby also harboring the illusion of validity—in that they want an opportunity to prove themselves. These heuristics and biases emerge in low-validity environments such as medical school interviews.[4] A further discussion of low-validity environments is included in Box 5.1.

BOX 5.1: *Advocatus diaboli*: Low-validity environments

Daniel Kahneman who won the Noble Prize in Economic Sciences for his revolutionary work in cognitive psychology has challenged the rational model of judgment and decision making. Rational thought (the analytic system of cognition) is especially undermined in conditions of uncertainty or incomplete information such as in business, medicine, politics, psychology, and education. These conditions of uncertainty or incomplete information result in low-validity environments.[4] Under these conditions, non-rational or intuitive thought seems to predominate.

Many aspects of business (e.g., the job interview, stock market fluctuations), medicine (e.g., longevity of cancer patients, diagnosis of cardiac disease), politics (e.g., selecting candidates for office, success of social programs), psychology (e.g., diagnosis of mental illness, effectiveness of psychotherapy), and education (e.g., selection for medical school, assessing teacher effectiveness) occur in low-validity environments. Aspects of assessment and evaluation in medical and other health professions education frequently occur in low-validity environments as well. This includes assessing "professionalism," "communication skills," "team work," "interprofessional education," and even "clinical skills and procedures."

The overall conclusion from decades of research is that formulas in the form of algorithms are better for predicting outcomes than are experts especially in low-validity environments. Part of the reason for this is that experts attempt to be clever and consider complex combinations of features in making their predictions. Such enhanced complexity reduces validity. Another part of the reason is that experts attend to irrelevant stimuli and cues which further reduce validity.

(Continued)

BOX 5.1 (*Continued*): *Advocatus diaboli*: Low-validity environments

A number of studies have shown that human decision makers are inferior to a prediction formula even when they are given the score predicted by the formula[4]! In medical school admissions, the final determination is made by faculty members who interview the candidate. It appears that conducting the interview is likely to diminish the accuracy of the selection procedure when the interviewers also make the final admission decision, which is common practice in medical schools.[2] The interviewers tend to be overconfident in their intuitions thus assigning too much weight to their personal impressions and too little weight to other sources resulting in lowered validity. The same biases and heuristics are operative for residency selection. To echo Kahneman, the research in this area suggests a surprising conclusion: to maximize predictive accuracy, final decisions should be left to formulas, especially in low-validity environments. Expert judgment—with the illusion of apparent high face validity—muddies the waters and reduces validity.

In a different domain, forensic auditing by expert accountants, the results are eerily similar to medical expert judgment.[11] Grazioli et al. constructed a computer algorithm to detect fraudulent financial statements. The software correctly identified the frauds 87% of the time, while the expert auditors correctly identified only 45% of the cases. When reviewing the cases, the auditors articulated their thinking aloud which was audio recorded. On analyses of these talk-aloud protocols, Grazioli et al. discovered that many irrelevant cues (e.g., superficial similarity to previous cases such as age) effected judgment. A confirmation heuristic, "most people don't commit fraud so probably this one didn't either", also played a role. Moreover, emotions such as generosity or "giving the benefit of the doubt" were part of the mix. Notwithstanding their dismal performance, the auditors expressed a great deal of confidence of the correctness of their judgments. The accountant auditors were suffering from the illusion of validity of their judgments.

BOX 5.2: *Advocatus diaboli*: Expertise and confidence

Recent research indicates that most people are not very accurate in assessing their own performance, competence, or expertise in relation to either objective standards or peer assessments. Kruger and Dunning,[12] in a series of experiments employing undergraduate students, found that poor performers in a variety of intellectual and social domains tended to overestimate their competence or performance compared to objective measures or peer assessments. Conversely, high performers tended to underestimate their own performance compared to objective outcomes or peer assessments.

(Continued)

BOX 5.2 (*Continued*): *Advocatus diaboli*: Expertise and confidence

They concluded that the cognitive skills necessary to perform well in a domain are the same as those needed to recognize good performance in that domain. In other words, poor performers lack the meta-cognitive skills (self-appraisal, knowledge and organization of the task, standards of performance in the task, memory processing, etc.) to be competent or perform well but also to accurately assess their own performance. Most people—whether they perform well or not—express high degrees of confidence in their judgments or performance especially in the face of uncertainty.

A recent study[13] focused directly on the confidence (i.e., as self-assessed) expressed by medical students, residents, and faculty physicians on their diagnostic accuracy of clinical cases (correct vs. incorrect as objectively assessed). On a case-by-case basis, Friedman et al. found a weak relationship between confidence and diagnostic accuracy. Residents were overconfident (confidence was not related to correctness) in 41% of the clinical cases, faculty physicians in 36%, and medical students in 25%. Even experienced clinicians appear unaware of the correctness of their diagnoses at the time they make them. Practice improvement and reduction of medical errors cannot rely exclusively on clinician's perception of their performance or needs. Rather, external (peer or objective) feedback is required.

What factors characterize people who are so poor at self-assessments? Kruger and Dunning[12] suggested that the lack of knowledge and skills that lead to poor performance are the very same ones that are necessary for accurate self-assessment. Therefore, a paradox results: poor performers can only improve the accuracy of their self-assessments by improving their performance first. Kruger and Dunning have indicated that unskilled people are frequently unaware of their own "incompetence" because they lack the very skills needed to both perform well and self-assess accurately. Hodges et al.[14] have identified a similar phenomenon with novice physicians who were found to be unskilled and unaware of it.

The main conclusion is that even officially designated experts (e.g., physicians) who are unskilled are highly confident in their own judgments. In low-validity environments, the heuristics or biases of judgment are invoked. Experts are often able to produce quick answers to difficult questions by substitution thus creating coherence where in fact there is none. A classical substitution heuristic has been found in answering the following question: "How happy are you with your life these days?" In response to this question, people usually substitute (unconsciously) the following question: "What is my mood right now?"[4] When experts (and others) employ these cognitive heuristics to answer questions, they express a high level of confidence of their subjective judgment even though the judgment is likely wrong.

By way of summary then, face validity, while the most superficial sort of validity, can and does play a significant role in both educational and psychological assessment and evaluation. Indeed, classroom climate can be adversely or positively influenced by the face validity of a particular test. It is important, therefore, for the faculty to be aware of this fact and the "public relations" role of testing. Face validity, however, plays a secondary role to content validity.

CONTENT VALIDITY

Content validity concerns the extent to which an assessment adequately samples the domain of measurement—the content. A patient questionnaire which requires the patient to evaluate the physician's clinical skills and cognitive knowledge would lack content validity, because these are not areas in which a patient has sufficient expertise. A peer questionnaire to evaluate physicians' clinical skills and cognitive knowledge requiring that physicians complete it would have content validity. In the case of this questionnaire, the content refers to both what is sampled (i.e., clinical skills and cognitive knowledge) and who is the rater.

Content validity therefore involves sampling or selecting. The domain of measurement must be clearly defined and detailed. Not only must the content areas or subject matter be identified but so must the cognitive processes involved. The cognitive processes refer to the levels of Bloom's taxonomy[5] (knows, comprehends, applies, analyzes, synthesizes, evaluates/creates).* We must determine not only the content to be assessed but as well the cognitive processes or skills that have been specified by a task or performance analysis.

Enhancing content validity may be achieved most directly through the use of a TOS. Prior to developing a TOS, we must know what the instructional objectives of the program or course are.

INSTRUCTIONAL OBJECTIVES

Instructional objectives are goals of instruction that specify student or learner behavior as an outcome of instruction. These should specify overt student or learner performance during or at the end of instruction. Two types of instructional objectives are usually identified: (1) general and (2) specific.

General instructional objectives

A general instructional objective is an intended outcome of instruction that has been stated in general enough terms to encompass a domain of student

---

* Since the original the original publication there has been revisions of this taxonomy. The major and most controversial change is at levels 5 and 6. The revised version has demoted "evaluation" to level 5 and has substituted "creating" in level 6 as the highest level. See Table 5.1 for further details.

performance. A general instructional objective must be further defined by a set of specific learning outcomes to clarify instructional intent and describe the type of performance students are expected to demonstrate.

The following general instructional objectives that have been adopted by a number of medical schools from the AAMC physician competencies reference sets[6] describe domains of student performance.

All graduates when they receive an MD must be able to:

1. Demonstrate knowledge of the basic, clinical, and behavioral sciences and apply this knowledge to patient care (**Knowledge for Practice**).
2. Communicate and interact effectively with patients, their families, and members of the inter-professional healthcare team (**Interpersonal and Communication Skills**).
3. Function as a member of an inter-professional healthcare team and provide patient care that is compassionate, appropriate, and effective for the treatment of health problems and the promotion of health in diverse populations and settings (**Patient Care**).
4. Demonstrate a commitment to upholding their professional duties guided by ethical principles (**Professionalism**).
5. Demonstrate the ability to investigate and evaluate their care of patients, to appraise and assimilate scientific evidence, and to continuously improve patient care based on constant self-evaluation and life-long learning (**Practice-Based Learning and Improvement**).
6. Demonstrate awareness and understanding of the broader healthcare delivery system and will possess the ability to effectively use system resources to provide patient-centered care that is compassionate, appropriate, safe, and effective (**Systems-Based Practice**).
7. Demonstrate the skills to participate as a contributing and integrated member of an interprofessional healthcare team to provide safe and effective care for patients and populations (**Interprofessional Collaborative Practice**).
8. Demonstrate the qualities and commitment required to sustain lifelong learning, personal and professional growth (**Personal and Professional Development**).

Guidelines for stating general instructional objectives

- Begin each objective with a verb (demonstrates, knows, understands, appreciates, etc.)
- State at the proper level of generality (clear, concise, readily definable)
- State in terms of student performance (e.g., demonstrates knowledge of clinical sciences), not in terms of instructor performance (e.g., will teach clinical sciences)
- Include only one objective per statement

- State in terms of the performance outcome, or product (communicates effectively), not the learning process (acquires communication skills)
- State in terms of the skill or terminal performance (understands the ethics of a situation) not the specific subject-matter topics (ethics of end of life assistance)

Specific learning outcomes

These objectives are sometimes also referred to as specific objectives, performance/skill objectives, behavioral objectives, and measurable objectives. An intended outcome of instruction is stated in terms of specific, measurable, and observable student or learner performance. Specific learning outcomes describe the types of performance that learners will be able to exhibit when they have achieved a general instructional objective.

General instructional objectives:

1. Demonstrates knowledge of the basic, clinical, and behavioral sciences and applies this knowledge to patient care (**Knowledge for Practice**).
   Possible specific learning outcomes:
   1.1. Summarizes the normal structure and function of the human body and each of its major organ systems.
   1.2. Describes cell and molecular biology for understanding the mechanisms of acquired and inherited human disease.
   1.3. Identifies altered structures and function of major organ systems that are seen in common diseases and conditions.
   1.4. Explains clinical, laboratory, and radiologic manifestations of common disease and conditions.
   1.5. Integrates behavioral, psychosocial, genetic, and cultural factors associated with the origin, progression, and treatment of common diseases and conditions.
   1.6. Explains the epidemiology of common diseases and conditions within a defined population and systematic approaches useful in reducing the incidence and prevalence of these maladies.
   1.7. Applies knowledge of the impact of cultural and psychosocial factors on a patient's ability to access medical care and adhere with care plans.

2. Demonstrates competence in presenting information orally.
   Possible specific learning outcomes:
   2.1. Delivers a patient presentation to peers effectively.
   2.2. Projects voice and delivery.
   2.3. Uses time effectively.
   2.4. Fields questions about patient presentation effectively.
   2.5. Introduces topics in such a way to generate interest.
   2.6. Discusses topics using examples and illustrations.

2.7. Concludes topic by summarizing main ideas.

2.8. Uses visual and multimedia aides effectively.

2.9. Involves audience in the presentation of information.

2.10. Explains test results to patients at an appropriate level.

CHARACTERISTICS OF GOOD OBJECTIVES

When writing specific learning outcomes or objectives, the performance or observable learner behavior must be clearly identified. The specific learning outcome, or objective, can be further defined and clarified by stating the conditions and criteria for that student performance.

Performance: an objective is useful to the extent it specifies clearly what students must be able to *do* when they demonstrate mastery of the objective.

Given ten clinical problems, the student will solve 90% correctly.

Condition: an objective is useful to the extent it clearly states the *conditions* under which the learning/performance must occur (i.e., circumstances and materials).

Given ten clinical problems, the student will solve 90% correctly.

Criteria: an objective is useful to the extent it specifies the *quality* or *expected level* of performance.

Given ten clinical problems, the student will solve 90% correctly.

Guidelines of stating specific learning outcomes

- Describe the **specific** performance or observable behavior expected
- Describe a performance or behavior that is **measurable**
- Begin each specific learning outcome with a verb that specifies definite **observable** performance (discusses, writes, projects, concludes)
- Describe the performance in the specific learning outcome so that it is **relevant** to the general instructional objective
- Include only one learning outcome per statement (writes a case history) not multiple learning outcomes per statement (writes and presents a case history)
- Specific learning outcome should be free of course content so it can be used with various units of study

For example:

This is good: diagnose diabetes.

This is poor: diagnose diabetes in the case of Mr. Smith who is a 53-year-old obese white male.

TAXONOMIES OF OBJECTIVES

Various taxonomies or classification schemes have been developed for objectives. An important such taxonomy is the one developed by Benjamin Bloom for the cognitive domain. This is summarized in Table 5.1. The taxonomy is hierarchically organized into six categories ranging from verbatim recall or

Table 5.1 Bloom's taxonomy of instructional objectives in the cognitive domain

Classification	Definition	Example verbs
1. Knowledge/ **remembering**[a]	Recall or recognition of learned material	Define, describe, identify, list match, name, recall, recognize, remember
2. Comprehension/ **understanding**	Translation, interpretation, and extrapolation of information	Defend, explain, rewrite, paraphrase, infer, re-word, interpret, explain
3. Application/ **applying**	Apply knowledge to an unfamiliar or new situation	Predict, prepare, use, relate, solve, modify, operate, compute, discover, apply
4. Analysis/ **analyzing**	To break down into its constituent components and identify their interrelationships	Identify, differentiate, discriminate, infer, relate, distinguish, detect, classify
5. Synthesis/ **evaluating**[a]	Combining elements to form a new whole	Combine, compose, design, devise, organize, plan, revise, summarize, deduce, produce
6. Evaluation/ **creating**	Making judgments about the value of materials or methods	Appraise, compare, conclude, contrast, criticize, support, justify, compare, assess

Source: Anderson and Krathwohl[7]

[a] The words in bold have been added to the levels since the revisions of this taxonomy. The major and most controversial change is at levels 5 and 6. The revised version has demoted "evaluation" to level 5 and has substituted "creating" in level 6 as the highest level. All the levels are stated as verbs, suggesting that learning is an active process. Some debate continues on the order of levels 5 and 6 but this revised version has gained acceptance overall.

knowledge at the lowest level to the process of evaluation at the highest level. As well as a description of each level, each category contains examples and verbs that exemplify from which to construct instructional objectives. As well as specifying intended performance for students, instructional objectives should be written at the appropriate cognitive level. The information in Table 5.1 will help you both write instructional objectives and subsequently test items that measure the instructional objectives.

TABLE OF SPECIFICATIONS

A TOS is a blueprint of the assessment device or procedure. Just as an engineer develops a detailed plan of a bridge that is to be built and an architect draws a blueprint of the building that is to be erected, so to the researcher begins with a plan for the assessment device. This plan specifies the content areas to be assessed as well as the cognitive processes and skills that are to be measured. Thus, it is called a *table of specifications.*

A well-designed and carefully developed TOS will provide a sound plan for an assessment. The closer the match between the assessment in its accurate sampling of both the content and cognitive processes, the higher the content validity. If a researcher develops an assessment with high content validity, then a good measurement may result. Content validity concerns the extent to which the test adequately samples the domain of measurement, the content.

In a first-year medical school neurosciences course, 275 new terms have been introduced and students are required to know them. The domain of measurement refers to the definition of all the terms. You would probably not want to include all of these on a test, however, as it would be too long, tedious, and exhausting. Thus, you might randomly select 75 terms from the total domain of 275 terms to include in the test. The extent to which the 75 terms selected adequately represent the total number of terms, determines the content validity of the test. Content validity is usually the most important consideration in course, unit, or subject-matter tests.

Content validity involves sampling or selecting. The domain of measurement, therefore, must be clearly defined and detailed. Not only must the content areas or subject matter be identified but so must the cognitive processes involved. The cognitive processes refer to the levels of Bloom's taxonomy (knows, comprehends, applies, analyzes, synthesizes, evaluates). You must determine not only the subject matter to be tested but as well the cognitive outcomes that have been specified by the instructional objectives. Enhancing content validity may be achieved most directly through the use of a TOS.

An assessment device that is constructed without a TOS results in a poor quality test lacking in content validity. A similar result would be obtained by constructing a bridge or building without blueprints. The TOS is a chart where, by convention, the content area to be measured is itemized along the vertical axis, while the cognitive outcomes are specified along the horizontal axis. Use the following steps to construct the TOS:

1. Prepare a heading on a blank sheet of paper or file. Write the subject (e.g., cardiovascular), date, and educational level (e.g., Year 3) of the test.
2. Identify all of the content areas to be tested and list these on the left-hand margin in the order they were taught.
3. Across the horizontal, specify the levels of learning outcomes specified in the instructional objectives.
4. Determine the total number of items that will be on the test.
5. In the right-hand margin, write the number and percentage of items that will be devoted to each specified content area and do the same for the objectives.
6. In each cell (intersection of content area and level of learning outcome), write the number of items and percentage of the total test that these items represent (some cells may be blank).

7. Carefully consider the percentage of test items in each cell and ensure that this accurately reflects the emphasis and time spent in the teaching and learning of this content. If only 10% of the total time was spent learning names of scientists and their discoveries, then only 10% of the test items should be devoted to this.

8. Each item should be carefully checked to ensure that it indeed measures at the intended cognitive outcome (Chapters 11 and 12 contain detailed discussions of item construction). If, for example, a mathematics problem intended to measure application outcomes is given but the problem has been previously presented in class, then the item probably only measures at the knowledge level, since the students may have simply memorized the answer.

A well-designed and carefully developed TOS will provide a sound plan for your test. The closer is the match between the test's accuracy in sampling of the content and learning outcomes, the higher is the content validity. If a professor or course committee develops a test with high content validity, then a good test usually results. Examples of tables of specifications are presented in Tables 5.2 and 13.4.

As we have already seen, Table 5.2 contains a TOS of a Year 3 cardiovascular exam. Table 13.4 contains a TOS for a 12 station OSCE assessing clinical, communication, and counselling skills employing standardized patients. The OSCE stations are classified by content area (patient presentation) and level of assessment (e.g., physical exam/diagnosis/management). As OSCEs refer to "clinical exams"—history taking, physical exam, counselling a patient, ordering tests, etc., they frequently, but not always, involve a standardized patient. This TOS covers the content and levels of assessment in medicine and some pediatrics, illustrating the use of a TOS for clinical, communication, and counselling skills.

Table 5.3 is the published "table of specifications" from a standardized test, Step 1 of the United States Medical Licensing Exam (www.usmle.org/step-1/#content-outlines). Notice that it is called "Test Specifications" but essentially specifies the content of the test (left-hand margin) and the percentage ranges of items number of items in each cell. There is no indication of the cognitive levels of measurement. Therefore, this not a true TOS but only a partial one although the content is classified as "System" and "Process."

DELPHI PROCEDURE

A Delphi procedure may be used to further enhance the content validity of a test or other assessment. This name derives from the 8th century BC Oracle of Delphi, who gave prophecies about important future events. Today, the Delphi is a method employing a systematic procedure to achieve consensus of group judgments where expert input is required. It is assumed that input from several experts is more valid than individual judgments. In testing and assessment, this method seeks agreement from experts on the content and processes of an assessment.

Table 5.2 Table of specifications (test blueprint)

Cardiovascular, Year 3

Date_____

Content area	Level of understanding				Total
	Knowledge	Comprehension	Application	Higher	
1. Examination of the patient					10 (13%)
a. History	1	2	0	0	3 (4%)
b. Electrocardiography	1	2	1	0	4 (5%)
c. Echocardiography	1	1	0	1	3 (4%)
2. Heart failure					15 (20%)
a. Clinical aspects	2	3	0	0	5 (7%)
b. Pathophysiology	2	1	1	1	5 (7%)
c. Management	2	1	1	1	5 (7%)
3. Arrhythmias, sudden death and syncope					12 (16%)
a. Genesis of arrhythmias	1	1	0	0	2 (3%)
b. Genetics	1	1	0	0	2 (3%)
c. Diagnosis	1	2	1	1	5 (7%)
d. Management	1	1	0	1	3 (4%)
4. Preventive cardiology					20 (27%)
a. Vascular biology	1	2	1	0	4 (5%)
b. Risk for cardiac disease	2	2	1	2	7 (9%)

(Continued)

Table 5.2 (**Continued**) Table of specifications (test blueprint)

Cardiovascular, Year 3

Date____

Content area	Level of understanding				
	Knowledge	Comprehension	Application	Higher	Total
c. Treatment of Hypertension	1	2	0	1	4 (5%)
d. Obesity, diet and nutrition	2	2	1	0	5 (7%)
5. CV disease and other organ systems disorder					18 (24%)
a. Heart in endocrine	1	2	0	0	3 (4%)
b. Rheumatic fever	1	2	0	0	3 (4%)
c. Oncology and CV diseases	1	2	1	2	6 (8%)
d. Renal and CV diseases	1	2	1	2	6 (8%)
Total	23 (31%)	31 (41%)	9 (12%)	12 (16%)	75

Table 5.3 Information provided by the United States medical licensing exam on the website

USMLE Step 1 test specifications[a]	
System	**Range (%)**
General principles of foundational science[b] immune system	15–20
Blood & lymphoreticular system	
Behavioral health	
Nervous system & special senses	
Skin & subcutaneous tissue	
Musculoskeletal system	
Cardiovascular system	
Respiratory system	
Gastrointestinal system	
Renal & urinary system	
Pregnancy, childbirth, & the puerperium	
Female reproductive & breast	
Male reproductive	
Endocrine system	60–70
Multisystem processes & disorders	
Biostatistics & epidemiology	
Population health	
Social sciences	
Process	**Range (%)**
Normal processes[c]	10–15
Abnormal processes	55–60
Principles of therapeutics	15–20
Other[d]	10–15

Source: www.usmle.org/step-1/#content-outlines (accessed April 15, 2016).

[a] Percentages are subject to change at any time. See the USMLE Web site for the most up-to-date information.

[b] The general principles category includes test items concerning those normal and abnormal processes that are not limited to specific organ systems. Categories for individual organ systems include test items concerning those normal and abnormal processes that are system-specific.

[c] This category includes questions about normal structure and function that may appear in the context of an abnormal clinical presentation.

[d] Approximately 10%–15% of questions are not classified in the normal processes, abnormal processes, or principles of therapeutics categories. These questions are likely to be classified in the general principles, biostatistics/evidence-based medicine, or social sciences categories in the USMLE Content Outline.

Gabriel and Violato[8] illustrated this procedure in a recent study by developing and testing an instrument for assessing knowledge of depression of patients with non-psychotic depression. A TOS was created for three levels of cognitive outcomes of Bloom's taxonomy: knowledge, comprehension, and application. It was decided to write 27 multiple-choice questions (MCQs) to cover the content areas and level of measurement. The initial items and the TOS were developed based on empirical evidence from an extensive review of literature, theoretical knowledge, and in consultation with national and international psychiatry experts. The MCQ items were written following basic rules for item construction so as to avoid common technical item flaws (see Chapter 11).

A volunteer panel of experts met on three occasions to review the items for the following: (1) appropriateness of difficulty and relevancy for patients as examinees, (2) concise, clear language free from medical or psychiatric jargon at the appropriate level (Grade 9), (3) knowledge to be demonstrated in a specific area of depression or its treatment, and (4) at least three experts agreed on the correct answer for each question. Additional experts were asked to rate the relevance of each MCQ in sampling patient knowledge of depression and its treatment on a 5-point scale (1 = irrelevant, 2 = slightly relevant, 3 = moderately relevant, 4 = significantly relevant, and 5 = highly relevant).

The 12 psychiatrists (mean of 22 years' experience) included both men and women experts in mood disorders. There were nine at the rank of professor, two at associate professor, and one at assistant professor. Three of the experts were invited for an informal panel discussion of the instrument and an in-depth review of the individual items. Each of the remaining nine experts independently rated each item for its relevancy in testing depression knowledge and its treatment on the five-point scale.

The experts achieved consensus of the relevance of each item for testing patient knowledge of depression. There were no significant differences between men and women in ratings of experts or based on their years of experience. There was a very high overall agreement (88%) among experts about the relevance of the MCQs to test patient knowledge on depression and its treatments. The majority of the items were rated as highly or significantly relevant (mean = 4.4, SD = 0.67, range = 1–4).

There was significant positive relationship ($r = 0.35$, $p < 0.01$; $r = 0.33$, $p < 0.05$), between having the necessary knowledge about the *risks of relapse* (subscale #2) and being aware of the *symptoms of depression* (subscale #4), on the one hand, and having knowledge of different *biological and psychological treatments* (subscale #5), respectively. It is assumed that when patients understand the causes of depression, they will be able to think of treatment options more rationally. There was also positive correlations ($r = 0.30$, $p < 0.05$; $r = 0.27$, $p < 0.05$) between subscale #5 "understanding biological and psychological treatments" and subscale #3 "knowledge of etiology and triggers of depression," and subscale #4, "knowledge of symptoms", respectively. There were no correlations of the subscales with subscale #1, "definition of terms."

The evidence for content validity therefore is supported by two main factors. First, the MCQ test was initially developed based on empirical evidence from extensive literature review and from consultations with experts in the field of depression. Second, a very high degree of agreement was achieved among experts on the relevancy of its contents to measure patient knowledge of depression and its treatments (very high mean = 4.4) using a Delphi procedure. The formal inclusion of external experts illustrates the Delphi procedure for enhancing content validity.

UPDATING CONTENT VALIDITY: THE 2015 MEDICAL COLLEGE ADMISSION TEST

The Medical College Admission Test (MCAT) has been widely used by most medical schools in the United States, Canada, and elsewhere for more than 80 years. In 1928, F.A. Moss created an early version, the Moss Scholastic Aptitude Test, to improve selection and reduce high failure and attrition rates. It remained until 1946, when the first revision was undertaken by the American Association of Medical Colleges and was subsequently renamed twice to the Professional Aptitude Test and finally the MCAT in 1948.[9] The Moss version, 1928–1946 was criticized for its lack of breadth and its focus on the recall or recognition of facts.

The post-World War II versions were thought to be an improvement and provided a better prediction of medical student success beyond the first 2 years of basic sciences or preclinical performance in medical school. Subsequent revisions have been composed of four subscales, measuring basic sciences and social or verbal reasoning ability. The objectives of early versions concentrated heavily on designing a reliable and valid assessment that would not only aid in selection but also produce estimates of future success, namely predictive validity. Minor revisions occurred in 1962, followed by changes that emphasized a focus on the sciences in 1977, the introduction of a Writing Sample subtest in 1991, and finally a major over haul for 2015. The new version consists of four sections:

- Chemical and physical foundations of biological systems
- Critical analysis and reasoning skills
- Biological and biochemical foundations of living systems
- Psychological, social, and biological foundations of behavior

According to AAMC documents,[10] "the blueprints [i.e., TOS] for the new exam shift focus from testing what applicants know to testing how well they use what they know." This new TOS is presumably based on accumulated scientific evidence over the past one or two decades of both the changing healthcare system and advances in testing and psychometric theory and practice. The content validity of assessment devices should be updated as science, assessment, and psychometrics evolve and change.

SUMMARY AND CONCLUSIONS

This chapter dealt with the two forms of validity, logical and content, commonly referred to as face and content validity. Face validity has to do with appearance: does the test appear to measure whatever it is supposed to measure? Face validity provides an initial impression of what a test measures but can be crucial in establishing rapport, motivation, and setting classroom climate.

An issue with face validity is that many educators, psychologists, and others judge assessments only on the basis of face validity. Nearly every medical school uses the personal interview as a major criterion for selection into the school, for example. How can such massive effort continue with such a useless activity?

One of the explanations is face validity. When people—even experts—are faced with complex judgment without complete information, they typically rely on the intuitive system of judgment versus the analytic cognitive system. When judgments are made under uncertainty, a number of cognitive biases and heuristics involving superficial aspects of the assessments result in an overreliance on face validity.

Content validity concerns the extent to which an assessment adequately samples the domain of measurement—the content. Content validity therefore involves sampling or selecting. The domain of measurement must be clearly defined and detailed and must sample the cognition processes involved, and the levels of Bloom's taxonomy (knows, comprehends, applies, analyzes, synthesizes, evaluates).

Enhancing content validity may be achieved most directly through the use of a table of specifications. Prior to developing a TOS, we must know what the instructional objectives of the program or course are. Instructional objectives are goals of instruction that specify student or learner behavior as an outcome of instruction.

A TOS is a blueprint of the assessment device or procedure. The educator begins with a plan for the assessment device. This plan specifies the content areas to be assessed as well as the cognitive processes and skills that are to be measured. A well-designed and carefully developed TOS will provide a sound plan for your test. The closer is the match between the test's accuracy in sampling of the content and learning outcomes, the higher is the content validity.

The Delphi procedure may be used to further enhance the content validity of a test or other assessment. It is a method employing a systematic procedure to achieve consensus of group judgments where expert input is required. In testing and assessment, this method seeks agreement from experts on the content and processes of an assessment. Evidence for content validity therefore is supported from consultations with experts in the relevant field and a high degree of agreement among experts on the relevancy of the contents to measure the domain of interest. Content validity needs to be updated based on evolving scientific and societal changes and needs.

REFLECTIONS AND EXERCISES

Reflections 5.1: Face validity

1. Briefly define face validity.
2. Why is it so important that educational tests have high face validity?
3. Construct four questions at the application level of knowledge that measures basic concepts in arithmetic (e.g., area, percentage). Write several versions of each question so that it has face validity for four groups of

people (e.g., physicians, carpenters, mechanics, bank tellers, teachers, carpet layers, etc.). A particular question should measure the same concept for everyone but should be stated so as to have face validity for each group (e.g., If 12 cm are cut from a board 80 cm long, what percentage is removed?—application for carpenters. If six students leave a class of 40 students, what percentage has left the class?—application for instructors).

4. Discuss the aspects of the test that you would examine to improve face validity when developing a first-year medical school test on immunology.

Reflections 5.2: Content validity

1. Briefly define content validity.
2. How can a table of specifications be used to enhance content validity?
3. Construct a table of specifications for a test in a subject area in which you have some expertise. Make the test 50 items long and use at least four levels of learning outcomes from Bloom's taxonomy. Break the content areas into appropriate subdivisions.
4. Identify two assessments in health sciences education that may have content validity problems (e.g., in training evaluation reports—ITERS). Specify what these shortcomings are.

Exercise 5.1: Instructional objectives

18 marks

Purpose: to study the nature of instructional objectives and to practice writing both general instructional objectives and specific learning outcomes. Objectives enable instructors to plan and execute instruction and to fairly assess and evaluate student achievement and performance.

DIRECTIONS

1. Write three general instructional objectives in any content/subject area of your choice. Indicate the cognitive level of each according to Bloom's taxonomy. **(3 marks)**
2. For each of the general instructional objectives, list five specific learning outcomes that describe **observable** student performance as a result of instruction. Indicate the cognitive level of each according to Bloom's taxonomy. **(15 marks)**

SUBMIT TO THE INSTRUCTOR

One page with three general instructional objectives, each followed by five specific learning outcomes (also indicating the level of Bloom's taxonomy).

Exercise 5.2: OSCE table of specifications assignment

20 marks

Purpose: to study the nature of tables of specifications for objective structured clinical exams (OSCEs) utilizing standardized patients.

DIRECTIONS

1. Design and develop a table of specifications/blueprint for an OSCE in any specialty of interest (e.g., surgery, psychiatry, obstetrics/gynecology, internal medicine, etc.)
2. Using the template in Table 13.4: patient and presentation, assessments, differential diagnoses and/or management

SUBMIT TO THE INSTRUCTOR

One page with five stations **(10 marks)**, each with a patient name and condition, followed by assessments **(5 marks)** and possible differential diagnoses and/or management **(5 marks)**.

Exercise 5.3: Delphi procedure

10 marks

Purpose: to develop the plans for a Delphi procedure.

DIRECTIONS

1. Design and develop a Delphi procedure for enhancing content validity of an assessment (use the TOS in Exercise #1 or #2 or design a new one)
2. Identify experts (e.g., surgeons, etc.) who will participate in your Delphi study.
3. How many experts will you include?
4. Design the questionnaire for the Delphi procedure (provide some examples (at least 3) of the items that will be in your assessment) and the multi-point scale that you will use.

SUBMIT TO THE INSTRUCTOR

One page with three items **(6 marks)** and the rating scale that the experts will use **(4 marks)**.

REFERENCES

1. Violato C. Effects of Canadianization of American-biased items on the WAIS and WAIS-R information subtests. *Canadian Journal of Behavioural Science*. 1984; 16(1):36–41.
2. Patterson F, Knight A, Dowell J, Nicholson S, Cousans F, Cleland J. How effective are selection methods in medical education? A systematic review. *Medical Education*. 2016; 50(1):36–60.

3. Tversky A, Kahneman D. Judgment under uncertainty: Heuristics and biases. *Science.* 1974; 185(4157):1124–1131.

4. Kahneman D. *Thinking Fast, Thinking Slow.* Macmillan: New York, 2011.

5. Bloom BS, Engelhart MD, Furst EJ, Hill WH, Krathwohl DR. *Taxonomy of Educational Objectives: The Classification of Educational Goals. Handbook I: Cognitive Domain.* David McKay Company: New York, 1956.

6. Englander R, Cameron T, Ballard AJ, Dodge J, Bull J, Aschenbrener C. Toward a common taxonomy of competency domains for the health professions and competencies for physicians. *Academic Medicine.* 2013; 88:1088–1094.

7. Anderson L, Krathwohl DA. *Taxonomy for Learning, Teaching and Assessing: A Revision of Bloom's Taxonomy of Educational Objectives.* Longman: New York, 2001.

8. Gabriel A, Violato C. The development of a knowledge test of depression and its treatment for patients suffering from non-psychotic depression: A psychometric assessment. *BMC Psychiatry.* 2009; 9:56. doi:10.1186/1471-244X-9-56.

9. Donnon T, Paolucci EO, Violato C. The predictive validity of the MCAT for medical school performance and medical board licensing examinations: A meta-analysis of the published research. *11th Ottawa International Conference,* Barcelona Spain, July, 2004.

10. Association of American Medical Colleges. The new score scales for the 2015 MCAT exam, 2015. Available at www.aamc.org/mcat2015/admins.

11. Grazioli S, Johnson PE, Jamal K. A cognitive approach to fraud detection. *Journal of Forensic Accounting.* 2006; VII(1):65–88; University of Alberta School of Business Research Paper No. 2013–676. Available at SSRN: http://ssrn.com/abstract=920222 or doi:10.2139/ssrn.920222.

12. Kruger J, Dunning D. Unskilled and unaware of it: How difficulties in recognizing one's own incompetence lead to inflated self-assessments. *Journal of Personality and Social Psychology.* 1999; 77(6):1121–1134.

13. Friedman CP, Gatti GG, Franz TM, Murphy GC, Wolf FM, Heckerling PS, Fine PL, Miller TM, Elstein AS. Do physicians know when their diagnoses are correct? Implications for decision support and error reduction. *Journal of General Internal Medicine.* 2005; 20(4):334–339.

14. Hodges B, Regehr G, Martin D. Difficulties in recognizing one's own incompetence: Novice physicians who are unskilled and unaware of it. *Academic Medicine.* 2001; 76(10 Suppl):S87–S89.

6

Validity II: Correlational-based

Validity—the extent of which a test measures whatever it is intended to measure—is usually classified into four types: (1) face, (2) content, (3) criterion-related, and (4) construct.

The topic of this chapter, criterion-related and construct validity both require empirical evidence (primarily correlational) for their support. Criterion-related validity involves concurrent and predictive forms both of which require validity coefficients. Construct validity subsumes all forms of validity plus a further determination of the psychological and educational processes involved in the construct.

1. When we are interested in how performance on a test correlates with performance on some other criterion, we are concerned about criterion-related validity. There are two categories of this kind of validity: (1) predictive (How well does a test predict some future performance), and (2) concurrent (How well do two tests intercorrelate concurrently).
2. The determination of a test's criterion-related validity requires empirical evidence in the form of correlation coefficients (r). Interpreted in the context of validity, r is called a validity coefficient. The validity coefficient can be transformed into the coefficient of determination (r^2) which in turn is used to determine the percentage of variance in the criterion that is accounted for by the test.
3. In predictive validity, individual scores on the criterion can be estimated using regression techniques. This strategy allows the prediction of individual scores on some future criterion.
4. Construct validity focuses on the truth or correctness of a construct and the instruments that measure it. A construct is defined as an entity, process, or event which is itself not observed and can be measured only indirectly. Establishing the validity of constructs also requires determination of the

validity of relevant instruments. Establishing construct validity is a complex process.

5. One of the most widely researched and readily measureable constructs in education and psychology is intelligence. Systematic measurement and research in the area has been going on nearly 100 years beginning with the work of Alfred Binet in France. Much controversy, however, continues to surround the validity of the construct of intelligence.

6. A number of factors influence the validity of tests. Some of these factors are internal to the tests such as the directions on the test. Others such as noise or distractions during test administration are external to the test. We summarized 12 such factors in this chapter.

CRITERION-RELATED VALIDITY

When we are interested in how performance on a test correlates with performance on some other criterion, we are concerned about criterion-related validity. The criterion may be any performance on some other measure. There are two subcategories of criterion-related validity: (1) predictive and (2) concurrent. Predictive validity refers to how current test performance correlates with some future performance on a criterion and thus involves the problem of prediction. Concurrent validity refers to how test performance correlates concurrently (at the same time) with some criterion. If you develop a test which will be used for screening and hiring management personnel, you are dealing with a prediction problem because it is the future performance of the candidate as manager that is at question. A pencil-and-paper test of knowledge of computers represents a concurrent validity problem where the simultaneous criterion is actual skills in computer use. Since the empirical procedures used in both predictive and concurrent validity are essentially the same (correlation), and since each involve a criterion external to the test, they are classified together under criterion-related validity and involve the use of validity coefficients.

VALIDITY COEFFICIENTS

Evaluating the criterion-related validity of a test requires examining the magnitude of the correlation coefficient, which is referred to as the validity coefficient. Validity coefficients are merely correlations that are interpreted within the context of validity. Interpretations can be aided further by using the coefficient of determination (r^2) and then determining the percentage of variance (a statistical summary of the total differences in test scores—see Chapter 4) that is accounted for in the criterion by the test. The percentage of variance accounted for is derived by multiplying the coefficient of determination by 100 ($r^2 \times 100$ = percent of variance accounted for). When the correlation is used within the context of predictive validity, it is called the predictive validity coefficient. In the context of concurrent validity, it is called the concurrent validity coefficient.

PREDICTIVE VALIDITY

How well does test performance predict some future performance? Figure 6.1 schematically represents this problem. Generally, a criterion (also the dependent variable) and a predictor (independent variable) are identified and their intercorrelations are called the predictive validity coefficient. The arrow in the Figure which points from the predictor to the criterion indicates that interest is unidirectional from the predictor to the future. Six examples are given in Part A of Figure 6.1.

In the Medical College Admissions Test (MCAT) example, the correlation between this predictor and medical school test scores, which is the criterion, is approximately $r = 0.61$.[1] This indicates that 37% of the variance ($0.61^2 \times 100 = 37\%$) in medical school test scores is accounted for by performance on the MCAT. The correlation between the Law School Admissions Test (LSAT) scores as a predictor and law school Grade Point Average (GPA) as the criterion is approximately $r = 0.51$ ($0.51^2 \times 100 = 26\%$ of the variance in law school GPA is accounted for by performance on the LSAT).

The correlation between the Reading Readiness Test (given to preschool children) and performance on a standardized reading achievement test given at the end of grade one is $r = 0.60$. Therefore, 36% of the variance ($0.60^2 \times 100 = 36\%$) in reading achievement is accounted for by reading readiness before children begin school. Finally, in example six of Figure 6.1, Infant Tests (vocalization, locomotion, manipulation skills of hands and fingers, attention span, goal directedness) correlate with childhood IQ at approximately $r = 0.20$. This accounts for 4% ($0.20^2 \times 100 = 4\%$) of the variance. Given the above data, are the predictors good, moderate, or poor? How large does the predictive validity coefficient have to be?

Part A: Predictive Validity

1. MCAT scores ⟶ Board test scores during medical school (r = .61)

2. Medical school GPA ⟶ Residency directors ratings (r = .18)

3. GRE scores ⟶ Graduate school GPA (r = .48)

4. LSAT scores ⟶ Law school GPA (r = .51)

5. Reading Readiness Test scores ⟶ School achievement test scores (r = .10)

6. Infant Tests ⟶ Childhood IQ (r = .20)

Part B: Concurrent Validity

1. IQ scores ⟷ Achievement test scores (r = .47)

2. Personality scores ⟷ Achievement test scores (r = .30)

3. Attitude scores ⟷ Achievement test scores (r = .10)

Figure 6.1 Schematic representation of criterion-related validity.

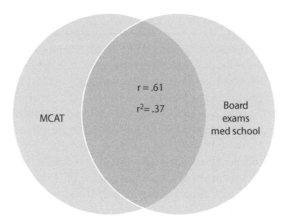

Figure 6.2 Venn diagram of the correlation between MCAT and board exams.

Interpreting the predictive validity coefficient

Figure 6.2 is a schematic of the correlation and overlap between the MCAT and board exams taken during medical school. It is quite rare to derive a predictive validity coefficient greater than $r = 0.61$. This is because the criterion we wish to predict is extremely complex (e.g., achievement, IQ, marital satisfaction, managerial skills), and because people and situations are continuously changing. The factors determining whether or not a validity coefficient is large enough depends on the benefits obtained by making the predictions, the cost of testing, and the cost and validity of alternative methods of prediction. Obviously, the higher the predictive validity coefficient, the better is the prediction. In some circumstances, a validity coefficient of $r = 0.60$ may not justify an extremely expensive and time consuming examination, while in others, a coefficient of $r = 0.20$ may make an appreciable difference.

In the predictive validity examples in Figure 6.1, the LSAT, SAT, RRT, and GRE are moderate to good predictors of their respective criteria (16%–36% of the variance is accounted for). The Infant Tests, however, are poor predictors of childhood IQ as only small amounts of the variance is accounted for (4%). Determining the efficacy of a predictor, therefore, is based on a number of factors including the magnitude of the validity coefficient, the variance accounted for in the criterion, the cost of testing, and the financial and social costs of alternative procedures.

So far the discussion has focused on judging the overall predictive validity of the test. But how can we predict an individual's score on the criterion, given a score on the predictor?

Regression: Predicting individual scores

If the correlation between two variables is known, as in the case of predictive validity, a person's outcome on the criterion can be predicted using regression

Regression Analysis of MCAT and USMLE Step 1

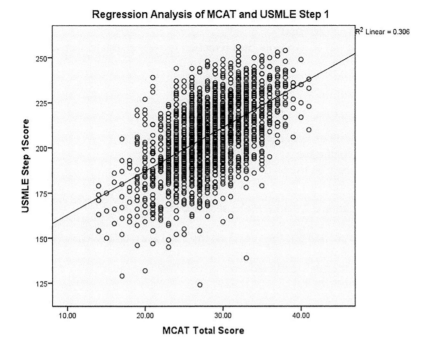

techniques. There are two regression approaches: simple and multiple regression; the latter one builds on the former (see Chapter 4).

A particular student, Jason, has an MCAT total score of 30 and his average science GPA of 3.7. To predict Jason's Step 1 score based on MCAT alone, we would use the simple regression (regression results from Chapter 4): $Y' = 2.422 \times \text{MCAT} + c \left[Y' = 2.422 \times 30 + 138.655 = 211.315 \right]$

To improve the prediction of a particular student, Jason's performance in Step 1, we now use the results from the multiple regression and equation 4.3 (Chapter 4). Jason's MCAT total score of 30 and his average science GPA of 3.7 for performance on Step 1 of the USMLE becomes: $Y' = 2.422 \times \text{MCAT} + 9.171 \times \text{GPA} + c$

Substituting the values for Jason: $Y' = 2.422 \times 30 + 9.171 \times 3.7 + 112.972 = 219.56$

This is a 13% improvement in predictive validity by employing a second variable, average science GPA over the simple regression of only MCAT total. These results indicate that average science GPA contributes unique variance beyond the one predicted by the MCAT alone. The percentage of variance accounted for with both variables ($0.345 \times 100 = 34.5\%$) is an improvement over the percentage with only the MCAT ($0.306 \times 100 = 30.6\%$).

Such predictions also have course and classroom applications. Suppose that a professor of Biochemistry knows that the correlation between a Quiz (Mean = 15; SD = 2) given in September and the Final exam (Mean = 68; SD = 10) given in

December is $r = 0.72$. If Katherine achieves a score of 8 on the Quiz, what is her predicted score on the Final?

The simplest way to carry out the prediction is using standard scores:

$$z_{criterion} = r \times z_{predictor} \qquad (6.1)$$

where

$z_{criterion} = z$ score on the criterion
$r =$ validity coefficient
$z_{predictor} = z$ score on the predictor

Employing equation 3.7, Katherine's z score on the Quiz is $z = \dfrac{8-15}{2} = -3.5$

Now using equation 6.1, the z score on the Final is $z = 0.72 \times -3.5 = -2.52$

To derive Katherine's predicted score on the Final, use equation 3.7 $z = \dfrac{X - M}{SD}$

$$-2.52 = \frac{X - 68}{10}$$

Re-arranging,

$$X = 68 + (-2.52)10 = 43$$

All things remaining equal, Katherine's predicted score on the Final may mean that she will fail the course. Now is the time, of course, for the professor to intervene and make sure "that all things do not remain equal." The prediction has allowed the teacher to identify Katherine as a student at risk.

CONCURRENT VALIDITY

A similar problem to predictive validity is that of concurrent validity. Part B of Figure 6.1 depicts the concurrent validity problem. Compared to predictive validity (Part A), concurrent validity has no predictor. Both variables are called criteria (independent variables). The line with an arrow at both ends is used to indicate a simultaneous, reciprocal relationship. The two tests or measures are taken simultaneously. In predictive validity, on the other hand, time (months or years) separates the two measures.

The concurrent validity problem arises most frequently when we wish to identify the correlations between two theoretically related but separate domains, such as IQ test scores and achievement test scores that are given more or less at the same time. Theoretically, we expect these two domains to be related. Similarly—though perhaps less obvious—we might expect attitude test scores and personality test scores to be related to achievement test scores. To determine the validity of these tests, research must be carried out. The personality and attitude tests must be given simultaneously (e.g., within a few days) to determine their intercorrelations. Used in this context, the correlation is called a concurrent validity coefficient.

Interpreting the concurrent validity coefficient

When examining the correlation between the tests, the magnitude of the correlations requires considerable interpretation. The actual magnitude required depends on the theoretical relationship between two domains. We would expect, for example, that the correlations between IQ and achievement should be higher than those between personality and achievement. The higher correlation between IQ and achievement ($r = 0.47$) compared to personality and achievement ($r = 0.30$) makes theoretical sense. Therefore, the pattern of correlations in Figure 6.1 Part B provides evidence for the overall concurrent validity of achievement. If the correlations are too high between the two tests, it suggests that the two tests are measuring the same variable.

CONSTRUCT VALIDITY

Construct validity is a multifaceted and complex idea that has undergone much discussion, debate, and revision since its elegant definition by Cronbach and Meehl.[2] They proposed the nomological network approach that identifies, defines, and operationalizes constructs, contains theoretical propositions, and specifies linkages between constructs as a central idea for construct validity. The linkages maybe correlation based (Pearson's r, regression, factor analysis, etc.) or experimentally based hypothesis testing specifying between group differences (analyses of variance, etc.).

Construct validity focuses on the truth or correctness of a construct and the instruments that measure it. What is a construct? A construct is an "entity, process, or event which is itself not observed" but which is proposed to summarize and explain facts, empirical laws, and other data.[3] In the physical sciences, gravity and energy are two examples of hypothetical constructs. Gravity has been proposed to explain and summarize facts such as planets in orbit, the weight of objects, and mutual attraction between masses. Gravity, defined as a process or force, cannot be directly observed or measured; only its effects can be identified and quantified. Energy, also an abstraction or construct, is used to explicate such disparate phenomena as photosynthesis in plants, illumination from a light bulb, and the engine that propels a jet liner.

In psychological and medical educational measurement, examples of constructs include intelligence, scholastic aptitude, communications, clinical competence, honesty, clinical reasoning, and creativity. These constructs have been proposed to explain, summarize, and organize empirical relationships and response consistencies. Clinical competence, like gravity, cannot be directly measured; its existence must be inferred from behavioral measurements. Similarly, anxiety is indicated by behavioral and physiological markers, while creativity is indexed by products (e.g., paintings, novels, inventions) though it is thought to be a process. In any case—whether gravity, clinical competence, honesty, or anxiety—construct validity requires the gradual accumulation of information from a variety of sources. In effect, it is a special instance of the general procedure of validating a theory in any scientific endeavor. The ultimate purpose of validation is explanation, understanding, and prediction.

Cronbach[4] has proposed that all forms of validity are really construct validity. Content and criterion-related evidence are pieces of the puzzle on which we can focus our attention. In many tests, it follows that all forms of validity should be considered and synthesized to produce an explanation and understanding. Therefore, all data from the test or data relevant to it are pertinent to its construct validity. There are, however, specific procedures that contribute to construct validity. These are explicated below.

In general, several important steps and procedures are central to establishing construct validity. These may be summarized as follows:

1. Identify and describe the meaning of the construct.
2. Derive theoretical support for the construct.
3. Based on the theory, develop items, tasks, or indicators of the construct.
4. Develop a theoretical network for the construct that can be empirically established by correlation. If, for example, the test is to measure neuroticism, then it should correlate with clinical ratings of neuroticism made by psychologists and psychiatrists. A test of mechanical aptitude as another instance should correlate with measures such as ability to fix an engine or assemble machinery.
5. Conduct research to obtain the data necessary to investigate the correlations between the variables in the theoretical framework.
6. Design experiments based on the construct, theory, and correlations to test for causal relationships.
7. Evaluate all of the relevant evidence and revise the theory, construct, and measures if necessary.
8. Fine-tune the measures of the construct by eliminating items and revising the tasks.
9. Return to Step 3 and proceed again.

Probably the best developed, most widely researched, and readily measureable construct in psychology and education is intelligence. The process of establishing construct validity of intelligence will be summarized here since it serves as an excellent illustration.

The construct validity of intelligence

The concept of intelligence has its roots in antiquity. The early Greek philosophers such as Plato and Aristotle speculated about and debated the nature of intelligence. More recently, Charles Darwin offered an analysis of intelligence in his book, *The Descent of Man* (1871), as did his cousin, Sir Francis Galton in his book, *Hereditary Genius* (1869). These original but crude conceptions involved equally crude measures such as reaction time and attention span.

With the work of Alfred Binet in France at the beginning of the twentieth century, understanding of intelligence and its measurement underwent considerable advances. In 1904, Binet was appointed by the French government to a committee to investigate the causes of intellectual disability among public school children. Binet decided to refine the concept on intelligence and develop a test which measured important aspects of it. Based on rational and logical analyses (procedures for establishing content validity), Binet constructed a test which measured verbal and numerical reasoning. By giving the test to large numbers of children at different ages, Binet was able to develop norms of mental age (MA). Binet then identified various criteria (school performance, reading ability) that were relevant to the test and gathered data to see if the test is correlated with these. These early tests did show impressive results, both as concurrent and predictive measures. It was the German psychologist Wilhelm Stern who took the next logical step and divided MA (as determined by the test) by chronological age and multiplied this quotient by 100 to produce the familiar Intelligence Quotient (IQ). That is,

$$IQ = \frac{MA}{CA} \times 100$$

The French psychiatrist, Theodore Simon, joined Binet in his later work in revision of the test to produce the Binet–Simon Intelligence Tests. These were valuable beginnings in the measurement of intelligence.

In 1916, the Stanford University psychologist Lewis Terman, using the Binet–Simon test as a model, produced a test for use in the United States. This is now called the Stanford–Binet Tests of Intelligence. Terman et al. gave the tests to many thousands of participants and studied the nature of the distribution of the scores, correlations between the scores and other criteria (school success, memory ability, reading ability, etc.), and the internal consistency of the subtests across different populations. In addition, Terman launched a longitudinal study (which is still ongoing) that has produced important data relevant to the stability/instability of intelligence over the life span. Many thousands of other researchers have since administered the tests to many millions of people and have empirically studied its relationships to other theoretically relevant variables. A number of other measures of intelligence have since been developed by other psychologists such as David Wechsler (the Wechsler Intelligence Scales) as well as others (e.g., the Otis–Lennon, Full-Range Picture Vocabulary Test).

The data that has accumulated over the course of the past century or so involving thousands of scientists, millions of subjects, and many different measures are all relevant to the construct validity of IQ, intelligence, and the tests which are used to measure it. Based on this research and these data, the following general conclusions can be made[5]:

- MA (as measured by the original Binet scales) increases steadily until cognitive maturity is reached in late adolescence or early adulthood. Thereafter, it stabilizes. This is in keeping with the general principles of growth (height for example).
- People who score poorly on IQ tests generally also have difficulties in theoretically related tasks such as reading, memory, arithmetic, and abstract reasoning. Conversely, those who achieve high scores on IQ tests do well on these tasks.
- Children who achieve high scores on IQ tests tend to do well in school; those who achieve low scores tend to do poorly.
- Subjects with clinical abnormalities affecting brain growth and organization (e.g., Down's syndrome, Phenylketoneuria) do very poorly on IQ tests.
- IQ scores show stability over a number of years and even over the entire life span.
- The IQs of identical twins show very high correlations even when the siblings are raised apart.
- Experiments to alter or increase IQ have yielded inconsistent results. While this last conclusion still remains controversial, some psychologists have concluded that intervention attempts have demonstrated that IQ is not very malleable and represents a stable trait.

The above results are in substantial agreement with logical, theoretical, and empirical expectations of intelligence. Thus, current evidence provides support for the construct validity of intelligence and some tests which measure it (Wechsler tests, Stanford–Binet). Even so, the construct of intelligence as it is currently formulated and operationalized is constantly undergoing critical scrutiny and is the center of much controversy in the continuing process of construct validation.

Factors that influence validity

A number of test characteristics, administration, and other factors can seriously affect the validity of a test. Twelve such factors are summarized below.

1. Directions of the test. If the directions are vague, misleading, or unclear, this can have detrimental effects on test performance. Students may run out of time to complete the test, for example, if the directions about the time allotted are unclear or misleading. Long complicated directions may similarly distract and confuse test-takers and reduce validity.
2. Reading level. If many of the candidates cannot understand the questions, because the reading level is too difficult, validity is compromised. A reading level that is appropriate for graduate students may be too difficult for second-year nursing students.

3. Item Difficulty/Ease. If the items on a test are either too difficult or too easy for the student's in question, then validity is compromised.

4. Test items inappropriate for the instructional objectives. If the items fail to correspond to the objectives, content validity is undermined. Items that measure synthesis are inappropriate for comprehension level objectives. Conversely, items that measure knowledge are not appropriate for application objectives. A public health question on a pharmacology exam where there were no public health instructional objectives compromises validity.

5. Time problems. Insufficient time to take the test will reduce its validity. This is because students may fail to complete some portion of the test or because they may be so rushed that they give only superficial attention to some items. In an OSCE, requiring a detailed patient history and complex neurological physical exam in 10 min, validity may be undermined.

6. Test length. A test which is too short will fail to sample adequately the domain of measurement and thus reduce content validly. Essay tests or other constructed response type tests (e.g., short answer) frequently suffer from this problem because a few essay items may not adequately sample the relevant domain.

7. Unintended clues. Wording of questions which provide clues to the answer reduces test validity. These can take the form of word associations, grammatical errors, plural-singular connections, and carryovers from previous questions.

8. Improper sampling of content/outcomes. Even when the test length is adequate, there may be improper sampling of content and outcomes such as too much emphasis on a content area (or too little). This will reduce content validity. A typical student comment illustrates this: "Biochem/genetics course was poorly organized with unclear objectives and material tested somewhat unfairly."

9. Noise or distractions during test administration. External noise or distractions within the examination room can affect performance and thus validity.

10. Cheating and copying. Students who cheat or copy from others do not provide their own performance and thus invalidate their results.

11. Scoring of the test. Careless or global scoring strategies by the assessor can influence test validity in a negative fashion.

12. The criterion problem. Tests which are to predict some future performance or which are to relate to some other measure of performance concurrently must correlate with some measure called the criterion. Frequently, the criterion is very difficult to define, operationalize, and measure. This is called the criterion problem. Consider, for example, a test which is to predict future performance in "professionalism." How can this criterion be defined, operationalized, and measured? What content and processes should be included on this test? How do you determine the relevant aspects of professionalism to correlate the test to?

These interrelated issues constitute the criterion problem. When the criterion is general and abstract, it is difficult to construct a test which will show correlations to the criterion. Conversely, the more specific and precise the criterion is, the easier it is to sample on a test. The problem is one of criterion-related validity.

Factor analysis and construct validity

The following study illustrated the use of factor analysis for evidence of construct validity. Multisource feedback questionnaires including self-assessments are a feasible means of assessing the competencies of practicing physicians including surgeons in communication, interpersonal skills, collegiality, and professionalism. In a study of 201 surgeons, data were collected on a 34 item instrument with a five-point scale. There were 25 general surgeons, 25 orthopedic surgeons, 24 obstetricians and gynecologists, 24 otolaryngologists, 24 ophthalmologists, 20 plastic surgeons, 20 urologists, 15 cardiovascular and thoracic surgeons, 13 neurosurgeons, 6 general practice surgeons, and 5 vascular surgeons. The data were entered into SPSS.

To run a factor analysis with SPSS, use the following.

Select "Dimension Reduction," then select "Factor." The following dialogue window should be open.

Select Items 1–34 and click over to the "Variables:" pane as below.

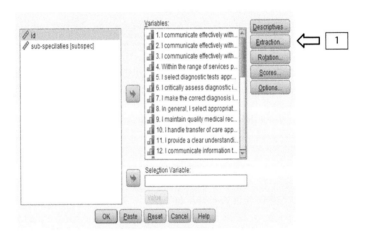

1. Select "Extraction." The following dialogue window should open.
2. The default "Method" should be "Principal components." If not, select it.
3. "Extract" should be "Based on eigenvalue." Eigenvalue greater than 1 should be the default. If not, select it. (You could use any number of factors by selecting "Fixed number of factors" if you had a good reason—theoretical or practical—to extract a particular number of factors which may not correspond to Eigenvalue greater than 1.)
4. The maximum number of iterations for this iterative process is 25. Leave this as the default, unless you have a very good reason to change it.

5. Click on "Continue."

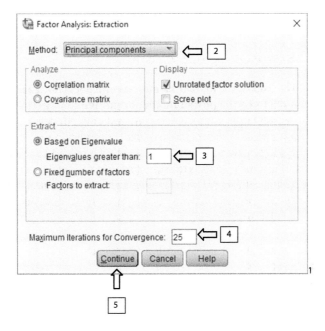

Select "Rotation" button in the dialogue box.
6. Under "Method," select "Varimax"
7. In "Display," "Rotated Solution" should be selected. If not, select it.
8. The maximum number of iterations for this iterative process is 25. Leave this as the default, unless you have a very good reason to change it.
9. Click on "Continue."

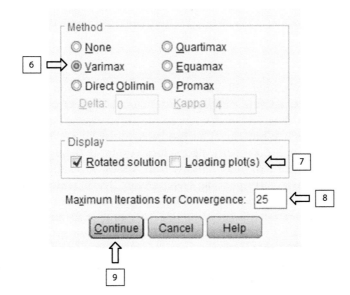

Click on "Options" in the Dialogue box.
10. For "Missing Values," "Excluded cases listwise" should be selected.
11. Under "Coefficient Display Format" the "Absolute value below:" should be set at 0.40.
12. Click on "Continue."

Now you should be back at the main dialogue box and the factor analysis is ready to run. Click on "OK" and the procedure should execute.

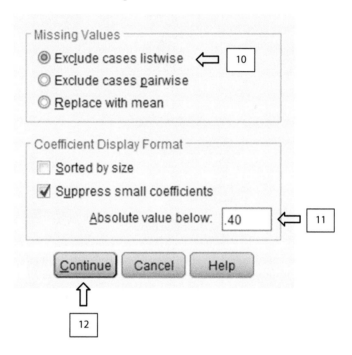

Output from SPSS

A large amount of output will ensue from analysis. The key is to identify and interpret the output relevant for the present analysis and problem.

We begin with Table 6.1 which contains the initial eigenvalues and the variance accounted for. While this table has been edited for brevity (Items 7–28 are missing), there are as many eigenvalues output as there are items (34). The eigenvalues are listed hierarchically from largest to smallest. Notice that Component 1 has a corresponding eigenvalue of 17.939 which accounts for 52.761% of the variance in the data. The magnitude of the next several eigenvalues decreases markedly accounting small amounts of the variance. A close inspection of Table 6.1 reveals that there are four eigenvalues greater than 1 and that accounts for 65.660% of the variance. Additionally, the table contains how much of the variance in this solution is accounted for by each component; e.g., Component 2 accounts for 18.639% of the common variance as determined by

Table 6.1 Total variance explained—Principal component extraction

Component	Initial eigenvalues			Rotation sums of squared loadings		
	Total	Variance (%)	Cumulative %	Total	Variance (%)	Cumulative %
1	17.939	52.761	52.761	6.668	19.613	19.613
2	1.649	4.850	57.612	6.337	18.639	38.252
3	1.507	4.433	62.045	4.940	14.530	52.782
4	1.229	3.615	65.660	4.378	12.877	65.660
5	0.974	2.863	68.523			
6	0.934	2.747	71.270			
29	0.157	0.462	98.523			
30	0.125	0.368	98.891			
31	0.118	0.346	99.238			
32	0.100	0.295	99.532			
33	0.090	0.263	99.796			
34	0.069	0.204	100.000			

the rotation sums of squared loadings. Therefore, four factors are selected in this analysis.

Interpreting the factors

Table 6.2 contains the varimax (orthogonally) rotated factors; convergence occurred in 11 iterations. Based on the factor loadings, theoretical meaning, and coherence, the next task is to name the factors. Factor 1 is *Clinical Performance* because the main large loadings (0.677–0.715) are from items:

4. Within my range of services, I perform technical procedures skillfully
5. I select diagnostic tests appropriately
6. I critically assess diagnostic information
7. I make the correct diagnosis in a timely fashion
8. In general, I select appropriate treatments

Many other relevant items load on this factor (Table 6.2).

Similarly, Factors 2 (*Patient Care*), 3 (*Communication & Humanist*), and 4 (*Professional Development*) are named based on the factor loadings, theoretical meaning, and coherence. There are many "split-loadings" (items load on more than one factor) in Table 6.2. For example, Item #14 (I maintain confidentiality of patients and their families) loads both on Factor 1 (*Clinical Performance*) at 0.600 and Factor 2 (*Patient Care*) at 0.523. This split makes theoretical sense as confidentiality is part of both clinical performance and patient care. The many other split-loading also make theoretical sense since they are part of more than one factor.

Table 6.2 Varimax-rotated component matrix[a]

	Factor			
	1 Clinical performance	2 Patient care	3 Communication & humanist	4 Professional development
1. I communicate effectively with patients			0.839	
2. I communicate effectively with patients' families			0.798	
3. I communicate effectively with other health care professionals			0.558	
4. Within my range of services, I perform technical procedures skillfully	0.677			
5. I select diagnostic tests appropriately	0.692			
6. I critically assess diagnostic information	0.714			
7. I make the correct diagnosis in a timely fashion	0.715			
8. In general, I select appropriate treatments	0.704			
9. I maintain quality medical records		0.446		
10. I handle transfer of care appropriately		0.482		
11. I make it clear who is responsible for continuing care of the patient		0.463	0.576	
12. I communicate information to patients about rationale for treatment	0.569		0.634	
13. I recognize psychosocial aspects of illness		0.488	0.505	
14. I maintain confidentiality of patients and their families	0.600	0.523		

(Continued)

Table 6.2 (*Continued*) Varimax-rotated component matrix[a]

	Factor			
	1 Clinical performance	2 Patient care	3 Communication & humanist	4 Professional development
15. I co-ordinate care effectively for patients with health care professionals	0.438	0.499		
16. I co-ordinate the management of care for patients with complex problems		0.405		0.436
17. I respect the rights of patients	0.553			
18. I collaborate with medical colleagues	0.467	0.549		
19. I am involved with professional development				0.717
20. I accept responsibility for my professional actions	0.627	0.402		
21. I manage health care resources efficiently		0.614		
22. I manage stress effectively		0.647		
23. I participate in a system of call for care for my patients when unavailable	0.467	0.580		
24. I recognize my own surgical limitations	0.567	0.471		
25. I handle requests for consultation in a timely manner		0.747		
26. I advise referring physicians if outside of scope of my practice	0.440	0.629		
27. I assume appropriate responsibility for patients	0.519	0.514		
28. I provide timely information to referring physicians about mutual patients		0.616		

(*Continued*)

Table 6.2 (*Continued*) Varimax-rotated component matrix[a]

	Factor			
	1 Clinical performance	2 Patient care	3 Communication & humanist	4 Professional development
29. I critically evaluate the medical literature to optimize clinical decisions				0.675
30. I facilitate the learning of medical colleagues and co-workers				0.733
31. I contribute to quality improvement programs and practice guidelines				0.763
32. I participate effectively as a member of the health care team		0.429		0.506
33. I exhibit professional and ethical behavior to my physician colleagues		0.428	0.473	
34. I show compassion for patients and their families	0.402		0.618	

Source: Violato et al.[6]
[a] Convergence in 11 iterations.

Construct validity

The results of this factor analysis provide evidence of construct validity of the self-report assessment of surgeon competence.

1. A large number of items (34) are reducible to a few basic underlying elements, latent variables, or factors
2. Based on the eigenvalues >1.0 rule, there are four clear factors
3. The four factors account for two-thirds (65.66%) of the total variance, a good result
4. The magnitude of the variance accounted for by the factors themselves provide theoretical support for construct validity. *Clinical Performance* accounts for the largest proportion of the variance—52.761%, while the other factors are much smaller. This is expected in surgical practice.
5. The factors overall provide theoretical support and are meaningful and cohesive. The split-loadings also provide supporting evidence since it is expected that some items are part of more than one factor. Other items load on only one factor as expected. Item #30 (I facilitate the learning of medical colleagues and co-workers) loads only on factor 4 (*Professional Development*) at 0.733 as theoretically expected.

The overall factor analysis then provides evidence of construct validity of the self-report assessment of surgeon competence.

SUMMARY AND MAIN POINTS

Validity—the extent of which a test measures whatever it is intended to measure—is usually classified into four types: (1) face, (2) content, (3) criterion-related, and (4) construct.

Face and content, which are the most important types on teacher-made tests, are non-empirical forms of validity. Criterion-related and construct validity both require empirical evidence (primarily correlational) for their support. Criterion-related validity involves concurrent and predictive forms both of which require validity coefficients. Construct validity subsumes all forms of validity plus a further determination of the psychological processes involved in the construct. Finally, there are a number of factors, some inherent to the test and some due to the administration which affect validity.

1. Three critical factors characterize educational tests: validity, reliability, and usability.
2. Validity, at its most general level, is the extent to which the test measures whatever it is supposed to measure.
3. There are four main types of validity: (1) face, (2) content, (3) criterion-related, and (4) construct.

4. Face validity has to do with the appearance of the test. It can affect classroom climate and mood, as well as influence testees' motivation.
5. Content validity, usually the most important consideration in classroom tests, is defined as the extent to which the test adequately samples the domain of measurement. This form of validity can be enhanced by the use of a table of specifications.
6. When we are interested in how performance on a test correlates with performance on some other criterion, we are concerned about criterion-related validity. There are two categories of this kind of validity: (1) predictive (How well does a test predict some future performance), and (2) concurrent (How well do two tests intercorrelate concurrently).
7. The determination of a test's criterion-related validity requires empirical evidence in the form of correlation coefficients (r). Interpreted in the context of validity, r is called a validity coefficient. The validity coefficient can be transformed into the coefficient of determination (r^2) which in turn is used to determine the percentage of variance in the criterion that is accounted for by the test.
8. In predictive validity, individual scores on the criterion can be estimated using regression techniques. This strategy allows the prediction of individual scores on some future criterion.
9. Construct validity focuses on the truth or correctness of a construct and the instruments that measure it. A construct is defined as an entity, process, or event which is itself not observed and can be measured only indirectly. Establishing the validity of constructs also requires determination of the validity of relevant instruments. Establishing construct validity is a complex process.
10. One of the most widely researched and readily measureable constructs in education and psychology is intelligence. Systematic measurement and research in the area has been going on nearly 100 years beginning with the work of Alfred Binet in France. Much controversy, however, continues to surround the validity of the construct of intelligence.
11. A number of factors influence the validity of tests. Some of these factors are internal to the tests such as the directions on the test. Others such as noise or distractions during test administration are external to the test. We summarized 12 such factors in this chapter.

REFLECTION AND EXERCISES

Reflection 6.1 Defining criterion-related and construct validity

1. Briefly define criterion-related validity (250 words maximum)
2. Briefly define construct validity (250 words maximum)

Exercises 6.1 Criterion-related validity

1. From the *Exercise 4.2: Clerkship Clinical Scores* (Chapter 4), compute the validity coefficient (i.e., *r*) for Peds as a predictor of the GPA. Treat the GPA as the criterion and Peds as the predictor.
2. Compute the validity coefficient for a composite predictor (sum of Peds, Surgery, IM, MCQ) of GPA. Is there a significant increase in predictive efficiency by combining the results of Peds, Surgery, IM, MCQ rather than just Peds? Explain your answer.
3. Compute the predicted scores on the GPA for students who achieve the following scores on Peds: 12, 17, 8, 10, 14, 16, 9, 15, 7, 11.
4. A researcher developed a new test of clinical reasoning, the *Clinical Reasoning Test* (CRT). This test consists of two subscales, Processing Speed and Quantitative Reasoning, and provides a total score as well. In order to investigate the validity of the CRT, the researcher gave the test to 86 third-year clinical students. He also obtained the students' MCAT Verbal Reasoning scores and their cumulative GPA. These data are summarized below. Enter the data into an SPSS file. Is there any evidence of the criterion-related validity of the CRT? What kinds? Are there any sex differences in the CRT or other variables? Explain your answer.
5. From the CRT dataset is there any evidence for the validity of the GPA as a measure of academic achievement? What kinds of validity? Explain your answer.

Dataset from the Clinical Reasoning Test (CRT), GPA, MCAT verbal reason, CRT processing speed, CRT quantitative reasoning, and total CRT for third-year clinical students

ID	Sex	Total GPA	MCAT verbal reason	CRT processing speed	CRT quantitative reasoning	Total CRT
1	Male	3.75	10	99.55	94.09	193.64
2	Male	3.68	9	95.45	95.45	190.91
3	Female	3.97	7	97.27	97.27	194.55
4	Male	2.84	9	90.00	88.64	178.64
5	Male	3.58	11	105.45	104.55	210.00
6	Female	3.62	9	98.18	97.27	195.45
7	Female	3.89	6	96.36	89.09	185.45
8	Male	3.39	13	88.18	93.64	181.82
9	Male	3.62	11	106.36	103.18	209.55
10	Male	3.12	11	98.18	105.91	204.09
11	Female	3.84	13	105.45	105.00	210.45
12	Female	3.42	9	98.18	97.73	195.91
13	Female	3.81	10	90.45	95.91	186.36

(Continued)

Dataset from the Clinical Reasoning Test (CRT), GPA, MCAT verbal reason, CRT processing speed, CRT quantitative reasoning, and total CRT for third-year clinical students

ID	Sex	Total GPA	MCAT verbal reason	CRT processing speed	CRT quantitative reasoning	Total CRT
14	Male	3.69	9	94.55	100.00	194.55
15	Female	3.72	12	97.73	90.00	187.73
16	Female	3.02	7	60.00	80.43	140.43
17	Male	2.94	8	74.55	81.36	155.91
18	Male	3.01	11	88.18	92.27	180.45
19	Female	3.56	9	93.64	90.45	184.09
20	Male	3.28	7	90.91	78.18	169.09
21	Male	3.47	10	85.91	90.45	176.36
22	Female	3.82	12	93.18	100.91	194.09
23	Female	3.41	6	90.45	93.64	184.09
24	Female	3.28	9	92.27	89.55	181.82
25	Male	3.38	9	103.64	90.91	194.55
26	Female	3.43	13	89.09	99.09	188.18
27	Female	3.05	9	100.00	97.73	197.73
28	Female	3.61	8	80.00	91.82	171.82
29	Female	3.65	8	97.27	90.91	188.18
30	Male	3.30	8	85.91	94.09	180.00
31	Female	3.37	11	89.55	101.82	191.36
32	Female	3.97	8	83.64	87.27	170.91
33	Female	3.60	9	102.73	100.45	203.18
34	Male	3.50	6	100.00	104.09	204.09
35	Male	3.72	9	86.82	82.73	169.55
36	Male	3.58	8	90.91	88.64	179.54
37	Male	3.69	11	80.18	76.36	156.55
38	Male	2.86	10	81.36	83.64	165.00
39	Female	3.52	8	83.18	80.45	163.64
40	Female	3.61	8	84.09	83.18	167.27
41	Male	3.08	10	90.00	96.82	186.82
42	Male	2.92	7	78.18	76.36	154.55
43	Male	4.00	9	79.09	94.09	173.18
44	Female	3.58	12	104.55	105.45	210.00
45	Female	3.49	10	95.00	94.09	189.09
46	Male	3.83	7	85.00	92.27	177.27
47	Female	3.67	9	81.82	85.45	167.27
48	Female	3.71	9	103.64	104.09	207.73
49	Male	3.90	7	75.45	85.45	160.91

(Continued)

Dataset from the Clinical Reasoning Test (CRT), GPA, MCAT verbal reason, CRT processing speed, CRT quantitative reasoning, and total CRT for third-year clinical students

ID	Sex	Total GPA	MCAT verbal reason	CRT processing speed	CRT quantitative reasoning	Total CRT
50	Female	3.31	9	96.36	96.82	193.18
51	Male	3.78	10	99.09	98.18	197.27
52	Female	3.33	10	94.09	101.82	195.91
53	Male	4.00	11	87.73	87.27	175.00
54	Male	3.45	11	100.00	109.55	209.55
55	Male	3.62	9	99.09	95.91	195.00
56	Female	3.14	11	95.00	93.18	188.18
57	Male	3.49	12	96.36	96.82	193.18
58	Male	3.25	10	81.82	77.27	159.09
59	Male	3.65	10	110.00	108.64	218.64
60	Female	3.93	9	101.36	98.18	199.55
61	Female	3.65	11	102.73	100.45	203.18
62	Male	3.75	9	80.91	94.55	175.45
63	Female	3.55	10	91.36	94.09	185.45
64	Male	3.63	9	109.55	98.64	208.18
65	Male	3.75	11	84.55	93.18	177.73
66	Male	3.11	7	90.91	89.55	180.45
67	Female	3.63	8	102.73	88.64	191.36
68	Male	3.38	7	95.91	101.82	197.73
69	Male	3.65	9	107.73	106.36	214.09
70	Male	3.08	11	105.00	100.91	205.91
71	Male	3.89	8	90.45	96.36	186.82
72	Female	3.69	11	95.45	102.27	197.73
73	Male	3.77	8	85.91	81.82	167.73
74	Male	3.01	10	104.09	109.55	213.64
75	Male	2.85	7	95.00	88.18	183.18
76	Female	3.92	10	94.09	96.82	190.91
77	Male	3.38	9	80.91	95.45	176.36
78	Male	2.00	10	81.82	82.73	164.55
79	Male	4.00	9	78.64	90.45	169.09
80	Female	3.55	11	93.18	104.09	197.27
81	Female	3.25	8	79.55	89.09	168.64
82	Male	3.68	10	83.18	88.64	171.82
83	Male	3.72	5	91.82	89.55	181.36
84	Female	3.61	11	85.91	94.55	180.45
85	Male	3.38	10	99.55	98.64	198.18
86	Male	3.96	6	89.55	100.45	190.00

Exercises 6.2 Construct validity

1. Briefly describe the general procedure for determining construct validity
2. Run a factor analysis on these data (Total GPA, MCAT Verbal Reason, CRT Processing Speed, CRT Quantitative Reasoning, Total CRT). Use the Kaiser rule for the number of factors and varimax rotation. Name the factors.
3. From the CRT dataset is there any evidence of the construct validity of the CRT? Discuss.

REFERENCES

1. Dunleavy DM, Kroopnick MH, Dowd KW, Searcy CA, Zhao X. The predictive validity of the MCAT exam in relation to academic performance through medical school: A national cohort study of 2001–2004 matriculants. *Academic Medicine*, 2013, 88, 666–671.
2. Cronbach LJ, Meehl P. Construct validity in psychological tests. *Psychological Bulletin*, 1955, 52, 281–302.
3. MacCorquodale K, Meehl PE. On a distinction between hypothetical constructs and intervening variables. *Psychological Review*, 1948, 55(2), 95–107. pp. 95–96.
4. Cronbach LJ. *Essentials of Psychological Testing* (6th ed). New York: Haper & Row, 1990.
5. Sternberg RJ, Kaufman SB (Eds.). *The Cambridge Handbook of Intelligence*. Cambridge: Cambridge University Press, 2011.
6. Violato C, Lockyer J, Fidler H. Multisource feedback: A method of assessing surgical practice. *British Medical Journal*, 2003, 326, 546–548.

7

Validity III: Advanced methods for validity

ADVANCED ORGANIZERS

- This chapter deals with advanced forms of validity, structural equation modelling (SEM), confirmatory factor analysis (CFA), multi-trait multi-method matrix (MTMM), systematic reviews and meta-analysis, hierarchical linear modelling (HLM), and a unified view of validity.
- Structural equation modeling is a family of statistical techniques used for the systematic analysis of multivariate data to measure underlying hypothetical constructs (latent variables) and their inter-relationships. It is a powerful statistical research tool in health sciences education research and in particular in investigating construct validity. SEM builds upon statistical techniques such as correlation, regression, and analysis of variance (ANOVA).
- CFA is an extension of exploratory factor analysis (EFA) and a subset of SEM. CFA provides a means by which researchers can model a priori latent variables or factors; this method identifies any variability (systematic and error variance) in a measured variable that is not associated with the latent construct. In addition, it can model the relationships between factors. The structural relations are the relations between the factors and are the core of SEM.
- MTMM is a method that involves correlating scores of different attributes (e.g., communication, physical examination) across different methods (e.g., patient questionnaire, direct observation); this gives a more comprehensive assessment of the construct measured than do correlations of traits assessed by single methods. The minimum requirement for using MTMM for a construct validity study is the use of two traits and two methods. The inter-correlations may thus provide evidence of convergent and divergent validity.

- Systematic reviews and meta-analyses are sometimes combined in a single study. A systematic review is a literature review of collecting and critically analyzing several research studies, using and explicitly specifying methods whereby the papers are located, identified, and selected. A meta-analysis is a statistical analysis that combines the results of multiple empirical studies. The purpose of meta-analysis is to use statistical approaches to derive a pooled estimate of the underlying regularities or constructs.
- HLM is an elaborated method of regression that can be used to analyze the variance in dependent variables when the independent variables are hierarchically organized such as students within courses within schools. Because of the shared variance, simple regression is inadequate and more advanced methods such as HLM is more appropriate. It can account for the shared variance in hierarchically structured data such as students within courses, which are within a school, which are within pedagogical approaches (e.g., organ systems vs. PBL curricula).
- Validity is a unitary concept called construct validity. A construct is a hypothetical entity (i.e., theory) that specifies the purpose or intent of the assessment and interpretation of relevant data. Evidence is gathered to support the interpretation of the construct and interpretation of scores. Several complex steps are required for validity evidence.

In the past several decades, several advanced methods for studying validity, particularly construct validity, have been developed and used. These include SEM modeling, CFA, MTMM approaches, HLM, meta-analysis, and a unified approach to validity. These are the subject of this chapter.

STRUCTURAL EQUATION MODELLING

Structural equation modeling (SEM) is a family of statistical techniques used for the systematic analysis of multivariate data to measure underlying hypothetical constructs (latent variables) and their inter-relationships. It is a powerful statistical research tool in health sciences education research and in particular in investigating construct validity. SEM builds upon statistical techniques such as correlation, regression, and ANOVA. It combines the strength of the confirmatory, data reducing ability of factor analysis with multi-regression techniques of path analysis to explicate the direct and indirect relationships between measured and hypothetical (latent) variables. The use of SEM has increased in psychological and educational research in the past few years but has not been widely applied in medical education research.

In this section, the basic tenets of SEM, the development of SEM as an integrated statistical theory, the central features of model creation, estimation, and model fit to data are outlined. The strengths and weaknesses are discussed together with an example of the use of SEM in medical education research. There is a discussion of areas where there are opportunities for the application of SEM for the study of validity.

Basics of SEM

SEM is a confirmatory approach that provides a mechanism to study the hypothesized underlying structural relationships between latent variables or constructs. The development of SEM was based on integration of three key components (1) path analysis, (2) factor analysis, (3) and the development of estimation techniques for model fit.

Path analysis employs models that represent the hypothesized casual connections among a set of variables and estimates the magnitude and significance of each connection. Path analysis moves beyond predicting whether independent variables predict a phenomenon (regression analysis) to examining the interrelationships between the variables.

CFA is an extension of EFA and allows a researcher to model *a priori* how measured variables identify latent constructs. CFA provides a means by which researchers can model latent variables; this method identifies any variability (systematic and error variance) in a measured variable that is not associated with the latent construct.

Integration of these statistical methods, which are referred to as measurement (factor analysis) and structural (path analysis) models, gave rise to the development of SEM described by researchers such as Karl Joreskog and Peter Bentler.[1] The structural relations are the relations between the latent variables and are the core of SEM. The measurement model (Figure 7.1) represents how the latent variables are measured by indicator variables and describes the measurement properties of the indicator variables.[2] The structural model defines the relationships between latent variables (and possibly observed variables that are not indicators

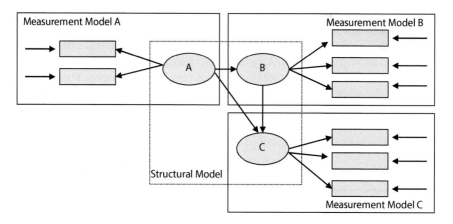

Figure 7.1 A structural equation model depicting three latent variables (*A*, *B*, and *C*) and the relationship between measurement models and a structural model. The path analytic model contains three variables, variable *A* has both a direct and indirect on *C*.

Source: Modified from Nachtigall et al.[3,4]

of latent variables) and allows for the determination of the extent of association between these variables.

COMPARISON OF SEM WITH OTHER STATISTICAL METHODS

SEM is a confirmatory approach which allows for the analyses of hypothesized inter-relationships between latent constructs. Use of SEM requires statistical tools which are based upon regression, ANOVA, and correlation. While regression and ANOVAs define the degree of significance between variables, it is difficult for researchers to model underlying constructs that independent variables might load upon.

SEM is built upon the multivariate techniques of factor and path analysis. While these methods are quite strong independently, SEM subsumes and allows for a higher level of abstraction, through the development of structural models of hypothesized constructs. Path analysis analyzes structural models between observed variables and depicts direct and indirect causal effects based upon hypotheses of causal effects. However, each variable is a single indicator and there is the assumption that the variables are measured without error. The strength of SEM over path analysis is that SEM allows for a structural model to be created between latent variables or a combination of measured and latent variables and the path coefficients in a SEM between latent factors are corrected for measurement error (observed variables have measurement errors), because the hypothetical constructs are measured by multiple indicators where measurement error is removed.

Factor analysis is a data reducing technique for explaining correlations among variables in terms of factors that are unobservable and superordinate to the measured variables. As we have seen, there are two major applications of factor analysis: exploratory (EFA) and confirmatory (CFA). EFA does not require a priori hypotheses regarding the number of underlying factors or the relationships between measured variables and factors. Because of its atheoretical nature, it is not typically used as an SEM procedure. CFA, on the other hand, requires a priori hypotheses and a proposed model (like SEM) about the number of factors and the nature of the relationships between measured and hypothetical constructs. Unlike SEM, CFA cannot model causality or the temporal relationships between variables. SEM subsumes CFA, in that CFA is the measurement model of a SEM, outlining the relationships between indicators and underlying hypothetical constructs.

SEM: AN INTEGRATED RESEARCH METHOD

SEM is a flexible and powerful statistical tool for the development, refinement, and validation of theories and hypothesized relationships between variables. SEM requires fundamental understanding of statistical methods and concepts. It is considered to be primarily confirmatory, in that models are specified a priori based upon theory and previous exploratory work. Nonetheless, it can also be exploratory in the sense that it provides a mechanism whereby competing models can be tested or models can be re-specified (i.e., re-drawn to improve fit).

The relationships among the variables should be justifiable, based on theory or based on previous research findings. A researcher must specify a model, or competing models, a priori, before any analysis is performed. Analysis and interpretation of a SEM, especially the underlying hypothetical constructs represented as the latent variables, depends on how those variables were measured. Therefore, SEM not only subsumes many statistical concepts (correlation, ANOVA, MR) it requires that the researcher understand measurement theory, meaning that the psychometric properties (reliability and validity) for each tool used to measure an underlying construct have to be elucidated. It is important to understand that SEM tests the **whole** model, for goodness of fit, and provides information as to the relevance of various measurement components as well as relationships between variables that can be reviewed based upon the theory that was used to create the model.

The development of a model occurs systematically. Bollen and Long[4] have outlined five steps that characterize most applications of SEM: (1) model specification, (2) identification, (3) estimation, (4) testing fit, and (5) re-specification. These operational steps are necessary in order to increase the likelihood that the observed data will fit the predicted model.

First, a research problem is outlined and a model is specified. This problem and subsequent questions influence and are influenced by the underlying theory that has surrounded the work in that area. The theory underlying the model should be supported by the presence of preliminary empirical evidence gathered by reliable and valid psychometric tools and analyzed by the appropriate univariate and multivariate techniques. SEM relies upon a priori hypotheses, and a researcher has to be able to define the theoretical underpinnings and how the research question was developed. The population under study also has an impact on the development of theory and research question(s) that are of interest.

A testable model, or competing testable models, is then developed based upon the research question and theory. The model is then specified, where the relationships between the variables must be explained and the measurement and the structural models are explicitly defined. Here the two component parts—the measurement model and the structural model—need to be explicated.

Second, the model is reviewed for identification. This determines whether it is possible to find unique values for the parameters of the specified model. In the measurement model, the data should contain multiple indicators of each latent variable (or at least two indicators). One indicator alone of a hypothesized latent construct would result in a biased measurement.[2,5] While some suggest that at least three indicators should be used to account for as much of the variance as possible in the latent variable, practically, most SEM models use two indicators at a minimum. The indicators must be selected carefully, and the reliability and validity of the psychometric tools used for the measured variables should be well described. Identification determines if there are more variables measured than parameters to be estimated.

For models to be properly empirically assessed, they should be identified or overidentified, meaning that the information in the data (which are the known values: variances and covariances) is equal to or exceeds the information being estimated (unknown values: parameter estimations, measurement error, etc.).

If the unknowns exceed the knowns, then the model is underidentified. For overidentification of a model, there should be two or more observed variables for a latent factor.[6]

Third, the model is estimated. Estimation techniques were developed to ascertain how a model fits the observed data based upon the extent to which the model implied covariance matrix is equivalent to the data derived covariance matrix. The most common methods for estimation are maximum likelihood (ML), generalized least squares (GLS), and asymptotic distribution-free (ADF). These estimation procedures are iterative, meaning that the calculations performed are iterative until the best parameter estimation is obtained.

ML is the default estimation technique in most SEM software and is the most widely used. ML assumes that variables are multivariate normal (i.e., distribution of the variables is multivariate normal) and require large sample sizes. ML estimates parameters which maximize the likelihood (the probability) that the predicted model fits the observed model based upon the covariance matrix. The covariance, defined as $cov_{xy} = r_{xy}SD_xSD_y$ (Pearson product–moment correlation between variables X and Y multiplied the standard deviation (SD) for X and Y), is the statistic primarily used in SEM. The covariance matrix used in SEM is meant to understand patterns of correlation among a set of variables and to explain as much of their variance as possible with the model specified by the researcher.

GLS is based upon the same assumptions as ML and used under the same conditions (it performs less well with smaller sample sizes, therefore, ML is recommended). GLS reduces the sum of the squared deviations (or variances) between the predicted model and observed model and is more popular in regression analyses.

Asymptotically distribution free (ADF) estimation techniques (such as arbitrary distribution least squares [ALS]) may be used if some measured variables are dichotomous and others are continuous and therefore multivariate normality cannot be assumed or if the distributions of the continuous variables are nonnormal. These estimation techniques are not as readily used.

The SEM study begins by collecting a sample from the population that the researcher wishes to generalize. Descriptive and univariate analyses are performed to determine whether the data meets the assumptions for SEM. The assumptions for SEM are similar to most statistical methods dealing with parametric data, in that SEM assumes multivariate normality, independence of observations (assumption of local statistical independence), and homoscedasticity (uniform variance across measured variables).

Fourth, the model fit is estimated. Generally, the estimation is based on testing the null hypothesis expressed as

$$\Sigma = \Sigma(\theta) \tag{7.1}$$

where
Σ is the population covariance matrix of the observed variables
$\Sigma(\theta)$ is the covariance matrix implied by the specific model
θ is a vector containing the free parameters of the model

A test statistic allows us to test the null hypothesis that the specified model leads to a reproduction of the population covariance matrix of the observed variables.

To assess goodness-of-fit of the observed data to the model, various fit indices have been developed. The following section describes the most common fit indices reported and the parameters associated with their use. There is no fixed rule as to which one to use or which combination to use, and there is still little agreement on what represents the best fit.[2]

Fit criteria indicate the extent to which the model fits the data. Only the χ^2 provides a significance test, while other measures are descriptive and are broken down into three categories: measures of overall model fit, measures based upon model comparisons, and measures of model parsimony.[2]

The χ^2 statistic as used in SEM assesses whether the calculated covariance matrix is equal to the model implied covariance matrix. It tests the null hypothesis that the differences between the two are zero. Therefore, a nonsignificant χ^2 value (p-value > 0.05) with associated degrees of freedom means that the null hypothesis is accepted and the model is considered to fit the data. In other words, we do not want a significant difference between the sample covariance matrix and the model implied covariance matrix.

There are problems with the χ^2 statistic in SEM. Theoretically, it has no upperbound and therefore the values are not interpretable in a standardized way. It is also sensitive to sample size, as sample size increases, so does the χ^2 value which means that the model may be rejected, as sample size decreases so does χ^2 value which may provide non-significant results even though there may be considerable difference between the sample and model implied covariance. Using χ^2 can lead to an inflated Type I error rate for model rejection. To reduce the sensitivity of the χ^2, some have suggested that the χ^2 be divided by the degrees of freedom (χ^2/df), and that the ratio be less than three in order for a good fit. Unfortunately, this still does not address the problem of sample size dependency.

Descriptive goodness of fit measures are used in conjunction with the χ^2 values to determine overall fit of the empirical data to the model. Descriptive measures of overall model fit measure the extent to which an SEM corresponds to the empirical data, based on the difference between the sample covariance matrix and the model-implied covariance matrix (measure of the average of the residual variances and co-variances between the sample matrix and the model implied matrix). Descriptive measures based on model comparisons assess the fit of a model compared to the fit of a baseline model. Baseline models are either an independence model where it is assumed that the observed variables are measured without error or a null model where all parameters are fixed to zero. Descriptive measures of model parsimony are used primarily when competing models are being compared. Typically, values of these measures range from zero (no fit) to one (perfect fit), while some provide a badness of fit with parameters of zero to one. Common fit indices include root mean square error of approximation (RMSEA), standardized root mean square residual (SRMR), goodness of fit index (GFI), Akaike Information criterion (AIC), the comparative fit index (CFI), and a number of others. The most reported index in the literature is the CFI which compares a predicted model with a baseline model (Table 7.1).

Table 7.1 A comparison of fit of three models of the development of medical expertise

Model	Goodness of fit indices					
	Goodness of fit index	Comparative fit index—CFI	Standardized root mean squared residual—SRMR	Root mean squared error of approximation—RMSEA	Chi square (χ^2)	Delta chi square (χ^2_D)
Knowledge Encapsulation (full model with no constraints on the covariance among BSA, CC and AFM)	0.973	0.968	0.038	0.063	88.11 (df = 29) [i]	—
Independent Influence (reduced model: estimate the covariance between BSA and CC to 0)	0.886	0.811	0.163	0.191	443.91 (df = 29)	355.80 ($df_D = 1$)
Distinct Domain (reduced model: estimate the covariance between BSA, AFM, and CC to 0)	0.856	0.779	0.225	0.170	514.93 (df = 29)	462.82 ($df_D = 3$)

AFM, aptitude for medicine; BSA, basic science achievement; CC, clinical competency.

Is there a consensus as to what constitutes an adequate fit? Some have suggested that a model fit is dependent upon more than the fit indices. The recommendation is that a model should be identified (parameters = observations), the iterative estimation procedure converges using ML or another technique, the parameter estimates for the model are within the range of permissible values, standard errors of the parameter estimates have a reasonable size, and the residual matrix (observed covariances—predicted covariances) should have residuals that are approximately zero.[7] Furthermore, as mentioned above, the χ^2 test for fit should not solely be used to assess goodness of fit. Usually several indices are provided which represent the different classes of fit criteria. It is suggested that χ^2 value and its p-value, χ^2/df, RMSEA, and its confidence interval (CI), SRMR, NNFI, and CFI. However, in practicality, usually the χ^2 value, CFI, SRMR, and RMSEA are presented as indicators of goodness of fit. For model comparisons, the χ^2 difference test and AIC should be provided. The literature strongly suggests that sample sizes of ≤250 should be treated with caution, the recommended procedure is to report multiple fit indices such as the CFI (≥0.95) in combination with SRMR (≤0.08) and RMSEA (≤0.06) as this combination tends not to reject models under non-robust conditions.[8]

Finally, as Bentler noted, model selection should be guided by the principles of parsimony, if several models fit the data, the simplest should be selected.[9] A model can only be rejected, it can never be proven to be valid. Models should not be re-specified based upon statistical criteria, they should be re-specified based upon theoretical criteria. If the fit is acceptable, the proposed relationships in the measurement model between the latent and the observed variables and the structural models between the latent variables is supported by the data.

The data collected are empirically assessed through estimation methods which attempt to fit the data to the hypothesized models; fit indices are calculated to assess the goodness of fit. Fit indices such as the CFI should be >.90. If the fit is poorer than this, then the model can be re-specified.

Fifth, the model may be re-specified. The first step is to re-specify the measurement model, which is then analyzed to assess fit. If the fit is acceptable, the SEM model can then be analyzed. The model is then assessed and re-specified if need be based upon statistical output and theoretical relevance. Finally, conclusions can be drawn from analyses and comparison against theory.

SAMPLE SIZE AND MODEL FIT

Sample size is important for goodness of fit as the estimation procedures used to calculate the model parameters require a sample size large enough to obtain meaningful parameter estimates.[10] Some have suggested that sample size needs to be more than 25 times the number of parameters with a minimum subject: parameter ratio of 10:1, the lower bound of total sample size should be approximately 100–200.[11] Bentler proposed that when sample sizes are small, multiple competing models must be tested, if some of the models are rejected using the fit indices, then the sample size is probably large enough because there is enough power to reject competing models.

STRENGTHS AND WEAKNESSES OF SEM

SEM is a theory strong approach. It supersedes other multivariate analyses because it can model the relationships between "error-free" latent variables by partialing out measurement error from multiple, "imperfectly reliable" indicators. Furthermore, SEM can be used for both cross-sectional and longitudinal studies.

A good fit does not imply a strong effect on the dependent variable. Even a high proportion of explained variance is no proof of causality; the best we can expect from SEM is evidence against a poor model but never proof of a good one. Well-designed, theory-strong longitudinal studies, however, can provide powerful evidence for the effect of one variable on another.

SEM does have a number of weaknesses. SEM is dependent upon a well-developed theory. If SEM is used for primarily exploratory purposes, then model fit may be more a function of statistical fit rather than theoretical fit. Furthermore, if the model is misspecified due to weak theory, unclear hypotheses or poor study design, the casual relationships between the variables will be misinterpreted.[11]

SEM, like other analytic procedures, cannot compensate for unreliable assessment (see Chapters 8 and 9). If measuring instruments with poor reliability are employed, the SEM will be laden with error. The use of only one measure to identify a latent variable is also a weakness, in that it reduces the amount of variability that can be identified in the latent variable thus producing a biased measurement. SEM cannot compensate for instruments with poor reliability and validity, poorly specified theoretical models, inadequate sampling, or misinterpretation of the fit indices.

WHERE SEM WOULD BE USEFUL IN MEDICAL EDUCATION RESEARCH

Although identified as a potentially powerful research tool, SEM has not been used much in health sciences education research. Some interesting SEM work has been done in medical education research such as CFA and path analyses. SEM has been used to test competing hypothetical models of how basic science knowledge and clinical knowledge are used in diagnostic reasoning to assess medical expertise,[12] to assess the predictive validity of various standard and non-standard selection criteria on medical school performance,[13] to assess students' motivation for choosing a specialization,[14] to assess a causal model of the influence of educational interventions and motivation in problem-based learning,[6] to assess the factor structure of a psychometric tool measuring readiness to engage self-directed learning, and to assess the stability of communication skills in medical students as measured in objective-structured clinical examinations (OSCEs) measured at different times,[15] but none of these approaches have employed the full SEM model of latent variable path analysis.

Researchers have created a LVPA assessing the predictive validity of the MCAT and UGPA on standardized outcome measures (USMLE Steps 1–3 examinations) as mediated through latent variables such as "undergraduate achievement," "aptitude for medicine," and "performance in medicine."[12]

Potential applications of SEM in medical education research could include, longitudinal measurement of student learning, verifying predictive power of selection process, predictive validity studies using cognitive and non-cognitive factors as predictors for student success, testing aspects of clinical performance, and test scale development.

LATENT VARIABLE PATH ANALYSIS

The following LVPA was performed as a confirmatory method to evaluate the findings of previous studies that have used correlation-based methods (e.g., Pearson's r, multiple regression) to test the predictive validity of the MCAT and other cognitive, achievement, and demographic variables on the performance of medical students on licensure examinations.

A total of 548 physicians (292 men—53.3%; 256 women—46.7%), who had graduated from Wake Forest School of Medicine from 2009 to 2014, participated. There were three types of data: (1) Admissions data that consists of undergraduate (GPA, MCAT) subtest scores (physical sciences, biological sciences, and verbal reasoning), (2) Course performance data (Year 1, Year 2, and Year 3), and (3) Performance on the NBME exams (i.e., Step 1, Step 2 CK, and Step 3).[12]

The data were used to test the fit of a hypothesized model using latent variable path analysis. In this model, the development of elaborate knowledge networks evolves through a process of biomedical knowledge acquisition, practical clinical experience, and an integration or encapsulation of both theoretical and experiential knowledge. The encapsulation process of basic science knowledge begins as soon as medical students are introduced to real patients through clinical encounters or presentations.[16]

Figure 7.2 shows the final three-latent variable model with parameter estimates and goodness-of-fit indices, GFI, CFI, SRMR, and RMSEA. In this ML estimation, the theoretical structure of the model is supported with the significant correlation ($r = 0.38$, $p < 0.01$) between the *Aptitude for Medical School* and *Basic Science Knowledge* latent variables. There are influences from both *Aptitude for Medical School* and *Basic Science Knowledge* latent variables to *Clinical Competency* with path coefficients at 0.76 ($p < 0.01$) and 0.45 ($p < 0.01$) respectively. In this model, the combination rules of cutoff score values are achieved for the GFI = 0.973, CFI at 0.968 and meet the criteria set for robustness and non-robustness conditions and values of SRMR at 0.04 and RMSEA at 0.06. This result represents and supports the encapsulation theory model. The findings support a theory where basic sciences and medical aptitude are direct, correlated influences on clinical competency that encapsulates basic knowledge.

The results support the integration of basic science with clinical knowledge and the construction of elaborate knowledge networks or illness scripts. This suggests that early exposure to patients for medical students is beneficial. Additionally, basic science knowledge could be revisited, in the relevant clinical

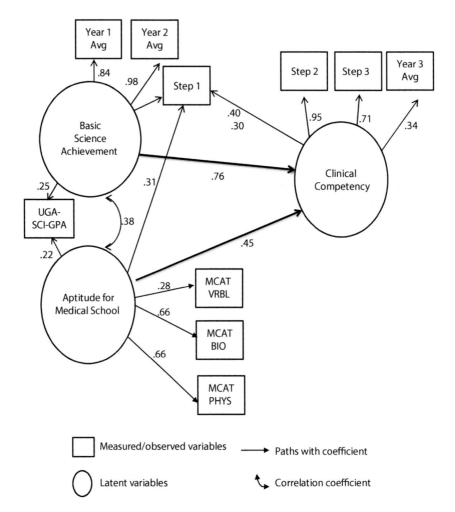

Figure 7.2 Maximum likelihood estimation of knowledge encapsulation latent variable path model (GFI = 0.973, RMSEA = 0.063; SRMR = 0.038; Bentler CFI = 0.968; n = 548).

context, during the whole of medical school, as an iterative process. Such pedagogy may facilitate the efficiency of knowledge encapsulation.

Summary for SEM

SEM is an integrated statistical method that allows researchers to test proposed theories through quantifiable measures. Models for SEM are composed of two basic parts, the measurement model and the structural model, which refers to the causal relationships between the latent variables. A good fit of the structural and measurement models to the data provides evidence that the hypothesized relationships in the model are consistent with the relationships in the observed data.

The research method underpinning SEM makes it a theory-strong approach. SEM is a useful statistical tool for medical education for longitudinal measurement of student learning, verifying the predictive power of selection process, predictive validity studies using cognitive and non-cognitive factors as predictors for student success, testing aspects of clinical performance, and test-scale development. However, it requires a strong conceptual understanding of the theory relevant to the research question which in turn influences the selection of the measured variables and the hypothesized causal relationships between the measured and latent variables.

MULTI-TRAIT MULTI-METHOD MATRIX

When we wish to assess a construct, it should be measured repeatedly and by different methods for evidence of validity. Additionally, it should be contrasted with other constructs that are independent of it. This is a process of "triangulation." The instruments designed to measure constructs have observable variables that are hypothetically linked to each other through the underlying phenomena or latent traits. The amount of empirical evidence required for construct validity is difficult to estimate as most of these attributes are complex and multifaceted. According to Kane,[9] this process of validation should be an attempt to clarify the interrelationships, interpretation, and use of scores on assessment instruments measuring observable attributes that are theoretical indicators of the construct.

Clinical competence is a complex, multi-faceted construct that requires a multi-faceted approach to its study. A variety of approaches including the following instruments have been implemented during and after supervised training for assessing competence: in-training evaluation reports (ITERs), clinical evaluation exercise (CEX and mini-CEX), and multisource feedback employing the Physician Achievement Review (PAR) instruments.

Most approaches to construct validity of high-stakes assessment instruments have not been researched extensively. The focus has been on reliability which is a necessary but not sufficient condition for validity. Some researchers that have attempted to investigate construct validity have employed methods like correlation, regression, and between group differences analyses (e.g., analysis of variance—ANOVA) of scores of candidates as empirical evidence for construct validity. Few have employed robust methods for investigating construct validity such as the MTMM approach introduced by Campbell and Fiske.[17] The MTMM method involves correlating scores of different attributes (e.g., communication, physical examination, clinical reasoning) across different methods (e.g., patient questionnaire, direct observation, test scores); this gives a more comprehensive assessment of the construct measured than do correlations of traits assessed by single methods. The minimum requirement for using MTMM for a construct validity study is the use of two traits and two methods. The inter-correlations may thus provide evidence of convergent and divergent validity.

In an ideal assessment, the variation in scores should be a reflection of the individual differences of the competence of the examinees and not related to the assessment method used (i.e., method specificity). Frequently, the method and/or the instruments employed (e.g., objective structured clinical exams, or OSCE, standardized patients, or SPs, multiple-choice questions, or MCQs, etc.) introduce error of measurement which may lead to variance in the scores of the candidates. The same trait measured with different instruments should yield similar scores for the examinees. If not, it is likely that the approaches used for assessing the trait on two methods contribute method variance. Conversely, different traits assessed by the same method should have low correlations. If not (the correlations are high), this is likely due to the method employed because of method specificity (e.g., MCQ examinations). MTMM is based on interpreting correlations of the same trait across different methods and correlations of different traits across the same methods. High correlations of the same trait assessed by different methods provide evidence of *convergent validity*, while low correlations of different traits assessed by the same methods provide evidence of *divergent validity*. The MTMM design isolates the correlations between traits and methods and variances attributable to them.

Forsythe, McGaghie, and Friedman used MTMM to assess construct validity of medical competence measures.[5] They assessed three attributes: cognitive abilities, interpersonal skills, and professional qualities in 166 residents from family medicine, internal medicine, and pediatrics. They used scores of the National Board of Medical Examiners (NBME) examination (for cognitive abilities), the California Psychological Inventory (CPI) (to measure interpersonal skills and professional qualities), and Resident Evaluation Forms (REF) (for peer and supervisor ratings). Their MTMM analysis provided convergent and divergent validity evidence for two traits (cognitive abilities and interpersonal skills) but not all three.

Hull et al.[10] interpreted the scores on assessment instruments to adduce evidence for construct validity of clinical competence employing three methods: (1) clinical evaluation form (CEF), (2) OSCE, and (3) NBME exam results. The evidence of constructs was collected for three traits: knowledge, clinical skills, and personal characteristics. In their study, the CEF had evidence for all the three traits, the NBME exams had evidence for one trait and the OSCE had evidence for two traits. According to Campbell and Fiske, their study met the minimal criteria for evidence of convergent and divergent validity. The method effect, however, accounted for a substantial amount of variance and the reliability of instruments was uneven.

The results of both the Forsythe et al. and Hull et al. studies underscore the importance of defining and investigating the validity of clinical competence with explicit details on the observable behaviors representing competence in a MTMM design. A construct as complex and multifaceted as competence requires further investigation employing MTMM approaches.

Baig et al.[18] improved and extended this prior work employing the MTMM to further investigate the construct of clinical competence. Three traits—doctor–patient relationship, clinical competence, and communication skills—were assessed with OSCE, in-training evaluation reports, and clinical assessments. These traits were inter-correlated in a MTMM. The results are presented in Figure 7.3.

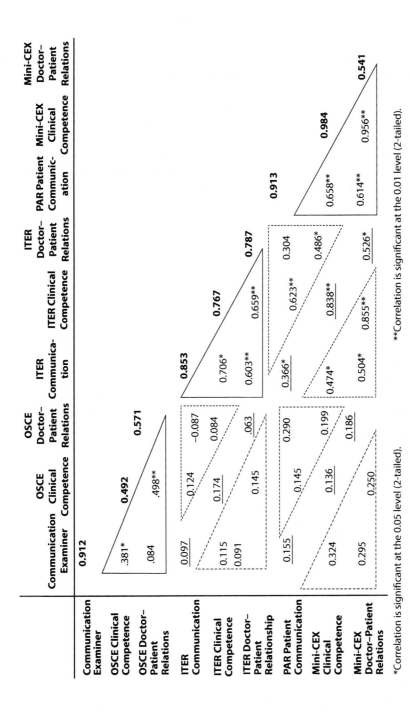

Figure 7.3 Multitrait multimethod matrix with four traits and three methods.

The reliability of assessments ranged from moderate to high. (Cronbach's alpha: 0.58–0.98; $Ep^2 = 0.79$). There is evidence for both convergent and divergent validity for clinical competence, followed by doctor–patient relationships and communications (validity coefficients = 0.12–0.85). The correlations between the same methods but different traits indicate that there is substantial method specificity in the assessment accounting for nearly one-quarter of the variance (23.7%).

The MTMM was constructed with the use of the Campbell and Fiske technique (Figure 7.3). In the matrix, the scores of different attributes across different methods are correlated and the correlation coefficient r across different methods for same trait is referred to as the validity coefficient (underlined in Figure 7.3). The reliability of the traits on each of the methods is also considered in the analysis of MTMM and is bolded in the matrix. The triangles with dashed lines are the heterotrait–heteromethod triangles, and the ones with solid lines are the heterotrait–monomethod triangles. The column and row headings represent the method and the trait used for the matrix from that instrument.

The reliabilities of the assessment instruments used for building the MTMM matrix were in the adequate to good range and are bolded in Figure 7.3. The several instruments produced the following reliabilities for the overall scores and for different traits wherever applicable: (1) MCQs Cronbach's $\alpha = 0.86$, (2) OSCEs $Ep^2 = 0.79$ for assessors, (3) ITERs Cronbach's α ranged from 0.34 to 0.85, (4) mini-CEX Cronbach's α ranged from 0.54 to 0.98, and (5) PAR Cronbach's α ranged from 0.86 to 0.96.

The correlations between all three constructs across all four methods are shown in the MTMM. Convergent validity is indicated by the underlined correlations in the diagonal. There is evidence of convergent validity for clinical competence, and doctor–patient relationship as assessed by the ITER, mini-CEX, and PAR but not with OSCEs. In the MTMM matrix for the communication trait, there is little convergence between the traits measured through OSCE, ITERs, and the PAR instruments. The large correlations enclosed in the solid-lined triangles suggest that there is substantial method specificity in the assessment. Conversely, the correlations enclosed in the dashed-lined triangles provide evidence of divergent validity of traits, especially as assessed by the ITERs, mini-CEX, and PAR four out of six (67%) of the correlations meet the Campbell and Fiske[17] criteria of discriminant validity. Overall, five out of six (83.3%) correlations meet the Campbell and Fiske criteria, thus providing evidence of discriminant validity. Clinical competence is the trait for which there is the most evidence for both convergent and divergent validity, followed by doctor–patient relationships and communications. There is evidence for the construct validity of all three traits across three methods.

This study further highlights the need for estimating the evidence of construct validity for instruments assessing competence in physicians, more specifically, clinical competence. The MTMM is a useful method; it can provide evidence for both the construct validity and the reliability of traits. MTMM can form a rigorous standard for validity evidence of complex traits.

SYSTEMATIC REVIEWS AND META-ANALYSES

A meta-analysis is a statistical analysis that combines the results of multiple empirical studies, while a systematic review is a systematic literature review of collecting and critically analyzing several research studies, using and explicitly specifying methods whereby the papers are located, identified, and selected. Systematic reviews and meta-analyses are sometimes combined in a single study. They are designed to provide a comprehensive and complete selection of current research relevant to a question or hypothesis.

The term "meta-analysis" was introduced by statistician and educational researcher, Gene Glass in 1976.[19] The results of multiple empirical studies are combined in a meta-analysis. The underlying assumptions behind meta-analyses are that there are common empirical commonalities of all conceptually similar studies. The results of all these studies are not identical because they contain variation in each study. The purpose of meta-analysis is to use statistical approaches to derive a pooled estimate of the underlying regularities or constructs. The research yields a weighted average from the results of the individual studies. The meta-analysis results in an estimate of the regularity, correlation, or effect size. Results from different studies can be contrasted and patterns identified among study results, sources of disagreement among those results or other relevant patterns that are discovered in the context of multiple studies.

Meta-analyses are frequently components of a systematic review. A meta-analysis, for example, may be conducted on several empirical studies of the predictive validity of an instrument. The objective is to better understand the correlation or regression equation of the predictor variables and the criterion. The results of several experiments on educational interventions are another example where meta-analysis may be used. Meta-analysis refers to statistical methods of combining empirical evidence such as correlation coefficients or effect sizes. Other aspects of research synthesis employing qualitative studies, for instance, are in the category of systematic reviews.

Direct observations have been widely accepted as one of the best ways to evaluate clinical competence. The mini-clinical evaluation exercise (mini-CEX) has been proposed to assess clinical competencies (e.g., medical interview, physical examination, professionalism, and communications) in the completion of a patient history within a medical training context. The mini-CEX for the assessment of medical students' and residents' clinical skill performance across a number of domains is an important advance in the use and recognition of the direct observation method of clinical evaluation. Accordingly, the mini-CEX has been adopted and used extensively as an instrument for the assessment of clinical skill performance in medical education programs in Canada, the United States, Europe, and in other countries. To date, the mini-CEX has proved to be a useful in-training assessment measure with some evidence of construct- and criterion-related validity. Alansari, Ali, and Donnon conducted a systematic review and meta-analysis of the validity evidence of the min-CEX as a direct observation measure of clinical competence.[20]

The systematic review

In this study, they searched several medical, health, and psychological databases. These included MEDLINE, PsychINFO, EMBASE, and CINAHL. To be included, a primary study had to meet the following criteria: (1) it used the original seven-item version of the mini-CEX, (2) it reported empirical findings on the use of the mini-CEX related to either medical students' or residents' clinical performance, (3) it employed psychometrically sound criterion measures (e.g., standardized instruments, summative in-training evaluations, objectively scored observational ratings), and (4) it was published in a refereed, peer-reviewed journal. The purpose for restricting the search of the articles to refereed journals was to enhance the inclusion of studies that are of high quality.

Studies were excluded if (1) the focus of the article was restricted to a generalizability analysis or investigation of the internal structure of the mini-CEX, (2) the review on the use of the mini-CEX did not provide any new empirical data, and (3) the analysis focused on differences related to rater stringency without reporting on actual student performance outcomes. The exclusion of studies in systematic review is nearly as important as the inclusion of the studies.

The meta-analysis

Depending on the empirical data reported in each of the primary studies, the authors used either the Pearson product–moment correlation coefficient (r) or mean differences (Cohen's d) as the effect size measures. They selected mini-CEX items or total mean score on the mini-CEX measures as the variables and either contrasted between groups (e.g., postgraduate or in-training year) or compared mini-CEX scores with other clinical skill measures (e.g., in-training evaluation report). A random-effects model in combining the unweighted and weighted effect sizes was used. Although a fixed effect model assumes that the summary effect size differences are the same from study to study (e.g., the consistent use of the mini-CEX instrument), the random-effects model calculation reflects a more conservative estimate of the between-study variance.

The mini-CEX has evidence of construct validity when used with residents across the years of a residency program. The effect size differences between performance levels within a peer group (superior/honors, marginal/high pass, poor/pass) ranged from $d = 0.43$ in one study on the total mean score of the mini-CEX up to $d = 1.86$ on the physical examination skills item. The rating differences of medical students on the mini-CEX between personnel (either residents or faculty members) showed an effect size differences that ranged from $d = 0.23$ on the clinical judgment item to $d = 0.50$ on the counseling skills item. The mini-CEX shows evidence of criterion-related validity when compared with other clinical skill achievement (e.g., certifying oral and written examinations) or performance (e.g., in-training evaluation reports, inpatient or outpatient write-ups) measures. There were large correlation coefficients with combined effect sizes ranging from $r = 0.26$ on the mean score of the mini-CEX to $r = 0.64$ on the overall clinical competence item.

The construct and criterion validity of the mini-CEX was supported by effect size differences based on measures between trainees' achievement and clinical skills performance, indicating that it is an important instrument for the direct observation of trainees' clinical performance. This meta-analysis therefore provides evidence of construct validity for the mini-CEX as a direct observational measure of clinical competencies.

Meta-analysis and forest plots

A common and effective method of representing the results of a meta-analysis is a forest plot (Figure 7.4). This graph shows the spread of results for each study. Horizontal lines indicate the results of a single study showing the length of the line representing the 95% confidence interval. The vertical line in the middle is where the effect size is zero. A confidence interval that crosses the line shows that the result is not statistically significant. The diamond at the bottom is the mean of the effect size.

Yammine and Violato[21] conducted a meta-analysis of the effectiveness of three-dimensional representational technology (3DVT) in teaching and learning anatomy compared to other methods: dissection, prosection, surface anatomy, textbooks, lectures, and two-dimensional (2D) digital images. Thirty-six studies met inclusion criteria including 28 (78%) randomized studies. The primary outcomes were *factual and spatial anatomy* knowledge acquisition. Secondary outcomes were *user satisfaction and learners' perception of the effectiveness* of the learning tool. Moderator variables were familiarity with computers/video games, prior anatomy knowledge, gender, age, and spatial abilities.

The meta-analysis was based on 2,226 participants including 2,128 from studies with comparison groups. Both random- and fixed-effects effect sizes were calculated. The analyses of the weighted mean difference effect sizes (d) are summarized in Figure 7.4 together with the forest plots for the spatial outcome. A visual inspection of Figure 7.4 shows that the studies are heterogeneous and, therefore, required a random effects weighted size calculation. This spatial knowledge $d = 0.50$ favoring 3DVT over all other traditional methods.

Other findings indicated superior results ($d = 0.30$) for factual knowledge, significant increase in user satisfaction ($d = 0.28$), and in learners' perception of the effectiveness of the learning tool ($d = 0.28$). There were generally no systematic significant effects of the moderator variables.

The major conclusions from this study is that given that anatomy teaching and learning in the modern medical school is approaching a crisis, 3DVT may be a potential solution to the problem of inadequate anatomy pedagogy.

HIERARCHICAL LINEAR MODELLING

HLM is an elaborated method of regression that can be used to analyze the variance in dependent variables when the independent variables are hierarchically organized. Medical students in a problem-based learning (PBL) group share variance based on their common instructor and common group. To assess the

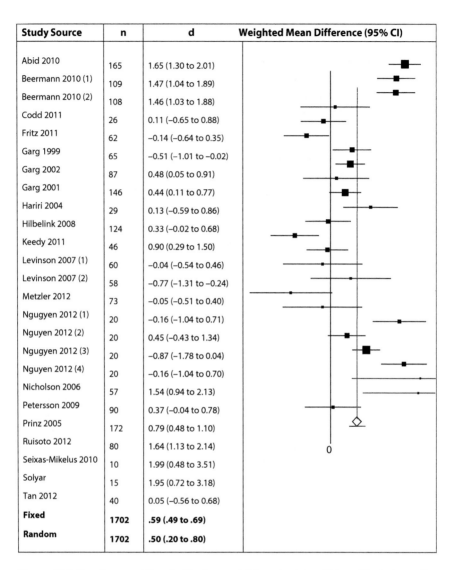

Study Source	n	d	Weighted Mean Difference (95% CI)
Abid 2010	165	1.65 (1.30 to 2.01)	
Beermann 2010 (1)	109	1.47 (1.04 to 1.89)	
Beermann 2010 (2)	108	1.46 (1.03 to 1.88)	
Codd 2011	26	0.11 (−0.65 to 0.88)	
Fritz 2011	62	−0.14 (−0.64 to 0.35)	
Garg 1999	65	−0.51 (−1.01 to −0.02)	
Garg 2002	87	0.48 (0.05 to 0.91)	
Garg 2001	146	0.44 (0.11 to 0.77)	
Hariri 2004	29	0.13 (−0.59 to 0.86)	
Hilbelink 2008	124	0.33 (−0.02 to 0.68)	
Keedy 2011	46	0.90 (0.29 to 1.50)	
Levinson 2007 (1)	60	−0.04 (−0.54 to 0.46)	
Levinson 2007 (2)	58	−0.77 (−1.31 to −0.24)	
Metzler 2012	73	−0.05 (−0.51 to 0.40)	
Ngugyen 2012 (1)	20	−0.16 (−1.04 to 0.71)	
Nguyen 2012 (2)	20	0.45 (−0.43 to 1.34)	
Ngugyen 2012 (3)	20	−0.87 (−1.78 to 0.04)	
Nguyen 2012 (4)	20	−0.16 (−1.04 to 0.70)	
Nicholson 2006	57	1.54 (0.94 to 2.13)	
Petersson 2009	90	0.37 (−0.04 to 0.78)	
Prinz 2005	172	0.79 (0.48 to 1.10)	
Ruisoto 2012	80	1.64 (1.13 to 2.14)	
Seixas-Mikelus 2010	10	1.99 (0.48 to 3.51)	
Solyar	15	1.95 (0.72 to 3.18)	
Tan 2012	40	0.05 (−0.56 to 0.68)	
Fixed	**1702**	**.59 (.49 to .69)**	
Random	**1702**	**.50 (.20 to .80)**	

Figure 7.4 Random and fixed effects model forest plots of the effect sizes of spatial knowledge.

efficacy of PBL versus other instructional methods (e.g., organ systems-based curricula), for example, simple linear regression has been commonly used in employing fixed parameters. Because of the shared variance, this method is inadequate, and more advanced methods such as HLM is more appropriate. It can account for the shared variance in hierarchically structured data such as students within classrooms, which are within a school, which are within pedagogical approaches (e.g., organ systems vs. PBL curricula).

HLM is nowadays used in education, health, social work, economics, and other areas. With HLM, we can simultaneously analyze associations within and between hierarchical levels of grouped data, so that we can account for variance among variables at different levels. We may ask the question, "Is PBL a better pedagogical method than large group lectures in an organ system-based course?"

To answer this question, we locate a medical school that employs PBL in the first 2 years of the curriculum and compare students' performance from another medical school where students attend lectures in the first 2 years in organ systems-based curriculum. This research question involves a hierarchy with three levels. School-related variables such as the school's budget, class size, and private versus public at the highest level of the hierarchy (level-3). In the middle level of the hierarchy (level-2) are class variables, such as instructors' assigned reading load, teaching style, and years of teaching experience. Level-2 variables are nested within level-3 and are influenced by level-3 variables.

Medical schools (level-3) that are private (level-3 variable) may have smaller class sizes (level-2) than publically funded schools. This may affect the interpersonal relationships between instructors and students and time that instructors can devote to individualized instruction. At the lowest level of the hierarchy (level-1), variables are nested within level-2 groups and share in common the impact of level-2 variables. In our example, student-level variables such as sex, MCAT performance, socioeconomic status, entry GPA, and learning styles, are in level-1. Thus, students (level-1) are situated within classes (level-2) that are located within schools (level-3). The dependent variable, performance on Step 1 of the USMLE, is also measured at level-1. In HLM, the dependent variable is always situated at the lowest level of the hierarchy (level-1).

In our example, the researchers wish to know if PBL students perform better on the Step 1 compared to large group lectures students. They would need to analyze the data within a hierarchical model, therefore, in order to determine the variance accounted for by student differences in MCAT scores (level-1), for example, within PBL versus lecture (level-2), within private versus publicly funded schools. The result in differences in Step 1 performance could account in the impact of these hierarchical variables in addition to the PBL versus lecture format.

In another application of HLM, researchers[22] wished to determine which admissions variables and curricular outcomes are predictive of being at risk of failing a performance measure in medical school: the Medical Council of Canada Qualifying Examination Part 1 (MCCQE1). Using data from five graduating cohorts (2011–2015), Schulich School of Medicine & Dentistry, Western University, they employed a two-level HLM to analyze performance outcomes on the MCCQE1 to account for the intrinsic hierarchal nature of the data (i.e., students were nested within cohorts). The HLM analyses identified sex, MCAT verbal reasoning score, two preclerkship course mean grades, and the Year 4 summative OSCE score as significant predictors of student risk.

The predictive accuracy of the models varied. Barber et al.[22] concluded that the predictive models developed suggest, that while it is not possible to identify student risk at admission, students within the first year can be identified and monitored. Programs may thus be able to identify and monitor students at risk quantitatively and develop tailored intervention and support strategies to mitigate their risk of academic failure.[22]

UNIFIED VIEW OF VALIDITY

As we have seen, validity research consists of several subtypes: face, content, criterion-related, and construct. It is also true that validity is a unitary concept, construct validity. A construct is a hypothetical entity (i.e., theory) that specifies the purpose or intent of the assessment and interpretation of the resulting data. The process of collecting validity evidence requires a precise definition of the assessments and an operational definition of the assessment and of score interpretation. Evidence is then gathered to support the interpretation of the construct and interpretation of scores. Several complex steps are required for validity evidence.

Evidence-based on test content (content validity)

Evidence for content includes use of a TOS which evolves from the construct and explicitly describes the domain, depth, and breadth of the content to be assessed, along with the type and number of assessment items defined for the content (Chapter 5). Content experts or specialists may also be involved for confirmation of the assessment content with the construct such as in a Delphi study (Chapter 5).

Evidence-based on empirical criteria (criterion-related and construct)

Empirical studies primarily based on correlational techniques such as Pearson's r, regression analyses, hierarchical linear modeling, factor analyses, structural equation modelling, discriminant analysis, and MTMM approaches are key for adducing construct validity evidence (Chapters 6 and 7). Techniques for analyzing between-group differences such as ANOVA and cluster analyses are also useful for investigating construct validity. Other useful social sciences techniques for exploring construct validity are systematic reviews and meta-analysis (Chapter 7) as well as item response theory and generalizability theory (Chapter 9). In short, all of these methods are used for scientific support for theories. Construct validity, therefore, more-or-less equals the process of supporting evidence for scientific theories.

CONSEQUENTIAL VALIDITY

Consequential validity refers to the social consequences of using a test for a particular purpose. The use of tests has consequential validity to the extent that society benefits or is harmed from the use of the test. Widespread use of tests such as the SAT (Scholastic Aptitude Test, later called the Scholastic Assessment Test, then the SAT Reasoning Test), LSAT, and the MCAT have consequential validity, because they are high stakes tests that are employed as screening devices for admissions to college, law school, and medical school, respectively. These tests are the preliminary screens for the country's university students, lawyers, and doctors. Given the large consequences of these tests, how well do we understand their predictive validity? Do higher scorers on these tests make better lawyers and doctors than lower scorers? The empirical evidence does not support this interpretation. People from higher socioeconomic status, particular racial groups, ethnic groups, and from some geographic areas score high on these tests and therefore have an advantage for entering law and medical school. Some testing experts believe that the social consequences of using these tests constitute a form of validity: *consequential validity*. Others, however, believe that important as the social consequences may be, they are not properly part of the concept of validity.

Messick has argued that "… it is not that adverse social consequences of test use render the use invalid but, rather, that adverse social consequences should not be attributable to any source of test invalidity such as construct–irrelevant variance."[23] According to this view, that some subgroups obtain lower scores on the LSAT and MCAT, and consequently do not get into law and medical school, does not render the test scores invalid. We do know, however, that these test scores do not have evidence of validity for identifying those that will be good lawyers or doctors. Accordingly, we could conclude that the adverse social consequences (e.g., rejecting candidates who might become better lawyers and doctors than those admitted) are caused by using the test scores that have sources of invalidity (e.g., cultural, racial, and socioeconomic biases). The validity of the test use (admissions decisions) is jeopardized in this case. A counter-argument is that this consequence is not a validity issue but rather a sociopolitical issue that needs to be addressed in that context rather than in the context of validity.

TRADITIONAL ORGANIZATION OF VALIDITY EVIDENCE

Throughout this textbook, advanced methods of approaches to construct validity have been elucidated, particularly in this chapter. At the same time, the traditional four categories of validity (face, content, criterion-referenced, construct) have been maintained as an organizational structure. This strategy is purposeful. While this text is intended as a comprehensive treatment of assessment—particularly directed toward assessing competence in the health professions—it is likely to be used by classroom-level instructors and researchers constructing local assessments. Most classroom teachers and course directors who construct the vast majority of locally made tests will have little knowledge and expertise in many of the construct validity methods described in this book.

Most of the assessment work of these users will be for the classroom or clinic. The focus of their tests and other assessments will be on face validity (does the test look valid) and content validity (does the test adequately sample the relevant content and learning processes). Most of the validity evidence that they will receive will be the test performance itself (item performance, difficulty of the test) and student feedback ("We never discussed Transfer RNA in class so why were there questions on it?", and "Numbers 15 and 24 were trick questions with 'A and B but not C' and 'None of the Above'"). These instructors are unlikely to ever approach their assessments for empirical evidence of validity, construct, or otherwise. Therefore, much of this book was written for them so as to elevate classroom assessment beyond so much of the amateurish errors that one finds in testing and assessments in the health professions education, and indeed post-secondary education as a whole.

For the professional and advanced users, there is a unified approach to validity. But they are in the minority of daily test constructors and users worldwide.

Even the *Standards for Educational and Psychological Testing*[24] dismiss face validity and don't do justice to content validity largely because the *standards* are aimed at professional test users and assessment experts. To re-iterate, the majority of test constructors and users (i.e., classroom instructors, professors, etc.) have never heard of and never will hear about "construct" validity. It is, therefore, important that they learn at least how to make and use tests that have face and content validity. There is little that will poison the educational environment in a course or classroom as an exam that is seen as "unfair" (i.e., lack face validity) and "tested just the last few weeks of the course" (i.e., lack of content validity). A great service will be done if the face and content validity of testing in health professions education and to post-secondary education as a whole if we can improve these aspects of testing.

SUMMARY AND MAIN POINTS

This chapter has dealt with advanced forms of validity, structural equation modelling, multi-trait multi-method matrix, systematic reviews and meta-analysis, hierarchical linear modelling, and a unified view of validity.

- Structural equation modeling is a family of statistical techniques used for the systematic analysis of multivariate data to measure underlying hypothetical constructs (latent variables) and their inter-relationships. It is a powerful statistical research tool in health sciences education research and in particular for investigating construct validity.
- CFA is an extension of EFA and a subset of SEM. CFA provides a means by which researchers can model a priori latent variables or factors; this method identifies any variability (systematic and error variance) in a measured variable that is not associated with the latent construct. In addition, it can model the relationships between factors. The structural relations are the relations between the factors and are the core of SEM.
- MTMM is a method that involves correlating scores of different attributes (e.g., communication, physical examination) across different methods (e.g., patient questionnaire, direct observation); this gives a more comprehensive assessment of the construct measured than do correlations of traits assessed by single methods. The minimum requirement for using MTMM for a construct validity study is the use of two traits and methods. The inter-correlations may thus provide evidence of convergent and divergent validity.
- Systematic reviews and meta-analyses are sometimes combined in a single study. A systematic review is a literature review of collecting and critically analyzing several research studies, using and explicitly specifying methods

whereby the papers are located, identified, and selected. A meta-analysis is a statistical analysis that combines the results of multiple empirical studies. The purpose of meta-analysis is to use statistical approaches to derive a pooled estimate of the underlying regularities or constructs.

- HLM is an elaborated method of regression that can be used to analyze the variance in dependent variables when the independent variables are hierarchically organized such as students within courses within schools. Because of the shared variance, simple regression is inadequate and more advanced methods such as HLM is more appropriate. It can account for the shared variance in hierarchically structured data such as students within courses, which are within a school and which are within pedagogical approaches (e.g., organ systems vs. PBL curricula).

- Validity is a unitary concept, called construct validity. A construct is a hypothetical entity (i.e., theory) that specifies the purpose or intent of the assessment and interpretation of relevant data. Evidence is gathered to support the interpretation of the construct and interpretation of scores. Several complex steps are required for validity evidence.

REFLECTIONS AND EXERCISES

Reflections

1. Compare and contrast SEM with regression, factor analysis, and path analyses (Maximum answer of 250 words)
2. What are the advantages of MTMM for construct validity studies? What are the disadvantages? (Maximum answer of 250 words)
3. Design a MTMM study to collect construct validity data for constructs of your choosing. (Maximum answer of 250 words)
4. Propose a systematic review and meta-analysis for any issue of interest to you. (Maximum answer of 250 words)

Exercise

1. Based on the results summarized in Table 7.1, which is the best fit between the data and the theory? Explain your answer. (Maximum answer of 250 words)

REFERENCES

1. Bentler PM. Linear systems with multiple levels and types of latent variables. In: Joreskog KG, Wold H, editors. *Systems under Indirect Observation Causality-Structure-Prediction.* New York: North-Holland; 1982. pp. 101–130.

2. Schermelleh-Engel K, Moosbrugger H, Muller H. Evaluating the fit of structural equation models: Tests of significance and descriptive goodness-of-fit measures. *Methods Psychological Research*, 2003;8(2):23–74.
3. Nachtigall C, Kroehne U, Funke F, Steyer R. (Why) should we use SEM? Pros and cons of structural equation modeling. *Methods of Psychological Research*, 2003;8(2):1–22.
4. Bollen KA, Long JS. (Eds.). *Testing Structural Equation Models*. Newbury Park, CA: Sage; 1993.
5. Forsythe GB, McGaghie WC, Friedman CP. Construct validity of medical clinical competence measures: A multitrait multimethod matrix study using confirmatory factor analysis. *American Educational Research Journal*, 1986;23:315–336.
6. Berkel HJM, Schmidt HG. Motivation to commit oneself as a determinant of achievement in problem-based learning. *Higher Education*, 2000;40(2):231–242.
7. Kline RB. *Principles and Practice of Structural Equation Modeling*. 2nd ed. New York: The Guilford Press; 2005.
8. Hu L-T, Bentler PM. Cutoff criteria for fit indexes in covariance structure analysis: Conventional criteria versus new alternatives. *Structural Equation Modeling*, 1999;6(1):1–55.
9. Kane M. Validating score interpretations and uses. *Language Testing*, 2011;29(1):3–17.
10. Hull AL, Hodder S, Berger B, Ginsberg D, Lindheim N, Quan J, Kleinhenz ME. Validity of three clinical performance assessments of internal medicine clerks. *Academic Medicine*, 1995;70(6):517–522.
11. Bentler PM. *EQS 6 Structural Equations Program Manual*. Encino, CA: Multivariate Software, Inc; 2004.
12. Violato C, Hong G, O'Brien MC, Grier D, Shen E. A test of three competing theories of the development of medical expertise: Distinct domains, independent influence and encapsulation models. *Advances in Health Sciences Education*, 2017. doi:10.1007/s10459-017-9784-z AHSE-D-16–00389.1.
13. Ferguson E, James D, O'Hehir F, Sanders A. Pilot study of the roles of personality, references, and personal statements in relation to performance over the five years of a medical degree. *British Medical Journal*, 2003;326:429–432.
14. Williams GC, Saizow R, Ross L, Deci EL. Motivation underlying career choice for internal medicine and surgery. *Social Science Medicine*, 1997;45(11):1705–1713.
15. Hoban JD, Lawson SR, Mazmanian PE, Best AM, Seibel HR. The self-directed learning readiness scale: A factor analysis study. *Medical Education*, 2005;39(4):370–379; Humphris GM. Communication skills knowledge, understanding and OSCE performance in medical trainees: A multivariate prospective study using structural equation modeling. *Medical Education*, 2002;36(9):842–852.

16. Schmidt HG, Rikers RM. How expertise develops in medicine: Knowledge encapsulation and illness script formation. *Medical Education*, 2007;41:1133–1139.
17. Campbell DT, Fiske DW. Convergent and discriminant validation by the multitrait-multimethod matrix. *Psychological Bulletin*, 1959;56:81–105.
18. Baig L, Violato C, Crutcher R. A construct validity study of clinical competence: A multitrait multimethod matrix approach. *Journal of Continuing Education in the Health Professions*, 2010;30(1):19–25.
19. Glass GV. Primary, secondary, and meta-analysis of research. *Educational Researcher*, 1976;5:3–8.
20. Al Ansari A, Ali SK, Donnon T. The construct and criterion validity of the mini-CEX: A meta-analysis of the published research. *Academic Medicine*, 2013;88(3):413–420.
21. Yammine K, Violato, C. A meta-analysis of the educational effectiveness of three-dimensional visualization technologies in teaching anatomy. *Anatomical Sciences Education*, 2014;8(6):525–538.
22. Barber C, Hammond R, Gula L, Tithecott G, Chahine S. In search of black swans: Identifying students at risk of failing licensing examinations. *Academic Medicine*, 2017. doi:10.1097/ACM.0000000000001938.
23. Messick S. The once and future issues of validity: Assessing the meaning and consequences of measurement. In: Wainer H, Braun IH, editors. *Test Validity*. Hillsdale, NJ: Lawrence Erlbaum Associates; 1988. pp. 33–45.
24. American Psychological Association; National Council on Measurement in Education; and the American Educational Research Association. *Standards for Educational and Psychological Testing*. Washington, D.C.: American Psychological Association, 2014.

8

Reliability I: Classical methods

- Reliability is a necessary but not sufficient condition for validity. Reliability is measured by an index called the reliability coefficient, r_{xx}.
- Classical methods of reliability are based on classical test theory. A test score is composed of the "real" score or true score plus error of measurement: X (Observed score) = T (True score) + e (error of measurement).
- There are four basic methods for deriving r_{xx}: test–retest, parallel forms, split-half, and internal consistency. Each method focuses on a somewhat different aspect of reliability.
- The Spearman–Brown prophecy formula describes the relationship between test length and reliability. Thus, once you know the reliability of a particular test, you can "prophesize" the effect on the reliability by either increasing the test length or decreasing it.
- The most practical and simplest method of determining reliability for classroom use is the Kuder–Richardson formula 21 (KR21), which is a general internal consistency method.
- The standard error of measurement (S_e) translates the test's reliability onto the actual test scale to estimate the error involved in actual scores that students receive. The S_e is most useful for interpreting an individual's performance on the test.
- The score a student actually obtains on a test is composed of the true score plus error of measurement. True scores are hypothetical entities estimated by the use of the S_e and a particular confidence interval. Thus, the true score falls within a band of error as circumscribed by the S_e with a specific degree of confidence.
- By convention, three confidence intervals are commonly used: 68% ($\pm 1 S_e$), 95% ($\pm 2 S_e$), and 99% ($\pm 3 S_e$).
- There are several common factors that directly influence a test's reliability. These include the test's length, the heterogeneity of the test-takers, whether or not the test is speeded, the length of the time interval in test–retest and parallel forms at different times, the difficulty of the test, and the objectivity of the scoring of the test.

INTRODUCTION

Reliability has to do with the consistency of measurement. It is a necessary condition for validity. While reliability is a precondition for validity, it does not guarantee it. That is, an assessment device that is reliable may not be valid. A clock that always runs 10 min fast is reliable since it is consistent, but it is not valid because it gives the incorrect time. It is evident then that reliability is a necessary, but not sufficient, condition for validity. Alternatively, an instrument that is valid must be reliable. The focus of this chapter is on reliability and its nature. Reliability deals with consistency of measurement.

What is meant by the consistency of measurement? What factors can lead to the inconsistency of measurement? How can you tell if a measurement is consistent or not? These questions are at the heart of the concept of reliability. A simple example can help to clarify the nature of reliability.

Suppose that you measured the length of your kitchen table with a ruler and it turned out to be 100 cm long. Later that day, you began to doubt this measurement so next morning you measured the table again. This time it turned out to be 82 cm long. Which is correct? To settle the matter, you measured the table a third time and this time it was 93 cm long. Still unsure, you measure the table several more times with a different result each time. What is the problem here? There are two possibilities: (1) the table keeps changing length every time it is measured or (2) something is wrong with your measurement instrument and the way you have applied it.

Under normal conditions, of course, tables do not change length; so in this case, the problem must be the measurement instrument. Upon closer examination, you discover that your ruler is made of rubber and the differential results are due to the inconsistency of the measurement. This is why of course, rulers are made from wood, plastic, or metal so that they don't stretch and shrink from time to time.

This example is not merely unlikely or trite. Many assessments in medical education and psychology do in fact behave like rubber rulers, because they produce inconsistent results or unreliable measurements. The concern with reliability in assessment in the behavioral sciences is paramount because of the difficulty of producing consistent measures of achievement and psychological constructs. In measuring physical properties of the universe, reliability is usually not a big problem (For example, think of measuring height, velocity, temperature, weight), while it is a central problem for assessing psychological characteristics or clinical competencies of medical students and physicians.

Reliability is a multifaceted concept rather than a singular idea. Indeed, there are several ways of thinking about and discussing reliability. While there are several approaches to understanding reliability such as generalizability theory (G-theory) and item response theory (IRT), one of the major theories for testing and measurement is classical test theory, which is the subject of this chapter. G-theory and IRT are the subjects of Chapter 9.

CLASSICAL TEST THEORY

Classical test theory is so-called because it was developed first in psychometrics. The premise is simple: any observed score (e.g., a test score) is composed of the "real" score or true score plus error of measurement: X (Observed score) = T (True score) + e (error of measurement). The early foundational work of scholars like Karl Pearson, Charles Spearman, EL Thorndike, and Fredrick Kuder was based on this idea.

$$X = T + e \qquad (8.1)$$

This theory has led to much of the work in testing in the past 100 or so years, including methods for establishing reliability. Four methods of establishing reliability are usually recognized. These are discussed in turn in the following section.

FOUR METHODS FOR DETERMINING RELIABILITY

The four methods or techniques for determining the reliability of a measurement instrument are listed as follows:

1. Test–Retest
2. Parallel Forms
   a. given at the same time
   b. given at different times
3. Split-Half
4. Internal Consistency

These techniques are not only different methods for establishing reliability, but each type produces a somewhat different type of reliability as well. While all forms of reliability focus on consistency, there are different aspects of the testing to which the consistency is relevant. The consistency on the test–retest method, for example, focuses on time. That is, does the assessment produce consistent results from one measurement to another at a different time?

Probably the simplest way to understand reliability is to think of it as consistency over different measurements. This is estimated by the test–retest method. In this method, a professor gives a test today, for example, and exactly 1 week later, the professor gives the same test to the same dental students. Suppose that Jaden, one of the students that took the test, is a very good student, studies diligently and works hard and so scored very well on the test. By contrast, Tracy is a lackadaisical student and thus scored poorly on the test. All things remaining equal, how would you expect Jaden and Tracy to score on the second administration of the test (assume no practice effects or further studying)? The most obvious answer is that Jaden should score well on the second administration, and Tracy should score poorly on the second administration of the test.

Test–retest rests on the ensuing assumption. Suppose that 75 students had taken the test in the above example. Those who did well on the first administration should do well on the second and those who did poorly on the first should do poorly on the second. Of course, the mediocre students are also expected to remain the same. The idea is that there should be consistency of performance across the two administrations. We determine the degree of consistency in the test–retest method by using correlation (See Chapter 4 for a discussion of correlation). Since, in our example, 75 students took the test, each one will have two scores (one on the first administration and one on the second). By treating each set of scores as a variable (say, X for time 1 and Y for time 2), we can compute the correlation (using the Pearson product–moment correlation computations) between the two sets of scores. This will be the estimate of the consistency or reliability of the test. This correlation, because it is interpreted within the context of reliability, is now called a reliability coefficient (r_{xx}).

A second type of reliability is estimated by parallel forms or equivalent forms method as it is also called. Here, the focus is on the consistency of measurement across different forms (parallel or equivalent) of the same test. Because the different forms can be given either simultaneously or at different times, stability of the assessment over time can also play a role in this method.

The third type of reliability—that is estimated both by split-half method and the internal consistency method—deals with the internal consistency of the assessment or the consistency of measurement across different items within the instrument. Thus, neither time nor form equivalence is relevant here. Split-half is a special version of internal consistency. Here, we are concerned about the extent to which each item (or group of items) consistently measures in the direction of the other items on the test. Each method and type of reliability is compared and summarized in Table 8.1.

Table 8.1 Classical methods of estimating reliability

Method	Reliability measure	Procedure
Test–retest	Stability over time	Give the same tests to the same group of subjects at different times (hours, days, weeks, months, etc.)
Parallel forms (same time)	Form equivalence	Give two forms of the same test to the same group at the same time
Parallel forms (different time)	Form equivalence and stability over time	Give two forms of the same test with a time interval between the two forms
Split-half, Cronbach's α, KR20, Guttmann	Internal consistency	Give the test once and apply the Kuder–Richardson formula, Cronbach's alpha coefficient formula, etc.

RELIABILITY COEFFICIENTS

Like validity coefficients, reliability coefficients are correlations but are now interpreted in the context of reliability. The reliability coefficient is computed using exactly the same procedures as for computing the validity coefficient. The interpretation, though, has some important differences.

In validity, the proportion of variance accounted for is derived by employing the coefficient of determination (r^2). This is because two different variables are correlated (r_{xy}, e.g., MCAT with GPA) and thus, r_{xy} must be squared in order to derive the proportion of variance accounted for in one variable by another. To distinguish it from a general correlation coefficient, the reliability coefficient is written as r with xx subscripts, r_{xx}, meaning a variable (assessment) correlated with itself. In reliability, the exact same variable is correlated with itself (the same test at different times) and thus there is no need to square r_{xx} to derive the proportion of variance accounted for in the two measurements. The correlation coefficient r_{xx} is a direct measure of the amount of variance accounted for in the measurement over two times. The difference from unity ($1-r_{xx}$) is the amount of inconsistency in the measurement over two occasions. The magnitude is a direct indication of the consistency or reliability of the test. Thus, the size of r_{xx} tells how good the reliability of the test is. How large must a reliability coefficient be?

INTERPRETING THE RELIABILITY COEFFICIENT

As in interpreting the validity coefficient, there are no fixed and firm rules for interpreting the reliability coefficient. To some degree, contextual factors need to be taken into account. There are, however, several useful rules of thumb, which can help to interpret the reliability coefficient. Different standards apply to different assessment situations.

For standardized tests (achievement, MCAT, USMLE step tests), reliability coefficients are generally expected to exceed $r_{xx} = 0.90$. This means that 90% of the variation in measurements is due to consistent and stable assessments. The remaining 10% ($[1-r_{xx}] \times 100 = 10\%$) is due to errors of measurement. A standardized test with a reliability of less than $r_{xx} = 0.85$ is considered inadequate as 15% of the variance is due to errors of measurements.

Different standards though, must guide the adjudication of research instruments or locally constructed instruments. Generally, any assessment—an instrument in development or otherwise—is considered poor if r_{xx} is less than 0.50. This means that only 50% of the variance in the measurement is consistent and a true measure, while 50% is error. An instrument with $r_{xx} = 0.40$ has 60% error of measurement and only 40% consistent measurement. Rating scales, self-report instruments, and attitude scales in development with reliabilities of 0.50 to 0.60 are adequate, of 0.61 to 0.70 are good, and with 0.71 and greater are very good and excellent. When r_{xx} exceeds .70, the error or measurement is less than 30%. Most researchers can realistically aim for reliabilities for their instruments in the order of $r_{xx} = 0.75$. On the other hand, technically sound tests like the MCAT have reliabilities of $r_{xx} > 0.90$.

The test–retest method is impractical for most purposes. There are several reasons for this. First, giving the exact same instrument twice is a waste of precious research or teaching time and resources. Second, respondents may consider this to be an odd practice and may react unfavorably to being assessed twice with the identical instrument. Third, it is simply inefficient practice to use test–retest methods for most purposes. Other methods for determining the reliability of assessment devices should be employed.

THE PARALLEL FORM METHOD

The main problem with the test–retest method is that participants receive *exactly* the same items on both assessment occasions. The solution to this problem might be to construct several different forms or versions of the instrument (e.g. Forms A, B, C) called *parallel forms* or *equivalent forms*. This means that on assessment occasion two, the participants would receive different items that measured the same thing as the instrument that was given on testing occasion one. The analogy here would be to measure the length of an object with one ruler on occasion one and a different ruler on occasion two and compare the results. The rulers are considered to be parallel or equivalent measures of length. The degree to which they produce equivalent results is an indication of their reliability (consistency across different forms or rulers).

To create parallel forms, the course director might proceed in the following way. First, the universe or domain of measurement is defined. This domain is defined by the instructional objectives that are to be assessed or by the table of specifications (see Chapters 5 and 6 for discussions of TOSs). Thus, the content area and the level of understanding of the content areas are defined. Second, for each cell in the TOS, the course director constructs a number of items. Many more items that will appear on any form of the test need to be constructed (perhaps 10 times as many). Third, the course director randomly selects the desired number of items from each cell in the TOSs to make up the whole test. This is called Form A. Fourth, the course director, using the same procedure, selects another set of items to make up Form B. Following the above steps, more forms can be constructed until the item pool is depleted. Forms A, B, and any other forms are called parallel or equivalent forms.

Suppose that Dr. Cooney, the course director, wanted to construct parallel forms of the first-year *Cardiovascular and Respiratory* exam. This assessment is to consist of 100 items. Dr. Cooney and the other course instructors now construct 1,000 items, 10% of which (100 items) deals with heart structure, 15% (150 items) with blood flow, 15% (150 items) with lung structure, and so on. To make Form A, Dr. Cooney now randomly selects 10 items from the heart structure (5 knowledge, 5 comprehension), 15 from blood flow (3 knowledge, 7 comprehension, 5 application), 15 from blood flow (3 knowledge, 6 comprehension, 6 application), and so on until all 100 items have been selected. A test has now been constructed according to the TOSs and therefore samples the universe or domain of measurement. Using the same procedures, Dr. Cooney can select another 100 items to construct Form B. Further forms can be constructed if necessary.

There are two options now available to Dr. Cooney. He can administer Forms A and B at the same time or with a time interval of, say, 1 week. These two procedures will yield somewhat different estimates of reliability. Let us examine both procedures beginning with administration at the same time.

Parallel forms administered at the same time

In this condition, Dr. Cooney has all his 170 first-year medical students write both forms at one sitting. Half of the students (85) are randomly selected to write Form A first and the other half will write Form B first. When they are finished, those that wrote Form A will write Form B, and those that wrote Form B will write Form A.

This procedure is to remove the possibility of order effects (doing one thing will have an effect on the thing that is to be done immediately after). Each student will now have two scores, one on Form A and one on Form B. Dr. Cooney can now correlate the two sets of scores using the Pearson correlation to derive a reliability coefficient, r_{xx}. This is an indicator of form equivalence. That is, it tells the extent to which the two test forms indeed measure the same thing. A very high index (close to 1.0) means that the two forms are highly equivalent, while a low index (close to 0.0) means that they are not at all equivalent. The second method is to administer the forms with a time interval.

Parallel forms administered at different times

The second option that Dr. Cooney had was to administer Form A first and 1 week later to administer Form B (as before to eliminate order effects, half of the students receive Form A and half Form B on testing occasion one and vice versa on occasion two). As before, each student will have two scores, one on Form A and one on Form B.

Using the Pearson correlation as before, Dr. Cooney can compute a reliability coefficient, r_{xx}. In this case, the reliability tells not only about form equivalence (since two forms are compared) but also about the stability of the forms, since a time interval has lapsed between the administration of the two forms. All things remaining equal then, we would expect the coefficient that was computed using the second method to be smaller than the one computed using the first method. Only one source of error of measurement is introduced in the first procedure (item equivalence), while two sources are introduced in the second situation (item equivalence and instability of the test over time). The second method is the most rigorous measure of the test's reliability, since both sources of measurement error are sampled. It is also more rigorous than the test–retest method, since in the parallel forms method, only instability over time contributes to measurement error (the items are identical so there is no issue of equivalence) in that condition.

It probably has become obvious that the parallel form method (either at the same time or at different times) is highly impractical for classroom use. This is true for a number of reasons. First, twice the testing time is required compared to a single administration of the test. Second, a tremendous amount of effort goes into test construction by the instructors since large numbers of items are required for this method. Third, students may anticipate the second administration and so may prepare or study the material sampled by the first form. Given these limitations, the parallel form method is rarely used in medical courses or other classroom practice.

Nevertheless, the parallel form method is widely used in standardized testing. Such well-known tests as the LSAT, SAT, MCAT come in multiple forms. These and many other tests have been developed, standardized, and are scored by professional organizations such as Educational Testing Services (ETS) and the American Association of Medical Colleges (AAMC). For several decades, these organization have been the foremost educational test developers in the world. As well, ETS is responsible for conducting research into testing and test development and has huge resources at its disposal such as a large campus-like physical plant, high-speed computers, and many hundreds of employees, many of which are psychologists and other specialists in testing and psychometrics.

With these abundant resources at their disposal, ETS can obviously do what the individual instructor cannot. The SAT, for example, has multiple forms on any given testing each of which has known form of equivalence reliability. ETS has many thousands of items that are designed for the SAT according to the general procedures described above. As well, new items are constantly developed, added to the tests, and tried out on forms of the test. The item bank, therefore, is constantly being replenished. Each form of the SAT is unique and will never be given as it is again. While these procedures employed by ETS approximate the ideal for test construction and development, they require such huge resources that it has not been practical for classroom use or at least hasn't been until recently.

Presently, test banks and test development software for personal, desktop, and laptop computers are widely available. Many of these software packages have the capabilities to store up to 100,000 items. Professors, therefore, can build item banks over time from which they can generate multiple forms of the same test by issuing a few simple commands to their computers. The ideal of the practice of ETS then is now becoming a real possibility for individual courses or at least groups of instructors in schools. Even so, however, the limitations of the parallel form method, which were described above, still hold. Thus, other methods for establishing the reliability of classroom tests have been developed. An important such method is the split-half technique.

THE SPLIT-HALF METHOD

Suppose that instead of giving his students Form A and then Form B of his test, Dr. Cooney simply had a single test made up of all of the items from the two forms. As far as the students are concerned, they received just one test. After the test was written, Dr. Cooney could split the test in half and derive a score for each student on each half. Then using the correlation procedures, he could compute the correlation between the scores on the two halves. This correlation is the basis for determining the reliability of the test. This procedure is the split-half method.

There are many ways of splitting an instrument into half. For a 50-item measure, for example, Items 1–25 could constitute the first half and Items 26–50 could constitute the second half. Alternatively, Items 1–7, 16–23, 32–43 could constitute the first half and the remaining items the second half.

The possibilities for splitting the instruments in half are staggering.* For a 25-item test, for example, there are 300 unique split-halves. A rule of thumb that has been developed is to use an *odd–even split*. The first half is made up of all the odd items (1, 3, 5, etc.) and the second half has all the even items (2, 4, 6, etc.).

This easy-to-remember rule allows for equivalent forms to be derived. Each respondent then receives a score on the even half and the odd half. These paired scores can now be correlated. A Pearson correlation can be computed for these scores although the result is not yet the actual reliability. This is because the reliability of the instrument is based on length, and by splitting it in half, the correlation that has been computed underestimates the actual reliability.

Instrument length and reliability

There is a relationship between the length of an instrument and its reliability (Figure 8.1). Generally, the longer, the more reliable it is. This is because a longer instrument samples more of the behavior of interest than does a short measure. Each item can be thought of as a sampling from an impression about the behavior—the more the behavior is sampled, the more reliable the results.

Consider an analogy of meeting new people to illustrate this principle of test length. When you meet a person for the first time for, say, 1 min, you form an impression about that person. This impression is probably not very reliable since the sampling of behavior that you have is highly limited. Now suppose that you meet that person again for another minute, your impression is likely to be more reliable than the first one but still is probably poor. The more you interact with that person, the more reliable your impression becomes—up to a certain point. Once you know someone very well, further interactions are not likely to change your impression of them very much.

This is the same with assessment devices. One item will not produce a very reliable measurement. Two items produces more reliability than one but still the reliability is low. As the number of items increases, so does the reliability. After a certain point, however, adding more items and thus sampling more behavior will not make much difference to the reliability just as your impression of a friend is unlikely to change with one further meeting once you have a very large sampling of their behavior (Figure 8.1).

---

* The number of combinations of n objects taken r at a time is given by the following equation:

$$\frac{n!}{r!(n-r)!}$$

The number of combinations of four objects taken two at a time therefore = 4!/2!(4−2)! = 3×3×2×1/2 × 1 (3 × 2 × 1) = 6. To calculate the number of possible split-halves of a test, the number of items (k) is treated as n in the equation, while r is half the number of items (k/2).

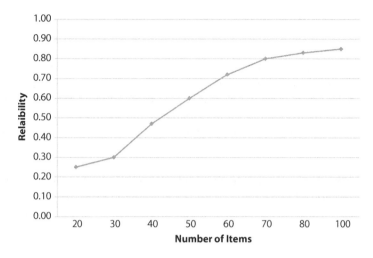

Figure 8.1 Test length and reliability.

The Spearman–Brown prophecy formula

The Spearman–Brown formula "prophesizes" the change in reliability of an instrument as a function of a change in length of the test. Thus, we can equally determine the new reliability whether we increase the length or decrease it. The formula is as follows:

$$r'_{xx} = \frac{Lr_{xx}}{1 + (L-1)r_{xx}} \tag{8.2}$$

where r'_{xx} is the adjusted reliability, L is the ratio in change in length of the test, r_{xx} is the known reliability.

Suppose, for example, that an instrument had a reliability of $r_{xx} = 0.60$ with 20 items. If we wish to know what the reliability will be, if we double the length to 40 items, using the above equation,

$$L = 40/20 = 2; r_{xx} = 0.60$$

Thus,

$$r'_{xx} = \frac{2 \, x \cdot 60}{1 + (2-1) \, x \cdot 60} = \frac{1.2}{1.6} = 0.75$$

Doubling the test length, therefore, will increase r_{xx} from 0.60 to 0.75, a substantial improvement. This is based on the assumption that the new items added are of equal quality to the original items. If the items are of better quality, the increase in reliability will be greater. If the items are of poorer quality, the increase will be less.

Figure 8.1 represents the relationship between test length and reliability. Notice that as the test length increases on short tests, the reliability increases sharply. When the test is longer, however, further increases in the length have little effect on the reliability. The "saturation" point on most tests is reached at about 75–80 items, and there is little increase in reliability after this. As far as reliability is concerned, this is the point of diminishing returns. The relationship between test length and reliability is not linear but rather is geometric and is described by a mathematical relationship, the Spearman–Brown formula.

The Spearman–Brown formula as given above is in its most general form and can be used to compute the change in reliability for any item number change, whether an increase or a decrease. All we need to know is the original reliability, r_{xx}, and L, the ratio change in length. L can be more precisely defined as k_2/k_1, where k_1 is the original length and k_2 is the new test length (k always refers to the number of items). Thus, if we wished to add 10 items to a 30-item test, the original test length, $k_1 = 30$ and $k_2 = 40$:

$$L = k_2 / k_1 = 40/30 = 1.33$$

Alternatively, if we had an instrument of 50 items and wished to shorten it to 40 items,

$$L = k_2 / k_1 = 40/50 = 0.80$$

In the split-half computations, however, we always want to know the result when we double the length and so L is always 2. Substituting 2 for L, the special version of the Spearman–Brown formula then becomes:

$$r'_{xx} = \frac{2r_{oe}}{1 + (2-1)r_{oe}} = \frac{2r_{oe}}{1 + r_{oe}} \tag{8.3}$$

where r'_{xx} is the adjusted reliability as before and r_{oe} is the correlation between the scores on the odd and even half of the instrument.

The general split-half method, and especially the odd-even split, is based on the assumption that the two halves of the instrument are equivalent. This assumption tends to be supported in most cases. If it is not, however, the reliability will be incorrect. This might happen, for example, if you were to give all of the items measuring clinical skills an even number and all items measuring interpersonal communication an odd number. In this case, an odd-even split would not result in equivalent forms since the even half would be measuring a different content and processes than the odd half.

The split-half method of determining reliability, despite its strengths, is somewhat impractical and labor intensive. In their continuing efforts to develop simple and practical methods for determining reliability, statisticians have invented several internal consistency methods.

THE INTERNAL CONSISTENCY METHODS

The odd-even split is just one of many possible split-halves. Indeed, there are a great many possible split-halves as we have seen, with a 25-item test producing 300 unique combinations. If you computed a correlation for each split-half, then you would have 300 correlations that would not be identical to each other. Taking the mean of these correlations, r, and adjusting this with the Spearman–Brown formula, will produce a reliability estimate, r_{xx}, which is called KR20.

This reliability computation was invented by Frederick Kuder and Marian Richardson in 1937, and there is a shortcut computation which fortunately avoids the necessity of calculating correlations at all. The formula of KR20 is:

$$KR20 = \frac{k}{k-1}\left(1 - \frac{\sum_{j=1}^{k} p_j q_j}{\sigma^2}\right) \tag{8.4}$$

where
  k = number of items
  p_j = proportion that got item j correct
  q_j = proportion that got item j incorrect
  σ^2 = variance of the test

Another more general internal consistency measure of reliability was developed by Lee J Cronbach (1951) and is called Cronbach's alpha or coefficient alpha. KR20 is a specific case of alpha (where items are scored dichotomously such as 1 or 0) which is the most general reliability coefficient. The formula for Cronbach's alpha coefficient is:

$$\alpha = \frac{k}{k-1}\left(1 - \frac{\sum_{i=1}^{k} \sigma_{Y_i}^2}{\sigma_X^2}\right) \tag{8.5}$$

where σ_X^2 is the variance of the total test scores and $\sigma_{Y_i}^2$ the variance of component i (e.g., items) for the current sample of persons.

The internal consistency methods, particularly the most general approach utilizing alpha coefficient, have been widely employed in instrument development. They provide a useful method for deriving internal consistency estimates from a single administration of the instrument. If stability is an important factor for the instrument, however, the internal consistency method is inappropriate.

Another way of thinking about reliability and utilizing the data is the error of measurement.

STANDARD ERROR OF MEASUREMENT

The unreliability of the measurement $(1 - r_{xx})$ is due to errors of measurement. In other words, the difference between the reliability coefficient and 1 is due to errors. This can tell the percentage or proportion of the variance in assessment that is due to error and not real individual differences.

If, for example, the variance on an assessment is 200 (SD = 14.1), how much of this is due to real differences among individuals and how much is due to errors of measurement? This question can be answered by using the reliability coefficient. An instrument with a reliability of $r_{xx} = 0.70$ leaves 0.30 due to errors of measurement $(1 - r_{xx})$. That is, 30% of the variance is due to errors of measurement. Therefore, 60 units of the variance (200 × 30/100) arise as a direct result of measurement error and not real differences in individual scores. The standard error of measurement (S_e) is the range on which we can be confident that a person's true score falls.

$$S_e = SD\sqrt{1 - r_{xx}} \qquad (8.6)$$

where
S_e = standard error of measurement
SD = standard deviation
r_{xx} = reliability coefficient

These concepts and data can be used more importantly to interpret individual test scores as well as group performance. What is of interest is how many points on the test are actually due to errors of measurement. This is called the standard error of measurement and is a direct function of the reliability of the test.

If a student received a score of 68 on this test $(k = 100)$, the student's real or *true* score on this test could be at least 7.7 points higher or 7.7 points lower, because these are how many test points are due just to errors of measurement (SD = 14.1).

$$S_e = 14.1\sqrt{1 - .70} = 7.7$$

The student's true score falls between 60.3 and 75.7 (68 ± 7.7).

This then is most useful for interpreting raw scores and deriving true scores.

CALCULATING RELIABILITY WITH SPSS

In SPSS, select "Analyze," then select "Scale" and then select, "Reliability". The window below should open.
1. Select Items 1–34 from the surgeon self-assessment data (see Chapter 7) and click them to the "Items" pane.

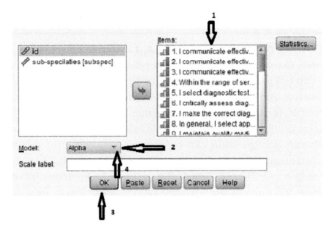

2. "Alpha" should be the selected model; if not, select it.
3. Click "OK"

Output from SPPS:

Reliability statistics	
Cronbach's Alpha	Number of items
0.971	34

4. To select other reliability, click on the down arrow. The following selection will appear:

Alpha
Guttman
Parallel
Strict Parallel

TRUE SCORES

A test writer receives an obtained or raw score, which is mixed with error. It is assumed that at the moment of writing the test, you have a theoretical entity called a true score, which is your error-free, measured level of performance. Since it is not possible to ever measure anything completely free of error, true scores cannot be measured directly. You can only estimate the range within which the true score falls at a particular level of probability. This idea is based on the fact that errors of measurement are normally distributed (See Chapter 3 for a description of the normal distribution.) with a mean of zero (this is the definition of error of measurement—random fluctuation).

For a test that has $S_e = 5$, the distribution of its errors of measurement is normal with a mean of 0 and SD of 5. Therefore, 68% of the time that this test is applied, it will produce raw scores that fluctuate within 1 standard deviation ($S_e = 5$) of the mean (0). Actual raw scores will fluctuate 10 points (0 ± 5) 68% of the time. Of course, 95% of the time, it will produce raw scores that fluctuate 20 points (0 ± 10; i.e. ± 2S) and 99% of the time, the raw scores will fluctuate 30 points (0 ± 15; i.e. ± 3S). These facts can be used in a slightly different version to help interpret test scores.

When a student receives a raw score of 54 on the above test, you can be confident at the 68% level that his true score fluctuates between 49 and 59 (54 ± 5; i.e., 54 ± 1S_e). While you can never know his true score (since true scores are error-free theoretical entities), you can construct confidence intervals around the raw score within which the true score falls. Recall that from equation 8.1, the relationship between raw score, true score, and error is given as:

$$X = T + e$$

The error of measurement in any given test is estimated by S_e and X is a known quantity for any given student. The three confidence intervals that are commonly used are defined by the SDs of the normal distribution (±1S, ±2S, ±3S), 68%, 95%, and 99%. For true score estimation, the confidence level and true scores are tabulated as follows:

Confidence level (%)	True score interval (S_e)
68	1
95	2
99	3

True scores, reliability, and standard error of measurement are all interrelated. Notice too that as the level of confidence increases (you are more confident about the range of true scores), the range of the true score becomes larger. Of course if you were to encompass the whole range of the test, you would be 100% confident that the true score falls in that range. The idea is to increase confidence without increasing the range of the true score interval. This can only be done by increasing the reliability of the test and therefore decreasing S_e. There are a number of factors that influence the reliability of tests.

Factors that influence reliability

Six main factors influence reliability.

1. Test Length. As already described, the length of the test is directly related to its reliability. A longer test not only provides a better sampling of the content area and cognitive outcomes of interest but it also tends to reduce the effects of chance factors such as guessing. If you had a test with only one true-false question, for example, the probability of selecting the correct answer by chance alone is 50%. Thus, a student who guesses wrong receives a 0 and is thought to know absolutely nothing about the content. Alternatively,

a student who guesses correctly receives a perfect score. Neither of the results, however, is indicative of any true knowledge, because the test is far too short to produce reliable results.

In general, tests should be longer if possible because of the reliability concern. Test length, however, reaches the point of diminishing returns as discussed previously (see Figure 8.1). Moreover, many other factors such as time available for testing, the amount of content to be covered by the test, the sophistication of the students, and so on will influence the determination of test length. Even taking all of these into account, a long test is usually more desirable than a short one.

2. Time Interval. In the test–retest and parallel form methods of estimating reliability, the time interval between testing sessions can vary from hours to days to months and even to years. The longer the time interval, the lower the reliability tends to be. This is because more time has elapsed between testing periods, the changes in the phenomenon that is measured (e.g., immunology, clinical skills) are likely to increase. Thus, the scores will likely be inconsistent across the testing periods producing low reliability estimates.

When instructors are using tests whose reliability are based on the test–retest or parallel form method, it is crucial that the time interval between the first and second administrations of the test is known. This is especially important when students' progress is measured using the same test (or parallel forms of it) over time. It is very common, for example, to assess clerkship students with the same instrument as a way of monitoring student progress. If you assess a student at the beginning of a 12-week rotation and then again at the end of it, it is crucial that you know the reliability of the test over at least a 2-month time span. Interpretations in the absence of this knowledge are likely to be incorrect. This may not be quite reliable over the period of assessment.

3. Heterogeneity of Test-Takers. The greater the heterogeneity of a group of test-takers, the more reliable the test tends to be. If you give a test to a group of Years 1, 2, and 3 nursing students, the reliability will tend to be higher than if you give the test to a same size group of Year 1 nursing students. The former group is more heterogeneous than the latter group and so will produce a greater spread of scores. Since reliability estimates are based on maintaining the relative position among test-takers, when the examinees are very similar (i.e., not very heterogeneous) chance factors can easily rearrange relative positions of scores because they are very close together in the first place. On the other hand, for examinees who are very heterogeneous, the spread of scores is great and chance factors have less influence on the relative position of the scores and thus the reliability of the test. All things remaining equal then, reliability estimates of a test will tend to be higher when they are based on a very heterogeneous group.

4. Speeded Tests. Speeded tests, in contrast to power tests, have time as a factor, and the items are uniformly easy. That is, they are designed so that most of the examinees will not finish the test in the time allotted although they will

get most of what they do correct. When internal consistency methods are used for computing reliability under these conditions, it has the effect of artificially increasing the reliability coefficient. This is because a series of items will be highly consistent in producing results—the last 10 items, for example, might be answered incorrectly by nearly all test-takers, perhaps because they ran out of time. While speed is rarely a factor in locally made tests, it can be an important consideration in standardized tests. Thus, when reliability coefficients are derived by the internal consistency method for standardized tests, you should check carefully if speed was used as a factor. If so, the coefficient is likely to be spuriously high.

5. Test Difficulty. Tests that are too difficult or too easy for the test-takers will have poor reliability. The concept of reliability is based on maximizing the variance of the group measured because you wish to detect individual differences as sensitively as possible. When a test is too difficult, most people score poorly and their differences are not detected by the test. Conversely, when a test is too easy, the same principle ensues. In norm-referenced test construction then, you should strive to write items of about average difficulty so as to maximize the reliability.

6. Objectivity in Scoring. Essay and short-answer tests cannot be objectively scored, as the procedure requires subjective judgments by the scorer. This lack of objectivity will tend to reduce the reliability of these tests. Multiple-choice tests have the advantage that they can be completely objectively scored by anyone in possession of the answer key or indeed, even by a machine such as an optical scanner. Due to validity considerations, however, it is frequently not possible to use objective type items for testing. This might be the case when higher-level cognitive outcomes such as synthesis, which require the organization and origination of ideas, are measured. Usually only essay-type items will suffice in these circumstances. By scoring the responses carefully according to pre-specified criteria, however, the subjectivity can be reduced with the effect that reliability will be improved.

Summary and main points

Reliability—defined as the consistency of measurement—is a necessary but not sufficient condition for validity. A test that is reliable is not necessarily valid, but a test that is valid must be reliable. Reliability is not a single, unitary concept, but rather is several related ideas. There are four basic ways to compute a reliability coefficient, r_{xx}: (1) test–retest, (2) parallel forms, (3) split-half, and (4) internal consistency. Each method focuses on a somewhat different aspect of reliability. Test–retest and parallel forms (administered at different times) both estimate the test's stability over time.

Parallel forms (administered both at the same and at different times) estimate form equivalence. Internal consistency—of which split-half is a special case— estimates the degree to which the items of the test "hang together" or measure in the same direction. In the split-half technique, the derived correlation coefficient must be adjusted using the Spearman–Brown prophecy formula which describes the relationship between test length and reliability. While reliability allows for the overall evaluation of a test, the standard error of measurement (S_e) gives an index of the band of error that exists on the total test scale. The S_e is especially useful for determining the band of error around an individual's obtained score and thus estimating the interval of that person's true score.

True scores are hypothetical entities that can never be measured directly but only inferred within a specified range on the test scale at a particular confidence level. Three confidence levels are generally used: 68%, 95%, and 99%. As the confidence level increases, the interval within which the true score falls also increases thereby losing precision. Confidence is gained at the expense of precision. Both precision and confidence can be increased by improving the reliability of the test.

A number of factors influence the reliability of the test. These include the length of the test, the heterogeneity of the students, the length of the time interval in test–retest, and parallel forms at different times, whether or not the test is speeded, the difficulty of the test, and objectivity of scoring of the test. There are a number of strategies that teachers can use to increase the reliability of their tests.

1. Reliability is a necessary but not sufficient condition for validity. A test can be reliable but not valid. A valid test, however, must be reliable.
2. Reliability is measured by an index called the reliability coefficient, r_{xx}.
3. There are four basic methods for deriving r_{xx}: test–retest, parallel forms, split-half, and internal consistency. Each method focuses on a somewhat different aspect of reliability.
4. The test–retest method involves administering the exact same test to the same group on two different occasions. The scores are then correlated to derive r_{xx}. This method is quite impractical for classroom use as it is inefficient, subject to practice and learning effects, and is wasteful of limited classroom time.
5. Parallel forms require that two or more forms of the test be constructed. Each form is thought to measure the same thing and they can be given at the same time or at different times. In the former situation, the second form is administered immediately after the first form is completed. The correlation between the scores on the two forms yields an index of form equivalence. When the forms are administered with a time interval, the resulting r_{xx} combines both form equivalence and stability over time. All things remaining equal, this is the most rigorous method of deriving reliability. Like the test–retest method, parallel forms have shortcomings (wasteful of time, requires that a very large number of items be constructed, is inefficient) that make it impractical for classroom use. It is a widely used technique, however, for standardized testing.
6. The split-half method is more practical for classroom use than either of the above methods. A single test is given and two separate scores are derived subsequently, usually one for the odd-numbered items and one for the even-numbered items. These scores are correlated to derive a coefficient that then must be adjusted with the Spearman–Brown prophecy formula to produce r_{xx}.

7. The Spearman–Brown prophecy formula, in its most general form (equation 8.2), describes the relationship between test length and reliability. Thus, once you know the reliability of a particular test, you can "prophesize" the effect on the reliability by either increasing the test length or decreasing it. To adjust the correlation coefficient in the split-half method, the specific version of the Spearman–Brown prophecy formula is used (equation 8.3) since you always want to know the results when the test is doubled (i.e., the ratio increase is two).

8. The most practical and simplest method of determining reliability for classroom use is the Kuder–Richardson formula 21 (KR21), which is a general internal consistency method. The KR21 method only requires that you know the number of items on the test, the mean of the test, and its variance. While KR21 is not as accurate an internal consistency measure of reliability, as some other methods (e.g., KR20, Cronbach's alpha), its simplicity of computation makes it the most preferred for classroom use.

9. The standard error of measurement, S_e, translates the test's reliability (equation 8.6) onto the actual test scale to estimate the error involved in actual scores that students receive. The S_e is most useful for interpreting an individual's performance on the test.

10. The score a student actually obtains on a test is composed of true score plus error of measurement. True scores are hypothetical entities estimated by the use of the S_e and a particular confidence interval. Thus, the true score falls within a band of error as circumscribed by the S_e with a specific degree of confidence.

11. By convention, three confidence intervals are commonly used: 68% ($1S_e$), 95% ($2S_e$), and 99% ($3S_e$). Notice that as the degree of confidence of the interval containing the true scores increases, precision decreases as the error band encompasses more of the test scale. Increasing the test's reliability will increase both confidence and precision.

12. There are several common factors that directly influence a test's reliability. These include the test's length, the heterogeneity of the test-takers, whether or not the test is speeded, the length of the time interval in test–retest and parallel forms at different times, the difficulty of the test, and the objectivity of the scoring of the test.

REFLECTIONS AND EXERCISES

Reflections: Methods of estimating reliability

1. What are the limitations of test–retest methods for determining the reliability of classroom tests?
2. Describe a measuring instrument and a situation in which test–retest would be appropriate. Be sure to discuss why this method would have to be used and how you would implement it.

3. Briefly discuss why parallel forms techniques of determining reliability are impractical for classroom use.
4. Under what conditions and how is it appropriate to use parallel forms methods to derive reliability?

Exercise 8.1

The following set of data is an odd-even split of test results from a 20-item test.

Student	Odd score	Even score	Total core
1	10	9	
2	8	8	
3	7	4	
4	10	8	
5	4	6	
6	8	8	
7	9	9	
8	9	7	
9	6	6	
10	5	5	
11	7	9	
12	6	4	
13	3	4	
15	7	8	
16	8	7	
17	5	6	
18	4	3	
19	9	8	
20	7	7	
21	4	2	
22	5	4	
23	6	8	

1. Compute the total score.
2. Compute the correlation between the odd and even halves.
3. Using this correlation, determine the reliability of the test (i.e., adjust r_{oe} with Spearman–Brown prophecy formula).
4. Compute S_e for the test data in Exercise 8.1 above (Hint: you will need the SD of the total test scores in addition to r_{xx} you calculated in Exercise 8.1).
5. For the test in Exercise 8.1 above, calculate the true score intervals for all 23 students at the 68%, 95%, and 99% level of confidence.

6. What would be the reliability of the test above if you doubled it in length to 40 items?
7. Using the above total score, compute the KR21 reliability.
8. Compute S_e for total score.

Exercise 8.2

Select any standardized test of your interest (e.g., IQ tests, Achievement tests, GRE, MCAT, SAT, Affective tests, etc.) and review it on the following: (1) reliability (What reliabilities are reported? Are these appropriate given the test's use? In what way is the test reliable? Are the reliabilities adequate given the intended use of the test?), (2) error associated with the test scores (i.e., S_e), and (3) the score reporting system (Are error bands drawn around raw score to indicate the S_e?).

Exercise 8.3

Dr. Yen gave her first-year nursing class a 40-item physiology test and got the following odd–even split results:

Student	Even score	Odd score	Total score
1	19	15	34
2	11	12	23
3	16	14	30
4	8	9	17
5	7	8	15
6	14	12	26
7	8	10	18
8	15	14	29
9	15	20	35
10	8	6	14
11	6	10	16
12	12	15	27
13	9	11	20
14	13	10	23
15	14	16	30
16	11	12	23
17	16	14	30
18	8	9	17
19	7	8	15
20	14	12	26
21	8	10	18
22	15	14	29

1. Compute the total score.
2. Compute the correlation between the odd and even halves.
3. Using this correlation, determine the reliability of the test (i.e., adjust r_{oe} with Spearman–Brown prophecy formula).
4. Compute S_e for the test data in Exercise 8.3 above (Hint: you will need the SD of the total test scores in addition to r_{xx} you calculated in Exercise 8.3).
5. For the test in Exercise 8.3 above, calculate the true score intervals for all 22 students at the 68%, 95%, and 99% level of confidence.
6. What would be the reliability of the test above if you increased the length to 60 items?
7. Using the above total score, compute the KR21 reliability.
8. Compute S_e for total score.

Exercise 8.4

Dr. Francs gave his third-year class a 30-item test and got the following test scores: 26, 8, 14, 14, 21, 23, 17, 14, 10, 11, 29, 11, 15, 14, 20, 18, 22, 12, 9, 9. He wanted to derive an internal consistency reliability measure so decided on KR21. Calculate this internal consistency reliability.

9

Reliability II: Advanced methods

ADVANCED ORGANIZERS

- Modern psychometrics consists of three major interrelated test theories: (1) classical test theory (CTT), (2) generalizability theory (G-theory), and (3) item response theory (IRT). All three theories are fundamental to the field.
- Classical methods of reliability are based on classical test theory: X (Observed score) = T (True score) + e (error of measurement).
- In CTT, each observed score has a single true score and a single source of error of measurement. G-theory is a statistical framework for conceptualizing and investigating multiple sources of variability in measurement.
- IRT is also known as latent trait theory. Like CTT and G-theory, it can be used for the design, analysis, and scoring of tests, questionnaires, and assessments measuring abilities, attitudes, or other variables. IRT is based on mathematical modelling of candidates' response to questions or test items in contrast to the test-level focus of CTT and G-theory.
- There are several statistics that can be used to calculate inter or intra-rater reliability. These coefficients include Cohen's kappa, Pearson's r, and Spearman's rho for inter-rater correlation and intra-class correlation (ICC).
- G studies are designed to assess the dependability of an assessment technique, while decision studies (D studies) are designed to gather data for decisions about individuals. D studies rely on the evidence generated by G studies to design dependable measures for a particular decision and a particular set of facets about which we would like to generalize. The goal is to design a measure that samples sufficient numbers of instances from different facets of a universe of observations to yield a dependable estimate of the universe score of the assessment.
- The actual design type that is most widely used is a one-facet, nested design. This is because it is rare for the same group of examiners to rate all of the candidates in the assessment; assessors rate some of the students,

and some students are rated by several of the assessors. This typically happens in a multi-station OSCE for example.

- Item response theory (IRT), also known as latent trait theory, is based on the relationship between performances on a test item and the ability or the trait that item was designed to measure. The items aim to measure the ability (or trait) that underlies the performance.

- IRT consists of one-parameter logistic (1PL) model that employs only a single parameter (item difficulty) in estimating ability, θ. The two-parameter logistic (2PL) model employs both the difficulty and discrimination and the three-parameter logistic (3PL) IRT model characterizes probability as a function of the examinee's ability, with three parameters representing the item's discriminating power, difficulty level, and guessing.

- An item's location (on the x-axis) is defined as the amount of the latent trait needed to have a 0.50 probability of correctly answering the item. The higher is the difficulty parameter (P in CTT), the higher the trait level an examinee needs in order to get the item correct. The item discrimination (D) indicates the steepness of the ICC at the items location.

- While G-theory and IRT have advantages compared to CTT, both have the disadvantage of low usability or feasibility in medical education because of their challenges in implementation.

INTRODUCTION

Modern psychometrics consists of three major interrelated test theories: (1) classical test theory (CTT), (2) generalizability theory (G-theory), and (3) item response theory (IRT). All three theories are fundamental to the field. This includes the objective measurement of attitudes, personality traits, skills and knowledge, abilities, and educational achievement. Psychometric researchers focus on the construction and adducing validity evidence of assessment instruments such as questionnaires, tests, raters' judgments, and personality tests, as well as with statistical research relevant to the measurement theories.

It is called classical test theory because it was developed first in psychometrics: any observed score is composed of the true score plus error of measurement. Thus, X (Observed score) $= T$ (True score) $+ e$ (error of measurement). The early foundational work of scholars like Karl Pearson, Charles Spearman, EL Thorndike, and Fredrick Kuder was based on this idea. This theory and its applications are detailed in Chapter 8.

G-theory was developed by Cronbach et al.[1] as an advance over CTT. In CTT, each observed score has a single true score and has a single source of error of measurement. G-theory is a statistical framework for conceptualizing and investigating multiple sources of variability in measurement.

An advantage of G-theory is that we can compute what proportion of the variation in test scores is due to factors that vary in assessment, such as raters, setting, time, and items. Anyone who has watched Olympic figure skating has observed the effect of different sources of variance. The variance of scores comes from the skaters' differences in performance, from the different judges, and the items (components of the performance—technical, artistic, etc.). The variation in scores, therefore, comes from multiple sources. In healthcare assessment, the same situation obtains when the student performs skills which are rated by two or more raters.

The third major theory, IRT is also known as latent trait theory. Like CTT and G-theory, it can be used for the design, analysis, and scoring of tests, questionnaires, and assessments measuring abilities, attitudes, or other variables. IRT is based on mathematical modelling of candidates' response to questions or test items in contrast to the test-level focus of CTT and G-theory. This model is widely used with multiple-choice questions (that are scored right or wrong) but can also be used on a rating scales, patient symptoms (scored present or absent), or diagnostic information in disease.

In IRT, it is assumed that the probability of a response to an item is a mathematical function of the person and item characteristics. The person is conceptualized as a latent trait such as aptitude, achievement, extraversion, and sociability. The item characteristics consist of difficulty, discrimination (how they distinguish between people), and guessing (e.g., on multiple-choice items). All three psychometric theories—CTT, G-theory, and IRT—have their relative advantages and disadvantages depending on their usability or feasibility.

INTER- AND INTRA-RATER RELIABILITY

In health sciences education, it is common practice to have more than one assessor rate a performance at the same time. An example is when two professors simultaneously rate students taking a case history from a patient. To what extent do the two raters agree with each other on the performance scores? This is inter-rater reliability, the degree of agreement among raters.

In other circumstances, the same rater may assess a student many times on the same performance. This may happen when students are taking a patient's vitals on several occasions and are assessed on this by the same professor. To what extent does the professor agree with her own ratings over time? This is an intra-rater agreement that is useful in refining instruments such as a scale, used by human judges, for assessing a variable. If raters cannot agree with themselves over occasions, either there is something wrong with raters or with the scale.

There are several statistics that can be used to calculate inter or intra-rater reliability. Different statistics are appropriate for different types of measurement. These coefficients include Cohen's kappa, Pearson's *r*, and Spearman's rho for inter-rater correlation and intra-class correlation (ICC).

Cohen's kappa can be used with two raters for nominal data. For continuous or rank-order data, Pearson's *r* and Spearman's rank correlation coefficient (rho), respectively, can be used. As described in Chapter 4, Pearson's *r* can be computed for pairwise correlation between two raters assessing on a continuous scale. Spearman's rho can be computed for pairwise correlation between raters using a scale that is ordinal. If more than two raters are used, an average level of agreement for the group can be calculated as the mean of the *r* or rho values from each possible pair of raters.

ICC is another way to determine inter-rater reliability. The ICC improves over Pearson's r and Spearman's rho, taking into account the differences in ratings for individual units, along with the correlation between raters. ICC describes how strongly units in the same group resemble each other. Unlike Pearson's r and Spearman's rho, ICC utilizes data structured as groups, rather than paired observations.

The ICC can be calculated as a ratio of variances as in equation 9.1:

$$ICC = \frac{\sigma_o^2}{\sigma_o^2 + \sigma_\varepsilon^2} \tag{9.1}$$

where
  σ_o^2 = variance of the dependent variable or the score of interest due to observers
  σ_ε^2 = error variance or residual (left over variance)

The ICC is used to assess the consistency of scores made by multiple raters on the same quantity. If several residents, for example, score the results of CT scans for signs of breast cancer, how consistent are the scores with each other? If the scan had already been scored by experts and the residents were being assessed for competency, then the residents scores could be compared to the know results. If the results were not known, ICC can reflect the similarity among the scores. There is both inter-rater and intra-rater variability. Inter-rater variability refers to differences among the raters. One resident may consistently score the CT scans positive for breast cancer compared to other residents or the known results. Intra-rater variability refers to fluctuations of a particular resident's score on a particular CT scan but may be part of systematic differences.

Table 9.1 contains student clinical scores assessed by three raters (professors) while the students were obtaining a history and performing a physical exam on patients. What is the degree of rater or observer agreement of the students' performance? To answer this question, we can compute the ICC from analysis of variance data summarized in Table 9.2:

1. $MS_{pxo} = \sigma_\varepsilon^2 = 9.40$
2. $MS_o = \sigma_\varepsilon^2 + n_p\sigma_o^2 = 44.40$
3. $ICC = 44.40/44.40 + 9.40 = 0.83$

All of the reliability coefficients described above range from 0 to 1.0. A value of 0 means that there is no agreement between raters and the variability of scores is entirely due to random fluctuations or error of measurement. A values of 1.0 indicates that there is no error whatsoever in the measurement and all of the variability is true score variance. Suppose in the example above, the ICC value was 0.75. This means that 25% of the variability in the scores assigned to the CT scans are due to error of measurement among the residents. Further training of the residents should improve the performance to a more acceptable value such as 0.90 or so.

GENERALIZABILITY THEORY

The reliability estimates of CTT such as Kappa, Pearson's r, ICC, Cronbach's α, and so on of a multidimensional measure tends to be low even when test–retest and parallel forms reliability estimates are high. This illustrates the limitations and contradictions of CTT.

G-theory reflects an advance on CTT. It focuses on the principle of generalizing from a sample of observations to a universe of observations from which the observations were randomly sampled. The reliability of an observation depends on the universe about which the inferences are to be made. A given score may generalize to several different universes; it may vary in how reliably it allows inferences about these universes. Accordingly, the score can be associated with different reliability coefficients. G-theory explicitly requires the specification of the universe of conditions over which observations can be generalized. This is referred to as generalizability, reliability, or dependability of observations. How different conditions are associated with different observations has implications on how dependable are the observations.

Generalizability theory utilizes some specialized vocabulary.

- **Universe score** supersedes the concept of true score in classic reliability theory. In G-theory, there is not a true score but a series of universe scores, where the universe of relevance is determined by the interests of the researcher.
- **Analysis of variance (ANOVA)**—this technique allows us to partition the variation in data into components and compares the relative sizes of these components. It provides insight into the factors that cause the variables to vary. ANOVA is a general statistical method of decomposing the variation of data into its various components. In the ANOVA model, specific observations vary due to differences between persons (i.e., person effects), differences between items (i.e., item effect), and other unaccounted for sources (i.e., residual).
- **Facets** in a generalizability analysis are similar to factors in ANOVA and include such things as observers, settings, test forms, items, and so on.
- **Mean squares** (MSs) and their expectations (EMS) are critical to the identification of variance components, which are required to calculate generalizability statistics.
- **G** (generalizability) studies and **D** (decision) studies are analogous to psychometric pilot study versus study proper. The G-study gives us information concerning how to conduct the D-study.
- **Residual**—unaccounted variance or "error" variance (leftover)
- **Variance components**

$$\sigma_\varepsilon^2 = \text{error}$$

$$\sigma_p^2 = \text{person (candidate)}$$

$$\sigma_o^2 = \text{observer (assessor)}$$

Example G and D studies

Table 9.1 contains student clinical scores assessed by three raters (professors), while the students were obtaining a history and performing a physical exam. How dependable are the score for this assessment? To answer this question, we conduct a single facet generalizability study.

Table 9.1 Ten medical students scored by three assessors on clinical skills performance

Person (Medical student)	Assessors (Professors)	Score (Clinical skills)
1	1	6
2	1	24
3	1	12
4	1	12
5	1	24
6	1	24
7	1	18
8	1	12
9	1	9
10	1	3
1	2	9
2	2	15
3	2	6
4	2	9
5	2	15
6	2	15
7	2	12
8	2	9
9	2	6
10	2	6
1	3	6
2	3	21
3	3	6
4	3	18
5	3	15
6	3	21
7	3	15
8	3	9
9	3	6
10	3	9

Table 9.2 Analysis of variance (ANOVA) summary table

Source	df	MS	E(MS)
Person	9	92.80	$\sigma_\varepsilon^2 + n_o\sigma_p^2$
Observers	2	44.40	$\sigma_\varepsilon^2 + n_p\sigma_o^2$
Residual	18	9.40	σ_ε^2

Steps in calculating generalizability coefficients

1. Run an ANOVA (e.g., with SPSS) on the raw data to produce a table like Table 9.2
2. Calculate the variance components
3. Determine which components contribute to universe and obtained score variance in D-study designs [using **E(MS)**]
4. Calculate ρ^2s (person variance components)

Calculate the variance components from this G-study

1. $MS_{pxo} = \sigma_\varepsilon^2 = 9.40$
2. $MS_p = \sigma_\varepsilon^2 + n_o\sigma_p^2 = 92.80$, so
3. $n_o\sigma_p^2 = 92.80 - 9.40 = 83.40$, and because
4. $n_o = 3, \sigma_p^2 = 83.40/3 = 27.80$
5. $MS_o = \sigma_\varepsilon^2 + n_p\sigma_o^2 = 44.40$, so
6. $n_p\sigma_o^2 = 44.40 - 9.40 = 35.00$, and because
7. $n_p = 10, \sigma_o^2 = 3.50$

The Variance Components are

$$\sigma_\varepsilon^2 = 9.40$$

$$\sigma_p^2 = 27.80$$

$$\sigma_o^2 = 3.50$$

The generalizability coefficients (ρ^2) for these analyses are summarized in Table 9.3. For all three assessors rating all ten students, the $\rho^2 = 0.86$. With two raters, the $\rho^2 = 0.75$ and with only one rater $\rho^2 = 0.68$. Recall that the ICC for all three assessors was 0.83, an underestimate of the ρ^2.

Additional facets

The single facet design study above could become increasingly complex by adding an additional facet. Each additional facet requires an additional factor in the G-study and in the analysis.

The simplest typical generalizability problem in health sciences education involves determining the reliability or dependability of scores when a constructed-response item (e.g., performing a physical exam) is scored by more

Table 9.3 Summary of the generalizability coefficients (ρ^2) for three D-study designs

D-study—same assessor rating all participants	$\rho^2 = \sigma_p^2 / \left[\sigma_p^2 + \sigma_\varepsilon^2 \right] = 27.80/[27.80+9.40]=0.75$
D-study—same two assessors rating each participant using their average rating	$\rho^2 = \sigma_p^2 / \left[\sigma_p^2 + \left(\sigma_\varepsilon^2/2 \right) \right]$ $= 27.80 / \left[27.80 + \left(9.40/2 \right) \right] = 0.86$
D-study—different observer rating each participants	$\rho^2 = \sigma_p^2 / \left[\sigma_p^2 + \sigma_\varepsilon^2 + \sigma_o^2 \right]$ $= 27.80 / \left[27.80 + 9.40 + 3.50 \right]$ $= 27.80/40.7 = 0.68$

than one rater (a facet). This is the design we employed in the above example. The universe of relevance here is the "skill of physical exam."

If we additionally want to know how scores generalize to the universe of "medical interviewing," two raters (Facet 1) would score candidates (Facet 2) on medical interviewing tasks with patients. If these two tasks (Facet 1) were conducted and assessed on ten patients (Facet 2) by 30 students (Facet 2) who were rated by two assessors (Facet 3), we would have a very complicated design.

The actual design type that is most widely used is a one facet, nested design. This is because it is rare for the same group of examiners to rate all of the candidates in the assessment; assessors rate some of the students and some students are rated by several of the assessors. This typically happens in a multi-station OSCE for example, when Dr. Renquart assessed 25 students in station 1 (chest pain) in the morning, but Dr. Jannard assessed 25 different students in station 1 in the afternoon. Dr. Norwenk rates a different 25 students in station 2 (asthma) in the morning and Dr. Billset rates a different 25 students in station 2 in the afternoon, and so on. This type of G-study requires a single facet, nested design (raters nested within students).

ASSESSING LANGUAGE PROFICIENCY IN ENGLISH AS A SECOND LANGUAGE (ESL) FOR NURSES

Communication is a necessary skill for all health professionals' competency. Nurses who have ESL are assessed for language proficiency. To assess for this in naturalistic conditions, we can sample spoken language, record it, and then have experts rate the language proficiency. The generalizability question is: how dependable are ratings of language proficiency made under naturalistic conditions to draw inferences about the universe consisting of all conditions? This can be computed directly in a G-study by deriving the generalizability coefficient, ρ^2.

A speaking assessment package consisted of 16 language samples of audio recordings of short narratives of a sequence of professional nursing tasks that were assessed by ten assessors. What is the ρ^2 for ten assessors across the 16

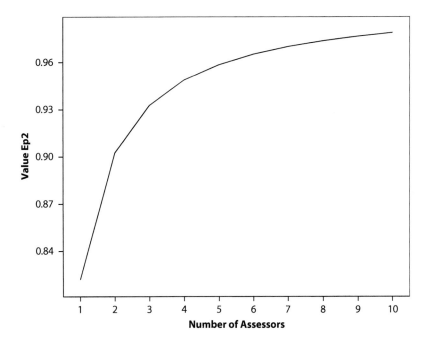

Figure 9.1 ρ^2 value as a function of the number of assessors for speaking.

samples in the spoken tasks? ANOVA of the data resulted in a variance component due to assessor ($n = 10$) of 81.33 and the error component was 1.76 resulting in a $\rho^2 = 0.97$, a very high dependability (Figure 9.1).

Ten assessors, however, is an inordinate number though this results is a very high ρ^2 it also is inefficient if high ρ^2 can be achieved with fewer assessors. From Figure 9.1, it is evident that there is a rapid increase in dependability of the data as the number of examiners increases to three ($\rho^2 = 0.93$) but very little increase by including more assessors. Three assessors are adequate for the speaking task to achieve high dependability.

In a writing task, the same ESL nurses provided 20 samples of written materials (memos and letters) that were assessed by three groups (four raters/group) of assessors. The variance component due to assessor ($n = 3$) was 67.11 and the error component was 1.30 resulting in a $\rho^2 = 0.97$.

What is the optimum number of group assessors for a dependable ρ^2 for the written tasks? There is a rapid increase in dependability of the data as the number of groups increases to three ($\rho^2 = 0.97$) but very little increase by including more groups (Figure 9.2). One group of assessors is adequate for the writing task to achieve high dependability.

What is the optimum number of raters to achieve dependability ($\rho^2 > 0.70$) across a variety of constructed response tasks? The graph in Figure 9.3 shows the theoretical relationship between these two variables. As can be seen from this, increasing either or both of these variables increases the dependability. To

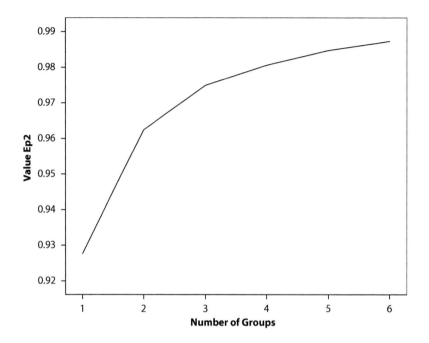

Figure 9.2 ρ^2 value as a function of the number of groups for writing.

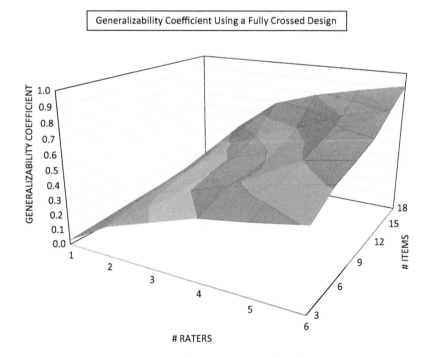

Figure 9.3 ρ^2 value as a function of the number of tasks and raters.

achieve $\rho^2 > 0.70$ with two raters, at least eight to nine tasks are required. With three raters, fewer tasks will be required (perhaps 4–5). The precise number of raters and tasks that are optimal will ultimately depend on the nature of the tasks (e.g., spoken language, clinical skills, etc.) and the competence and training of the raters.

G-studies are designed to assess the dependability of a particular assessment technique while decision studies (D-studies) are designed to gather data for decisions about individuals. D-studies rely on the evidence generated by G-studies to design dependable measures for a particular decision and a particular set of facet about which we would like to generalize. The goal is to design a measure that samples sufficient numbers of instances from different facets of a universe of observations to yield a dependable estimate of the universe score of the assessment.

ITEM RESPONSE THEORY

IRT, also known as latent trait theory, is based on the relationship between performances on a test item and the ability or the trait that item was designed to measure. The items aim to measure the ability (or trait) that underlies the performance.

In many medical education assessment situations, there is an underlying variable or latent trait, of interest that are easily intuitively understood, such as "professionalism" or "diagnostic reasoning." Latent traits (also called constructs) are not directly observable (see Chapter 7). Although such a trait can be easily described, and its attributes listed, it cannot be measured directly.

IRT models, in general, use with dichotomous items (e.g., MCQs scored as right-wrong), differ only in terms of the number of parameters describing the relationship between the examinee and the test item. The standard (i.e., unidimensional) IRT models include the one-parameter (Rasch), the two-parameter, and the three-parameter logistic models. Each of these allows us to compute the probability that an examinee will answer a specific test item correctly based on characteristics of the item and the examinee's knowledge or ability.

Item Characteristic Curves (ICC) are graphical functions that represent the examinee's ability as a function of the probability in getting the item correct. An item's location is defined as the amount of the latent trait needed to have a 0.50 probability of getting the item correct (Figure 9.4). The trait level is labelled ability (θ) with mean = 0 and a standard deviation = 1. Like z-scores, the values of θ typically range from −3 to +3.

IRT offers an important advantage of estimating an examinee's θ on the trait. IRT consists of one-parameter logistic (1PL) model that employs only a single parameter (item difficulty) in estimating ability, θ. The two-parameter logistic (2PL) model employs both the difficulty and discrimination and the three-parameter logistic (3PL) IRT model characterizes probability as a function of the examinee's ability, with three parameters representing the item's discriminating power, difficulty level, and guessing.

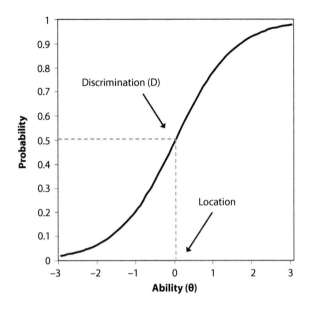

Figure 9.4 Item characteristic curve (ICC).

The difficulty of an item is the percentage or proportion of people who got the item correct. If everyone gets the item correct, it is an easy item; if very few test-takers get the item correct, it is a very difficult item. Item discrimination has to do with the extent to which an item distinguishes or discriminates between high-test scorers and low-test scorers. These item characteristics are discussed in detail in Chapter 15.

An item's location (on the x-axis) is defined as the amount of the latent trait needed to have a 0.50 probability of correctly answering the item. The higher the difficulty parameter (P—analogous to CTT), the higher the trait level an examinee needs in order to get the item correct.

The item discrimination (D) indicates the steepness of the ICC at the items location. It indicates how strongly related the item is to the latent trait. Items with high discriminations are better at differentiating examinees around the location point; conversely, items with low discriminations are poorer at differentiating.

Figures 9.5 and 9.6 illustrate ICCs with varying D and θ levels. Figure 9.7 shows two ICCs with different discrimination and θ and a guessing parameter (Curve 1) indicated by the lower asymptote. The inclusion of a guessing parameter indicates that examinees low on the trait may still get the item correct.

Analyses with more parameters tend to provide more information for the item than does fewer parameters as depicted in Figure 9.8. The one parameter ICC (1PL—right) is flatter and represents a more difficult item that the other two with 0.50 probability at about $\theta = 1.5$. The two parameter ICC (2PL—left) is sharper with a $\theta = -1.0$. Finally, the 3PL (middle) has the most information showing a lower asymptote with a sharp discrimination and for 0.5 probability, $\theta = 0$.

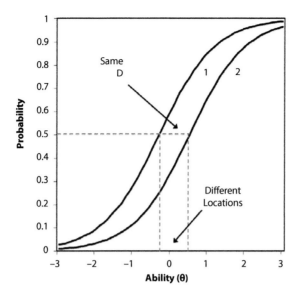

Figure 9.5 Two ICCs with the same discrimination but different θ.

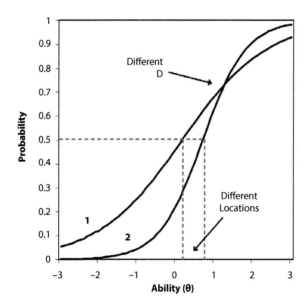

Figure 9.6 Two ICCs with different discrimination and different θ.

The nature ICCs with varying item discrimination and difficulty are summarized in Table 9.4. Item discrimination and difficulty are independent of each other. Graphically, discrimination is depicted as flat when it is low and S-shaped when it is high. Difficulty places the curve along the x-axis with difficult items to the left of 0 and easy items to the right of 0.

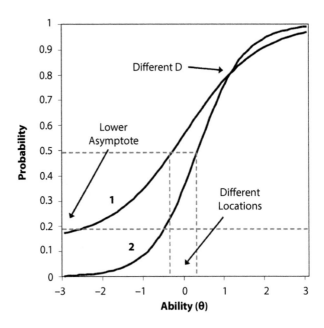

Figure 9.7 ICCs with different discrimination and θ and a guessing parameter (Curve 1).

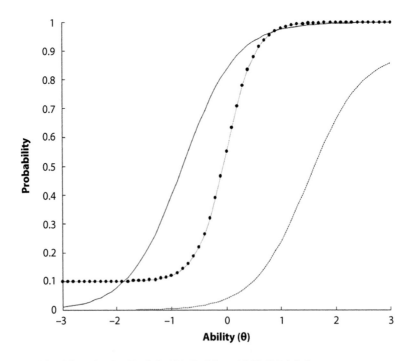

Figure 9.8 ICC with 1PL (Right), 2PL (Left) and 3PL (Middle).

Table 9.4 Summary of the item characteristic curve for difficulty and discrimination

Item discrimination	Item difficulty	Curve characteristic
Low	Easy item	Flat with $p(\theta) > 0.50$ ICC to the right of 0
Medium	Easy item	Sharper with $p(\theta) > 0.50$ ICC to the right of 0
High	Easy item	S-shape with $p(\theta) > 0.50$ ICC to the right of 0
Low	Moderate item	Flat with $p(\theta) \approx 0.50$ ICC around 0
Medium	Moderate item	Sharper with $p(\theta) \approx 0.50$ ICC around 0
High	Moderate item	S-shape with $p(\theta) \approx 0.50$ ICC around 0
Low	Difficult item	Flat with $p(\theta) < 0.50$ ICC to the left of 0
Medium	Difficult item	Sharper with $p(\theta) < 0.50$ ICC to the left of 0
High	Difficult item	S-shape with $p(\theta) < 0.50$ ICC to the left of 0

When an item has 0 discrimination, all difficulty levels result in the same horizontal line at a value of $p(\theta) = 0.50$, because the value of the item difficulty for an item with no discrimination is undefined. As summarized in Table 9.4, when an item is easy, $p(\theta) = 0.50$ occurs at a low ability level and when it is difficult, this value occurs at high ability level.

ADVANTAGES AND DISADVANTAGES OF IRT

All theories that are concerned with reliability, such as CTT, G-theory, and IRT, focus on measurement error. Central to all three theories is the nature of measurement error.

Advantages of IRT compared to both CTT and G-theory
- IRT provides several improvements in assessing items and people
- Difficulty of items and the ability of people are scaled on the same metric
- Difficulty of an item and the ability of a person can be compared
- IRT models can be test and sample independent thus providing greater flexibility where different samples or test forms are used
- These qualities of IRT are the basis for computerized adaptive testing.

Disadvantages of IRT compared to both CTT and G-theory
- Scoring generally requires complex procedures and understanding compared to CTT

- CTT provides simple to understand single reliability indices such as Cronbach's alpha
- In IRT analogous, indices such as the separation index are difficult and inaccessible
- It is difficult to decompose the specific sources of error in IRT while G-theory is designed, in part, for this purpose
- G-theory allows generalization of dependability to well-defined universes
- Compared to CTT, both G-theory and IRT have low usability or feasibility

REFLECTIONS AND EXERCISES

Reflections 9.1

The following analysis of variance table (Table 9.5) consists of the MS for 125 students assessed by three observers in an OSCE station assessing chest pain. This was a fully crossed design. Calculate the generalizability coefficients for assessors rating all 125 students.

- Three raters ρ^2
- Two raters ρ^2
- One rater ρ^2

Exercise 9.1 Steps in calculating generalizability coefficients

1. Calculate the variance components
2. Determine which components contribute to universe and obtained score variance in D-study designs [using **E(MS)**]
3. Calculate ρ^2s (person variance components)

Exercise 9.2 Calculate the variance components from this G-study

1. $MS_{pxo} = \sigma_\varepsilon^2$
2. $MS_p = \sigma_\varepsilon^2 + n_o\sigma_p^2$
3. $n_o\sigma_p^2$

Table 9.5 Analysis of variance summary table

Source	df	MS	E(MS)
Person	124	100.60	$\sigma_\varepsilon^2 + n_o\sigma_p^2$
Observers	2	53.40	$\sigma_\varepsilon^2 + n_p\sigma_o^2$
Residual	362	10.20	σ_ε^2

4. $n_o = 3, \sigma_p^2$

5. $MS_o = \sigma_\varepsilon^2 + n_p \sigma_o^2$

6. $n_p \sigma_o^2$

7. $n_p = 125, \sigma_o^2$

Exercise 9.3 The variance components are

1. σ_ε^2
2. σ_p^2
3. σ_o^2

Exercise 9.4 The generalizability coefficients are

1. Three raters ρ^2
2. Two raters ρ^2
3. One rater ρ^2

REFERENCE

1. Cronbach, L.J., Nageswari, R., & Glesser, G.C. (1963). Theory of general-izability: A liberation of reliability theory. *The British Journal of Statistical Psychology*, 16, 137–163; Cronbach, L.J., Gleser, G.C., Nanda, H., & Rajaratnam, N. (1972). *The Dependability of Behavioral Measurements: Theory of Generalizability for Scores and Profiles*. New York: John Wiley.

SECTION III

Test construction and evaluation

In Chapter 10, the various formats of testing for cognition, affect, and psychomotor skills are summarized. These include selection type items (multiple-choice questions, constructed response, checklists, and other item formats). There is a discussion of Bloom's taxonomies of cognitive, affective, and psychomotor skills, Miller's Pyramid and further work on the use of tables of specifications.

Chapter 11 deals specifically with multiple-choice items especially on how to write items, types of MCQs, number of options, how to construct MCQs and appropriate levels of measurement. MCQs are objective tests because they can be scored routinely according to a predetermined key, eliminating the judgments of the scorers. The multiple-choice item consists of several parts, the stem, the keyed-response, and several distractors. The keyed-response is the right answer or the option indicated on the key. All of the possible alternative answers are called options. The stems should include verbs such as define, describe, identify (knowledge), defend, explain, interpret, explain (comprehension), and predict, operate, compute, discover, apply (application).

In Chapter 12, constructed response items are detailed. These include essays, short answer, matching, and hybrid items such as the Script Concordance Tests. These item types are sometimes also called subjective tests because scoring involves subjective judgments of the scorer. Constructed-response questions are usually intended to assess students' ability at the higher levels of Bloom's taxonomy: application, analysis, synthesis, and evaluation. There are at least two types of essay questions, the restricted and extended response forms. The restricted response question limits the character and breadth of the student's composition.

There are two basic approaches to the scoring of constructed-response test questions: analytic scoring and holistic scoring.

Measuring clinical skills with the objective structured clinical exams (OSCE) is discussed in Chapter 13. The focus is on describing the OSCE and its use in measuring communications, patient management, clinical reasoning, diagnoses, physical examination, case history, etc. Additional issues of case development and scripts, training assessors, and training standardized patients are detailed. Content checklists and global rating scales are used to assess observed performance of specific tasks. Candidates circulate around a number of different stations containing various content areas from various health disciplines.

Most OSCEs utilize standardized patients (SPs), who are typically actors trained to depict the clinical problems and presentations of real issues commonly taken from real patient cases. OSCE validity concerns are (1) content based—defining the content to be assessed within the assessment; (2) concurrent based—this requires evidence that OSCEs correlate with other competency tests that measure important areas of clinical ability; and (3) construct based—one of the ways of establishing construct validity with OSCEs is through differentiating the performance levels between groups of examinees at different points in their education.

Chapter 14 deals with checklists, questionnaires, rating scales, and direct observations. Checklists, rating scales, rubrics, and questionnaires are instruments that state specific criteria to gather information and to make judgments about what students, trainees, and instructors know and can do on outcomes. They offer systematic ways of collecting data about specific behaviors, knowledge, skills, and attitudes and can be used at higher levels of Miller's Pyramid. A checklist is an instrument for identifying the presence or absence of knowledge, skills, and behaviors. Surgery has made extensive use of checklists to improve patient safety. A rating scale is an instrument used for assessing the performance of tasks, skill levels, procedures, processes, and products. Rating scales allow the degree or frequency of the behaviors, skills, and strategies to be rated. Rating scales state the criteria and provide selections to describe the quality or frequency of the performance. A five-point scale is preferred because it provides the best all-around psychometrics.

Chapter 15 is about evaluating tests and assessments using item analyses: conducting classical item analyses with MCQs (item difficulty, item discrimination, and distractor effectiveness), conducting item analyses with OSCEs, conducting item analyses with constructed response items, and computing the reliability coefficient and errors of measurement.

A complete analysis of a test requires an item analysis together with descriptive statistics and reliability. There are three essential features for an item analysis for multiple-choice questions: (1) difficulty of the item, (2) item discrimination, and (3) distractor effectiveness. All of these criteria apply to every other test or assessment form (e.g., OSCE, restricted essay, extended essay, survey) except for distractor effectiveness since there are no distractors in these test formats.

The difficulty of the item is the percentage or proportion of people who got the item correct. If everyone gets the item correct, it is an easy item; if very few test-takers get the item correct, it is a very difficult item. Item difficulty (P) is usually expressed as a proportion such as $P = 0.72$ (72% got it correct).

Item discrimination (D) is the extent to which an item discriminates between high-test scorers and low-test scorers. The point-biserial is commonly used for item discrimination, D. Distractor effectiveness refers to the ability of distractors in attracting responses.

Grading, reporting, and methods of setting cutoff scores (pass/fail) are discussed in Chapter 16. The focus is on norm-referenced versus criterion-referenced approaches, setting a minimum performance level (MPL) utilizing the Angoff method, Ebel method, Nedelsky method.

Grading systems can be based on norm-referenced (grading on the curve) or on criterion-referenced bases. All of these systems have some problems associated with them. The main and historically oldest symbols for grading are the letter grade, usually ranging from A to F. Substitutes have been attempted but have achieved little success because these usually involve reducing the number of categories (e.g., good, satisfactory, unsatisfactory). Numerical grades (percent or 1–10) have also met with limited success as have pass/fail systems and checklists of objectives, as well as empirical methods (borderline regression, cluster analyses, etc.).

The Dean's Letter or *Medical Student Performance Evaluation* employs multiple reporting systems dealing with the cognitive, affective, and skills domains. There are provisions for reporting learner achievement, effort, attitudes, interest, social and personal development, and other noteworthy outcomes. The wealth of information on the MSPE, however, should be balanced against the need for brevity and simplicity so that it can be readily understood.

10

Formats of testing for cognition, affect, and psychomotor skills

ADVANCED ORGANIZERS

- It is common practice to think of human behavior in three categories or domains: cognition (thinking), affect (feeling), and psychomotor (doing). Although we tend to discuss human behavior in these separate ways, most behavior involves all three aspects or domains.
- Thurstone's negative exponential or hyperbolic model learning curve represents a principle of learning in a variety of disciplines and for a variety of learners; learning increases rapidly with practice but attains an upper limit quickly and then flattens out.
- Notwithstanding scientific advances in the study of thinking, perception, memory, learning, much of assessment in medicine and the other health professions is based on lore, intuition, anecdotal evidence, and personal experience. The use of Bloom's taxonomies is helpful in systematizing assessment.
- Much of the testing in these domains involves selection items (e.g., multiple choice) or constructed response (e.g., essays) items.
- Jean Piaget's theory of intelligence is that we adapt to the world employing the dual cognitive processes of assimilation and accommodation. The theory both helps to explain key ideas such as deliberate and interleaved practice, retrieval practice, and learning styles and how to assess them.
- The script-concordance test (SCT) is used to assess the ability to interpret medical information under conditions of uncertainty, tapping Piaget's highest levels of cognitive functioning. There still remain a number of challenges to assess the processes of problem-solving, abstract reasoning, and meta-cognition.
- Students should be continuously tested so as to capitalize on the testing effect. Using retrieval practice with testing—working memory to recall or

retrieve facts or knowledge—is more effective than reviewing content or re-reading text.

- Both the experimental work and the correlational-based research suggest the need for purposeful, direct teaching for *integration* and *encapsulation* of basic sciences into clinical reasoning and clinical skills. This integration and encapsulation needs to be *assessed and tested dynamically* to determine the cognitive processes and outcomes of such pedagogy.

- Bloom is credited for developing a taxonomy in the affective (feeling) domain that provides a framework for teaching, training, assessing, and evaluating the effectiveness of training as well as curriculum design and delivery.

- In the affective domain, the structure of professionalism, aptitude, achievement, and personality are accounted by *Aptitude for Science* (cognitive variables, and Extraversion—a characteristic of working with people (e.g., medicine); *Aptitude for Medicine* (cognitive variables, and Conscientiousness and, inversely, Neuroticism); *Professionalism* is composed of the peer assessment and Openness; *General Achievement* is composed in almost equal parts of GPA and Agreeableness; and *Self-Awareness*.

- In health sciences education, psychomotor skills and technical skills—rarely defined in the health sciences literature—most commonly refer to motor and dexterity skills associated with carrying out physical examinations, clinical procedures, and surgery, and also using specialized medical equipment.

- Miller proposed a framework for assessing levels of clinical competence that encompasses the cognitive, affective, and psychomotor domains. In the pyramid, the lowest two levels test cognition (knowledge); this is the basis for initial learning of an area. The higher levels (shows, does) require more complex integration in the cognitive, affective, and psychomotor domains.

- Direct observations *in situ* or objective structured performance-related examinations (OSPREs) are methods to assess the higher levels of Miller's Pyramid.

INTRODUCTION

It is common practice in education and psychology to think of human behavior in three categories or domains: cognition (thinking), affect (feeling), and psychomotor (doing). Although we tend to discuss behavior in these separate ways, most behavior involves all three aspects or domains. The physician working with a patient, for example, is collecting information, arriving at a clinical impression and perhaps a diagnosis (thinking), making eye contact, nodding, smiling showing empathy (feeling), and palpating, percussing, and touching (doing). Aspects of all three domains are employed in complex, interactive ways. Nonetheless, for purposes of instructional design and assessment, we tend to approach these tasks in their separate domains.

While recognizing the interrelatedness of all three domains, in this chapter we will emphasize and discuss each in turn. Much of formal testing and assessment in education, in general, is in the cognitive domain (e.g., sciences, humanities, mathematics, etc.). Less formal testing occurs in the affective domain (e.g., music and art appreciation) and the psychomotor domain (e.g., lighting a Bunsen burner, keyboarding). In this chapter, we will in turn discuss assessment in the three domains with particular reference to medical and health profession education.

THE COGNITIVE DOMAIN

The cognitive domain has to do with thinking. We have learned a great deal about cognition, learning, and memory since Hermann Ebbinghaus' pioneering work more than 100 years ago.[1] His focus was on developing quantitative descriptions of psychological processes such as learning and forgetting and the precise mathematic assessment of these processes. Louis Thurstone was similarly preoccupied with systematizing the assessment of learning processes into mathematical equations, as well as the development of factor analysis (Chapters 4 and 6) and theories of intelligence. Thurstone's negative exponential or hyperbolic model learning curve represents a principle of learning in a variety of disciplines and for a variety of learners.[2] This model depicts learning as increasing rapidly with practice but attains an upper limit quickly and then flattens out. Figure 10.1 depicts data of the growth of aspects medical competence (physical exam, medical interview, clinical reasoning) during clinical clerkships.

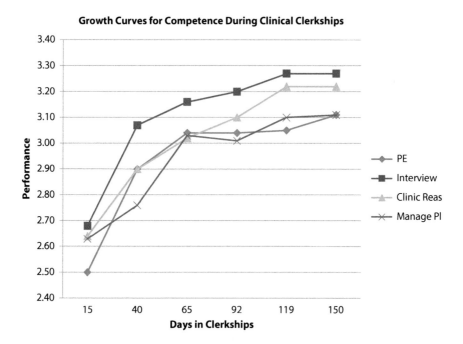

Figure 10.1 Negative exponential growth curves of competence.

Cognitive and educational psychologists have made scientific advances in the study of thinking, perception, memory, learning, and teaching in the past 100 years. Still, much of teaching and assessment in medicine and the other health professions is based on lore, intuition, anecdotal evidence, and personal experience. The use of Bloom's taxonomy is helpful in systematizing assessment.

Bloom's taxonomy of the cognitive domain is described in detail in Chapter 5. It is a simple, practical, and useful classification for assessment, learning, and teaching. Recall that there are six major categories, and the general objectives at each level provides the action verbs which are useful in writing objectives or constructing test items in each of these categories. It also helps to clarify cognition at high levels (i.e., analysis, synthesis, evaluation, creating) and more basic levels (i.e., knowledge, comprehension, application). While the knowledge can span all six categories, most assessment, teaching, and learning in medicine occurs at the first three levels. Much of the testing in these domains involves selection items or constructed response items.

Selection items

The most common type of selection items are multiple-choice questions (MCQs). Other forms of selection items include true-false and matching. In this item type, the answer is *selected* from a list following a prompt or a question; hence the term selection items. The construction and use of MCQs are detailed in Chapter 11. The other selection type items (true-false, matching) are so flawed from an assessment perspective that they are not used much and should be avoided in health sciences education.

Constructed response items

The most common type of constructed response items are essays. These are also referred to as open-ended items. Unlike MCQs, there is no list from which to select the answer. The student must *construct* the answer following a prompt or question. The major advantage that constructed response items have over selection item is that learning in the highest domains of Bloom's taxonomy can be assessed. In this item type, students can demonstrate fluency, flexibility, originality, elaboration, language mastery, and creativity in responses. The construction and use of constructed response items are detailed in Chapter 12.

Cognitive processes and development

Jean Piaget's theory[3] has several useful key ideas for learning and assessment in health sciences. His theory of intelligence is that we adapt to the world employing the dual cognitive processes of assimilation (the process by which material is taken into—subsumption—cognitive structures) and accommodation (the change made to cognitive structures as a result of assimilation). These cognitive structures are called schemas and are representations of perceptions, ideas, and/or actions, which go together. In its most practical sense then, Piaget's theory both helps to explain key ideas such as deliberate and interleaved practice, retrieval practice, and learning styles and how to assess them.

Assimilation takes in information through sensory input and attentional selection. This information is fit into existing schemas until the schemas no longer can hold new information. Accommodation occurs by restructuring, elaborating, or discarding the schema. Meaningful improvement in learning, therefore, results when the schemas or cognitive structures are altered. Such accommodating requires effortful learning. Organizations of schemas or cognitive maps help students organize their learning and facilitate the assimilation of new information and the subsequent accommodation by expanding, altering, or reorganizing schemas.

Piaget has proposed that human development proceeds in four stages of cognition: sensorimotor, preoperational, concrete operational, and formal operational period.

The sensorimotor stage is where infants construct knowledge and understand the world by sensorimotor interactions with objects (e.g., grasping, sucking, and tactile feeling). Infants progress from reflexive, instinctual action at birth to the beginning of symbolic thought (i.e. language) by age 18–24 months or so.

The second stage is the preoperational period where children's behavior is mainly categorized by symbolic play and manipulating symbols. This preoperational stage is characterized by intuitive, ego-centric behavior that lacks logic (ages 2–6 years). Behavior is intuitive and impulsive.

The third stage (ages 7–11 years), concrete operations, is characterized by the use of logic. At this stage, children apply logic mainly to concrete events or objects. They may be able to use inductive reasoning—drawing inferences from observations in order to make a generalization—but not deductive reasoning (using a generalized principle in order to try to predict the outcome of an event).

The final stage, formal operational stage (ages 11–13 years; adolescence and beyond), is characterized by logical use of symbols and abstract concepts. At this point, the person is capable of hypothetical and deductive reasoning. The adolescent or adult can employ hypothetical, counterfactual thinking (what-if), which is frequently required in science and healthcare. Other features of this stage include

- Abstract thought that considers possible outcomes and consequences of actions
- Metacognition, the capacity for thinking about thinking, allows reflection on one's own thought processes and monitors them
- Problem-solving with the ability to systematically solve a problem in a logical and methodical way

Most healthcare professionals and students should be functioning in the formal operational stage of cognitive development and therefore readily learn from symbolic content (speech, text, observation) and can be assessed accordingly. The SCT[4] is used to assess the ability to interpret medical information under conditions of uncertainty. It presents: (1) poorly defined clinical situations but respondents must choose between several realistic options; (2) the format allows flexible responses thus mirroring cognitive processes in problem-solving situations; and (3) scoring takes into account the variability of responses of experts to clinical situations.

This type of assessment is rooted in the highest stage of Piaget's cognitive reasoning. It is as important to assess or test the cognitive processes in this stage as the content of clinical reasoning as the SCT attempts to do. There still remain a number of challenges to develop assessments that measure not only the clinical content but also of the processes of problem-solving, abstract reasoning, and meta-cognition.

Continuous learning and assessment

With continuous learning, students acquire knowledge and increase learning intelligence (learning how-to-learn) through meta-cognition. The human brain is remarkably changeable. This phenomenon, known as neuroplasticity, refers to changes in neural pathways, synapses, and myelination due to learning, thinking, and changes in behavior. Although the architecture and gross structure of the brain are largely genetically determined, the detailed structure and neural networks are shaped by experience and can be modified.[5]

A recent naturalistic study has elegantly demonstrated this. To become a licensed taxi driver in London, trainees must learn the complex layout of London's streets over 4 years. Trainees that passed the tests of London streets had an increase in gray matter volume in their posterior hippocampi in brain scans. Controls and trainees that failed did not have structural brain changes.[6]

Continuous learning is valuable for its own sake and because it results in building new neural connections and intellectual capabilities. Students learn content and can increase their intelligence, both admirable educational outcomes. Both instructors and students need to work hard to form the cognitive structures and neural networks of meaningful learning that is deep and durable.

Additionally, students should be continuously tested so as to capitalize on the testing effect. Using retrieval practice with testing—working memory to recall or retrieve facts or knowledge—is more effective than reviewing content or re-reading text. Long-term memory is increased when some of the learning period is devoted to retrieving the information to-be-recalled. Testing practice produces better results than other forms of studying. Students who test themselves during learning or practice recall more than students who spend the same amount of time re-reading the complete information.

Retrieving information for a test will alter and strengthen it. Taking a test teaches students about a subject and they will perform better on a subsequent test than students who only reviewed or re-read the material. This is called the forward effect of testing.

A recent randomized study of neurology continuing medical education courses compared the effects of repeated quizzing—test-enhanced learning—and repeated studying on retention. A final test covering all information points from the course was taken 5 months after the course. Performance on the final test by neurologists showed that repeated quizzing led to significantly greater long-term retention (almost twice as much) relative to both repeated studying and no further exposure.[7]

THREE COMPETING THEORIES OF CLINICAL REASONING

Schmidt et al.[8] proposed a cognitive structure of medical expertise model based on the accumulation of clinically relevant knowledge about disease signs and symptoms referred to as illness scripts. In this model, the development of elaborate knowledge networks evolves through a process of biomedical knowledge acquisition, practical clinical experience, and an integration or encapsulation of both theoretical and experiential knowledge.

There is some support for the knowledge encapsulation theory, which postulates that basic science knowledge has an indirect influence on diagnostic reasoning by contributing directly to clinical knowledge. A large-scale study employing more than 20,714 medical graduates lent support to the encapsulation theory.[8] In this model, the biomedical or basic science knowledge in the first 2 years of medical school precedes and is eventually incorporated during the acquisition of clinical knowledge. Accordingly, basic science knowledge becomes encapsulated or reorganized into causal representations of illness scripts that lead to the formal process of diagnostic and clinical reasoning.

In the distinct world model, the relationship between basic science knowledge and clinical knowledge are unique domains with their own distinct structure and characteristics.[9] Diagnostic or clinical reasoning, from the clinical knowledge obtained from patient presentations of signs and symptoms, develops to taxonomy of disease. The activation of clinical knowledge is primary in the diagnostic or clinical reasoning process. Although this process rarely relies on the strict use of basic science knowledge, pathophysiological explanations can provide further support for the explanation of clinical phenomena.

Another theory of medical expertise is the independent influence model. Both basic science knowledge and clinical knowledge are independently related to diagnostic performance or clinical competency. Basic science knowledge provides a foundational basis in medical diagnosis. Clinical experience and knowledge are acquired temporally (second half of medical school and residency) and geographically (on the wards and clinics) separate from basic science knowledge (in the first half in classrooms and labs). As accurate diagnostic thinking develops with gained experience, students and residents draw on knowledge of the anatomy and physiology of the human body. In constructing clinical case representations, they recognize clinical phenomena and activate basic science knowledge to account for unexplained symptoms and to specify a diagnosis.

Experimental work

Several experimental studies have addressed the problem if and how basic sciences can become integrated into clinical reasoning or clinical skills. Employing medical students, physician assistant students, and nursing students, researchers compared a spatial and temporal proximity of clinical content to basic sciences versus a purposeful, explicit teaching model that exposes relationships between the domains. They concluded that proximity alone is insufficient for integration but that explicit and specific teaching may be necessary to facilitate integration for the learner. Integration requires teaching basic science information in a manner that creates a relationship between basic science and clinical science thus resulting in conceptual coherence—mental representations of clinical and basic science information that can help learners find meaning in clinical problems.[10]

In another study, undergraduate dental and dental hygiene students ($n = 112$) were taught the radiographic features and pathophysiology underlying four intrabony abnormalities with a test-enhanced (TE) condition (thought to enhance learning and cognitive integration) and a study (ST) condition. TE participants outperformed those in the ST condition group on immediate and delayed diagnostic testing, but there were no differences in a memory test between the groups. The inclusion of the basic science test appears to have improved the students' understanding of the underlying disease mechanisms learned and also improved their performance on a test of diagnostic accuracy.[11]

Both the experimental work and the correlational-based research (e.g., Pearson's r, regression, and latent variable path analyses) suggest the need for purposeful, direct teaching for integration and encapsulation of basic sciences into clinical reasoning and clinical skills. This integration and encapsulation needs to be assessed and tested dynamically to determine the cognitive processes and outcomes of such pedagogy. Such complex hypothesized models of medical expertise of aptitude for medical school, basic science achievement, and clinical competency employing longitudinal data can be studied within structural equation modelling (SEM). Accordingly, the development of medical expertise and clinical competency can be empirically verified.

AFFECTIVE DOMAIN

The affective domain has to do with feeling and emotions. The areas in psychology that generally deal with the affective domain are personality, motivation, interests, and attitudes.

Bloom is also credited for developing a taxonomy in the affective domain.[12] As with the cognitive domain, the affective domain provides a framework for teaching, training, assessing, and evaluating the effectiveness of training as well as curriculum design and delivery (Table 10.1).

Table 10.2 is a list of ten typical adjectives for healthcare professionals in the affective domain. Each is followed by some behavioral descriptors. Most of these are values at the higher levels of Bloom's taxonomy (levels 3, 4, 5).

Self-/peer assessment

Self- and peer assessment is used frequently as a tool to evaluate students, residents, and physicians as the basis of their professional behaviors. The Rochester peer assessment protocol (RPAP), a form consisting of 15 items, is an instrument

Table 10.1 Bloom's taxonomy in the affective domain

Category	Behaviors	Types of experience	Verbs that describe the activity
1. Receiving	Openness to experience and learning	Attend, focus interest learning experience, take notes, devote time for learning experience, participate passively	Ask, listen, focus, attend, take part, discuss, acknowledge, hear, be open to, retain, follow, concentrate, read, do, feel
2. Responding	React and participate actively	Participate actively, interest in outcomes, enthusiasm for action, question and probe ideas, make interpretations	React, respond, seek clarification, interpret, clarify, show motivation, contribute, question, present, cite, help team, write, perform
3. Valuing	Attach values and express personal opinions	Evaluate worth and relevance of ideas, experiences; commit to course of action	Argue, confront, justify, persuade, criticize, challenge, debate, refute
4. Organizing values	Reconcile internal conflicts; develop value system	Refine personal views and reasons, state beliefs	Build, develop, formulate, defend, modify, relate, reconcile, compare, contrast
5. Internalizing values	Adopt belief system and philosophy	Self-reliant; consistency with personal value set	Act, display, influence, solve, practice

Table 10.2 Professional behavior evaluation

1. Self-confidence—demonstrates the ability to trust personal judgment, an awareness of strengths and limitations; exercises good personal judgment
2. Communications—speaks clearly; writes legibly; listens actively; adjusts communication as needed to various situations
3. Integrity—consistently honest, can be trusted with confidential information, complete and accurate documentation of patient care and learning activities
4. Empathy—shows compassion and respect for others, calm, compassionate, and helpful demeanor toward those in need, be supportive and reassuring
5. Respect—polite to others, does not use derogatory or demeaning terms
6. Self-motivation—initiative to complete assignments, improve and/or correct behavior, following through on tasks, enthusiasm for learning and improvement, accepting constructive feedback in a positive manner, taking advantage of learning opportunities
7. Appearance and personal hygiene—clothing is appropriate, neat, clean and well maintained, good personal hygiene and grooming
8. Time management—consistently punctual, completes tasks and assignments on time
9. Teamwork and collaboration—places the success of the team above self-interest; does not undermine the team; shows respect for all team members; remains flexible and open to change; communicates with others to resolve problems
10. Patient advocacy—free from personal bias or feelings that interfere with patient care; places the needs of patients above self-interest; protects and respects patient confidentiality and dignity

commonly used to assess professional behaviors and attitudes in medical students and has been studied extensively for reliability and validity evidence.[13] Additional research on peer assessment in medical students reveals that there is high correlation in the pre- and post-test scores of the RPAP when administered longitudinally, and that there is no bias in rater evaluation of the students when the students being evaluated chose their assessors.[14]

Data in Table 10.3 contain typical assessment in the affective domains for both peer and self-ratings. A factor analysis was conducted for the peer questionnaire as the 15 items from the peer assessment were intercorrelated using Pearson product–moment correlations based on 120 students. The correlation matrix was then decomposed into principal components, and these were subsequently rotated to the normalized varimax criterion. Items were considered to be part of a factor if their primary loading was on that factor. The number of factors to be extracted was based on the Kaiser rule (i.e., eigenvalues > 1.0).

The factor analysis showed that the data on the peer questionnaire decomposed into two factors that accounted for 67.8% of the total variance: (1) work

Table 10.3 Peer and self-ratings on professionalism

Questionnaire items	Peer rating factor structure		Peer ratings	Self-ratings
	Work habits	Interpersonal habits	Mean (SD), Min-Max	Mean (SD), Min-Max
1. Is prepared for sessions	0.744		4.82 (0.45), 1–5	4.52 (0.57), 3–5
2. Identifies and solves problems using data	0.802		4.89 (0.37), 1–5	4.72 (0.49), 3–5
3. Able to explain clearly	0.745		4.87 (0.39), 1–5	4.56 (0.58), 3–5
4. Compassion and empathy		0.705	4.89 (.39), 1–5	4.85 (0.40), 3–5
5. Seeks to understand others' views	0.517	0.599	4.87 (0.39), 1–5	4.85 (0.36), 3–5
6. Initiative and leadership	0.747		4.67 (0.58), 1–5	4.40 (0.66), 3–5
7. Information or resource sharing	0.804		4.84 (0.43), 1–5	4.59 (0.59), 2–5
8. Assumes responsibility	0.753	0.407	4.88 (0.39), 1–5	4.73 (0.49), 3–5
9. Seeks and employs feedback	0.666		4.81 (0.48), 1–5	4.59 (0.59), 3–5
10. Presents consistently to superiors and peers—Trustworthy	0.416	0.787	4.91 (0.37), 1–5	4.90 (0.30), 4–5
11. Admits and corrects own mistakes—Truthful	0.521	0.642	4.90 (0.36), 1–5	4.82 (0.41), 3–5
12. Dress and appearance appropriate		0.803	4.95 (0.31), 1–5	4.89 (0.41), 2–5
13. Behavior is appropriate		0.862	4.90 (0.40), 1–5	4.80 (0.50), 2–5
14. Directs own learning—Think and work independently	0.784		4.88 (0.38), 1–5	4.71 (0.54), 3–5
15. I would refer family, patients, self to this future physician		0.766	4.81 (0.50), 1–5	—
Percent of variance	57.65	10.11	—	—
Cronbach's α	0.81	0.85	0.95	0.87

habits and (2) interpersonal habits but with work habits accounting for a large proportion of the variance (57.7% versus 10.1% for interpersonal habits—Table 10.3). Four items (#5—Seeks to understand others' views; #8—Assumes responsibility; #10—Presents consistently to superiors and peers—Trustworthy; #11—Admits and corrects own mistakes—Truthful) load on both factors (i.e., split loadings—see Table 10.3) as these items are relevant to both work and interpersonal habits.

Cronbach's α for internal consistency reliability indicated that both of the self and peer instruments' full scales had high reliability ($\alpha = 0.87$ and 0.95, respectively). The reliability for both factors (subscales) for the peer questionnaire had high reliability as well ($\alpha = 0.81$ and 0.85).

Personality and professionalism

One test that has been used to study medical student characteristics and performance is the NEO-PI, which is referred to as the Big Five Personality Inventory. This inventory measures five broad traits, domains, or dimensions in the affective domain. These are neuroticism (N), extraversion (E), openness (O), conscientiousness (C), and agreeableness (A). Conscientiousness has been found to be a predictor of performance in medical school and becomes increasingly important as students and residents advance through medical training. Other traits concerning sociability (i.e. extraversion, openness, and neuroticism) have also been found to be relevant for performance and adaptation in the healthcare environment.[15] The traits of neuroticism and conscientiousness are related to stress in medical school: low extroversion, high neuroticism, and high conscientiousness, results in highly stressed students (brooders), while high extroversion, low neuroticism, and low conscientiousness produces low-stressed students (hedonists).[16]

STRUCTURE OF PROFESSIONALISM, PERSONALITY, ACHIEVEMENT, AND APTITUDE

In order to explore the structure of personality, achievement, aptitude, and professionalism, a factor analysis was conducted employing the peer total score, self-total score, MCAT subtests scores, undergraduate grade point average (UGPA), and the five dimensions from the NEO-PI.

One-hundred-and-twenty medical students (64 men, 53.3% and 56 women, 46.7%) participated in a study. Data were obtained on (1) Rochester Peer Assessment Tool (RPAT), (2) a self-assessment survey contains the first 14 items of the peer assessment but adopted in the first person; (3) The NEO-PI is a 44 item personality inventory that describes five personality characteristics, and (4) MCAT scores and undergraduate GPA.

These variables were intercorrelated using Pearson product–moment correlations and the resulting matrix was decomposed into principal components and then rotated to the normalized varimax criterion (converged in eight iterations). The number of factors extracted was based partly on the Kaiser rule (i.e., Eigenvalues > 1.0) and partly on the theoretical meaning and cohesiveness of the factors. A close inspection of the results of this analysis in Table 10.4 shows

Table 10.4 Factor analysis of personality, peer assessment, self-assessment, aptitude and achievement

	Factor				
	Aptitude for science	Aptitude for medicine	Professionalism	General achieve-ment	Self-awareness
Extraversion	0.601				
Agreeableness				0.785	
Conscientious-ness		0.829			
Neuroticism		−0.660			
Openness			0.701		
MCAT VR score		0.478			0.435
MCAT PS score	0.559				
MCAT BS score	0.801				
Peer assessment			0.757		
Self-assessment					0.901
UGPA				0.755	
Percent of variance	17.5	15.9	12.1	10.3	9.2

five factors with their variance accounting properties: (1) Aptitude for Science, (2) Aptitude for Medicine, (3) Peer Professionalism, (4) General Achievement, and (5) Self-Awareness for a total of 64.9% of the variance.

STRUCTURE OF PERSONALITY, PROFESSIONALISM, AND COGNITIVE VARIABLES

The five factors for the structure of professionalism, aptitude, achievement, and personality accounted for more than two-thirds of the total variance. These factors are cohesive and theoretically meaningful. The first factor, Aptitude for Science, consists of MCAT Biological Sciences and Physical Sciences loadings as well as Extraversion, a characteristic of students with science aptitude who select to work with people (e.g., medicine). The second factor, Aptitude for Medicine, contains the MCAT Verbal score together with Conscientiousness and, inversely, Neuroticism—both important dimensions of personality consistent with high performance in medicine. The third factor, Professionalism, is composed of the Peer Assessment and Openness, which are theoretically cohesive characteristics. The fourth factor—General Achievement—is composed in almost equal parts of undergraduate GPA and Agreeableness, a factor that is important in achievement. The fifth factor, Self-Awareness, is composed of the Self-Assessment scores and MCAT Verbal score. Interestingly, the MCAT Verbal score has almost equal split loadings on Aptitude for

Medicine and Self-Awareness, possibly a result of verbal abilities for both of these dimensions.

Summary

The main findings are (1) the psychometric properties (response rates, descriptive statistics, reliability, validity evidence from factor analysis, feasibility) of the self–peer instrument are in accordance with theoretical expectations, (2) personality factors—Openness, Conscientiousness, Neuroticism—are significantly related to peer assessment of professionalism, and (3) factor analysis of personality, achievement, aptitude, and professionalism data results in five theoretically meaningful and cohesive factors.

PSYCHOMOTOR DOMAIN

The psychomotor domain has to do with doing or action. It was established to address skills development relating to the physical dimensions of accomplishing a task. Table 10.5 contains a classification of the psychomotor domain.

In health sciences education, psychomotor skills and technical skills—rarely defined in the health sciences literature—most commonly refer to the cognitive, motor, and dexterity skills associated with carrying out physical examinations, clinical procedures, and surgery by using specialized medical equipment. They also frequently include skills associated with conducting physical examinations, using specialized non-surgical equipment and administering medicines.

A recent study[18] sets out to determine which instruments exist to directly assess psychomotor skills in medical trainees on live patients and to identify the data indicating their psychometric and edumetric properties. This was to address the Accreditation Council for Graduate Medical Education (ACGME) Milestone Project that mandates programs to assess the attainment of training outcomes, including the psychomotor (surgical or procedural) skills of medical trainees. In a systematic review, researchers identified a total of 30 instruments used to assess psychomotor skills such as the following:

- sigmoidoscopy-generic skills; sigmoidoscopy-specific skills
- colonoscopy-generic skills, colonoscopy-specific skills
- laparoscopic skills (depth perception, bimanual dexterity, efficiency)
- epidural anesthesia
- laparoscopic cholecystectomy
- ophthalmic plastic surgical skills
- microsurgery skills

Construct validity was identified in 24 instruments, internal consistency in 14, test–retest reliability in five, and inter-rater reliability in 20. The modification of attitudes, knowledge, or skills was reported using five tools. Jelovsek et al.[18] concluded that while numerous instruments are available for the assessment of psychomotor skills

Table 10.5 Dave's psychomotor domain[17]

Category or stage	Behaviors	Types of experience	Verbs that describe the activity
1. Imitation	Copy action of another; observe and replicate	Observe instructor and repeat action, process or activity	Copy, follow, replicate, repeat, adhere, attempt, reproduce, organize, sketch, duplicate
2. Manipulation	Reproduce activity from instruction or memory	Follow written or verbal instruction	Re-create, build, perform, execute, implement, acquire, conduct, operate
3. Precision	Execute skill reliably, independent of help, activity is quick, smooth, and accurate	Perform a task or activity with expertise and to high quality without assistance or instruction; can demonstrate an activity	Demonstrate, complete, show, perfect, calibrate, control, achieve, accomplish, master, refine
4. Articulation	Adapt and integrate expertise to satisfy a new context or task	Combine elements to develop methods to meet varying, novel requirements	Solve, adapt, combine, coordinate, integrate, adapt, develop, formulate, master
5. Naturalization	Instinctive, effortless, unconscious mastery of activity and related skills at strategic level	Define aim, approach and strategy for use of activities to meet strategic need	Construct, compose, create, design, specify, manage, invent, project-manage, originate

in medical trainees, the evidence supporting their psychometric (i.e., reliability and validity) and edumetric (usability, training) properties is limited.

MILLER'S PYRAMID OF CLINICAL COMPETENCE: BRINGING THE DOMAINS TOGETHER

Miller proposed a framework for assessing levels of clinical competence (Figure 2.1)[19] that encompasses the cognitive, affective, and psychomotor domains. In the pyramid, the lowest two levels test cognition (knowledge) and this is the basis for initial learning of the area. Novice learners may know something about a neurological examination, for example, or they may know how to do a neurological examination.

The upper two levels test behavior or competence to determine if learners can apply what they know into practice. They can show how to do a neurological examination or do they actually do a neurological examination in practice. Doing such work includes both the affective domain (patient's focus, physician's empathy, etc.) and the psychomotor domain (physician skills in checking reflexes, muscle strength, etc.).

Cognitive performance (knows or knows how) does not generally correlate well with behavior performance (shows or does). A trainee who knows how to do something doesn't necessarily mean that they will be able to do it in practice. Nonetheless, the knowing is an important foundation for the "knows how" and "does" (Figure 10.2).

1. Knows: some knowledge
2. Knows how: to apply that knowledge
3. Shows: shows how to apply that knowledge
4. Does: applies that knowledge in practice

Miller's Pyramid model has been used to match assessment methods to the competency being tested. An MCQ test for students' examination of the shoulder might show they know about it but not that they can actually do it. The test shows

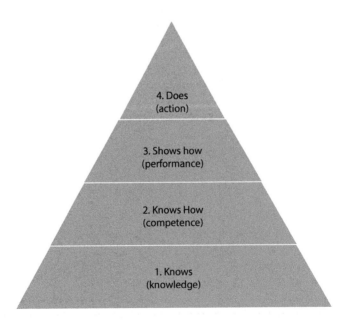

Figure 10.2 Miller's Pyramid of clinical competence.

how an OSCE type station to examine the shoulder might be used. Direct observation in the workplace itself would provide even better ecological validity.

The Miller model can also help formulate objectives for a particular assessment session: this requires careful articulation of the objectives to be achieved. A test of learner's ability to assess risk for a cardiac event, for example, might include the following objectives and the level of Miller's Pyramid being represented:

- Understands what is meant by risk for a cardiac event and why it is important (knows)
- Knows what to do if the risk is high (knows how)
- Can demonstrate the use of the cardiac risk calculator (shows)

To test at the does level, a practical workplace-based session would be most appropriate. Other methods might include a review of video consultations with real patients.

The model can also be used to create testing sessions at the appropriate level for learners. For instance, for assessing communication skills:

- Learners in their early stages of development may be tested on why it is important to solicit patient's ideas, concerns, and expectations and what the evidence says (knows)
- More experienced learners may be tested on how they might actually elicit ideas, concerns, and expectations: what phrases they might use (knows how)
- For advanced learners, direct observations *in situ* such as reviewing videos of actual consultations with patient may be employed (does)

Objective structured performance-related examination combining the domains

In a study of surgical residents, researchers[20] assessed surgical skills together with communication and professionalism in an objective structured performance-related examination (OSPRE). In this seven station OSPRE, they assessed skills in excision of a skin lesion, central line, chest tube insertion, enterotomy closure, tracheostomy, laparoscopic task, and acquiring informed consent (Table 10.6). Therefore, all levels of Miller's Pyramid were involved for this performance assessment of communication, professionalism, and surgical skills competencies.

The internal consistency reliability of the checklists and global rating scales combined was adequate for communication ($\alpha = 0.75-0.92$), surgical skills ($\alpha = 0.86-0.96$) but not for professionalism ($\alpha = 0$). There was evidence of validity as surgical skills performance improved as a function of PGY level but not for the professionalism checklist. Surgical skills and communication correlated in the two stations assessed ($r = 0.55$ and 0.57, $p < 0.05$). There is evidence for both reliability and validity for simultaneously assessing surgical skills and communication skills.

Table 10.6 Station name, content, and skills assessed for surgical residents

Station #	Name	Assessed skills	Mean (SD)	Cronbach's α
1	Excision of a skin lesion	Communication + surgical skills	82 (15.33)	0.87
2	Central line	Surgical skills	82 (16.20)	0.60
3	Chest tube insertion	Communication + surgical skills	83 (8.15)	0.19
4	Enterotomy closure	Surgical skills	80 (18.40)	0.58
5	Tracheostomy	Professionalism + surgical skills	80 (9.17)	0.68
6	Laparoscopic task	Professionalism + surgical skills	45 (19.74)	0.90
7	Acquiring informed consent	Communication in surgical context	61 (15.07)	0.69

Surgical skills performance

The performance of the residents (shows how—the 3rd level of Miller's Pyramid) in the surgical tasks was good in the first five stations (excision of a skin lesion, insertion of a central line, chest tube insertion, enterotomy closure, and tracheostomy) with a minimum mean score of 80%. The laparoscopic task (station 6) was to tie a square knot using an intracorporeal technique utilizing a laparoscopic simulator, a task that requires advanced technical skills. At this level, this task proved too difficult.

The correlation of the checklists and global rating scales within stations was high for most of the stations, with the exception of Station 3 (chest tube insertion). This was a very easy task for the residents thus producing low variability and a low correlation. Other easy tasks were in station 1, excision of a skin lesion, and station 5, tracheostomy.

In the present study, there was construct validity evidence for the OSPRE for assessing surgical skills. The year of enrollment of the resident was related to performance in surgical skills where PGY-4 residents outperformed PGY-1 residents. This finding is evidence of construct validity because of the known group differences; there was a clear difference in performance between junior and senior residents. There were no statistically significant differences between the four PGY levels and communication skills. This provides evidence of divergent validity as such differences would not be expected.

To assess at the highest level of Miller's Pyramid (does: applies knowledge and skills in practice), the surgical residents should be observed performing these task in the clinic with real patients. This would involve the use of a rating scale or checklist (e.g., min-CEX) while the resident was performing the task. The resulting data allows for assessment and evaluation of the trainee at the highest levels of competence.

SUMMARY AND MAIN POINTS

The various formats of testing for cognition, affect, and psychomotor skills are viewed independently but are integrated in practice. These include selection type items (multiple-choice questions, constructed response, checklists, and other item formats). Bloom's taxonomies of cognitive, affective, and psychomotor skills and Miller's Pyramid of clinical competence inform assessment practices across the domains.

- It is common practice to think of human behavior in three categories or domains: cognition (thinking), affect (feeling), and psychomotor (doing). Although we tend to discuss behavior in these separate ways, most behavior involves all three aspects or domains.
- Thurstone's negative exponential or hyperbolic model learning curve represents a principle of learning in a variety of disciplines and for a variety of learners; learning increases rapidly with practice but attains an upper limit quickly and then flattens out.
- Notwithstanding scientific advances in the study of thinking, perception, memory, learning, much of assessment in medicine and the other health professions is based on lore, intuition, anecdotal evidence, and personal experience. The use of Bloom's taxonomies is helpful in systematizing assessment.
- Much of the testing in these domains involves selection items (e.g., multiple choice) or constructed response (e.g., essays) items.
- Jean Piaget's theory of intelligence is that we adapt to the world employing the dual cognitive processes of assimilation and accommodation. The theory both helps to explain key ideas such as deliberate and interleaved practice, retrieval practice, and learning styles and how to assess them.
- The SCT is used to assess the ability to interpret medical information under conditions of uncertainty, tapping Piaget's highest levels of cognitive functioning. There still remain a number of challenges to assess the processes of problem-solving, abstract reasoning, and meta-cognition.
- Students should be continuously tested so as to capitalize on the testing effect. Using retrieval practice with testing—working memory to recall or retrieve facts or knowledge—is more effective than reviewing content or re-reading text.
- Both the experimental work and the correlational-based research suggest the need for purposeful, direct teaching for *integration* and *encapsulation* of basic sciences into clinical reasoning and skills. This integration and encapsulation needs to be *assessed and tested dynamically* to determine the cognitive processes and outcomes of such pedagogy.
- Bloom is credited for developing a taxonomy in the affective (feeling) domain that provides a framework for teaching, training, assessing, and evaluating the effectiveness of training as well as curriculum design and delivery.

- In the affective domain, the structure of professionalism, aptitude, achievement, and personality are accounted by *Aptitude for Science* (cognitive variables and extraversion—a characteristic of working with people (e.g., medicine); *Aptitude for Medicine*, (cognitive variables and Conscientiousness and, inversely, Neuroticism); *Professionalism*, is composed of the peer assessment and Openness; *General Achievement* is composed in almost equal parts of GPA and Agreeableness; and *Self-Awareness*.
- In health sciences education, psychomotor skills and technical skills—rarely defined in the health sciences literature—most commonly refer to motor and dexterity skills associated with carrying out physical examinations, clinical procedures, and surgery, and also using specialized medical equipment.
- Miller proposed a framework for assessing levels of clinical competence that encompasses the cognitive, affective, and psychomotor domains. In the pyramid, the lowest two levels test cognition (knowledge); this is the basis for initial learning of an area. The higher levels (shows, does) require more complex integration in the cognitive, affective, and psychomotor domains.
- Direct observations in situ or objective structured performance-related examinations (OSPREs) are methods to assess at the higher levels of Miller's Pyramid.

REFLECTIONS AND EXERCISES

Reflections

1. Compare and contrast the cognitive, affective, and psychomotor domains. (Maximum 500 words)
2. Critically evaluate Thurstone's negative exponential learning curve as a principle of learning in a variety of disciplines and for a variety of learners. (Maximum 500 words).
3. Respond to the statement "Notwithstanding scientific advances much of assessment in the health professions is based on lore, intuition, anecdotal evidence, and personal experience" (Maximum 500 words).
4. How does Jean Piaget's theory of intelligence explain key ideas such as deliberate and interleaved practice, retrieval practice, and learning styles and how to assess them? (Maximum 500 words)
5. Why is using retrieval practice with testing—working memory to recall or retrieve facts or knowledge—more effective than reviewing content or re-reading text? (Maximum 500 words)
6. Discuss direct observations in situ or objective structured performance-related examinations (OSPREs) as methods to assess at the higher levels of Miller's Pyramid (Maximum 500 words).

Exercises

1. Create an assessment for the cognitive, affective, and psychomotor domains for surgery in the OR (Maximum 250 words).
2. In a study, a large number of residents ($n = 300$) were assessed on multiple tests that assess in all three domains. Correlations (Pearson's r) among the tests from 0.30 to 0.54. Do these results provide evidence of validity? Explain. (Maximum 250 words).
3. Interpret the reliabilities for each station in Table 10.6 (Maximum 250 words).
4. In Table 10.4, the factor loading for Neuroticism on *Aptitude for Medicine* was −0.660. Interpret this result (Maximum 250 words)

REFERENCES

1. Ebbinghaus H. *Memory: A Contribution to Experimental Psychology.* New York: Dover, 1885.
2. Thurstone LL. The learning curve equation. *Psychological Monographs* 1919, 26, 114 pages.
3. Piaget J. *The Psychology of Intelligence.* Totowa, NJ: Littlefield, 1972.
4. Lubarsky S, Dory V, Duggan P, Gagnon R, Charlin B. Script concordance testing: From theory to practice: AMEE guide no. 75. *Medical Teacher* 2013, 35(3), 184–193.
5. Pascual-Leone A, Freitas C, Oberman L, Horvath JC, Halko M, Eldaief M, Bashir S, Vernet M, Shafi M, Westover B, Vahabzadeh-Hagh AM, Rotenberg A. Characterizing brain cortical plasticity and network dynamics across the age-span in health and disease with TMS-EEG and TMS-fMRI. *Brain Topography* 2011, 24, 302–315.
6. Woollett K & Maguire EA. Acquiring "the Knowledge" of London's layout drives structural brain changes. *Current Biology* 2011, 21, 2109–2114.
7. Larsen DP, Butler AC, Aung WY, Corboy JR, Friedman DI, Sperling MR. The effects of test-enhanced learning on long-term retention in AAN annual meeting courses. *Neurology* 2015, 84, 748–754.
8. Collin T, Violato C, Hecker K. Aptitude, achievement and competence in medicine: A latent variable path model. *Advances in Health Science Education* 2008, 14, 355–366.
9. Patel VL, Evans DA, Groen GJ. Reconciling basic science and clinical reasoning. *Teaching and Learning in Medicine* 1989, 1, 116–121.
10. Kulasegaram KM, Manzone JC, Ku C, Skye A, Wadey V, Woods NN. Cause and effect: Testing a mechanism and method for the cognitive integration of basic science. *Academic Medicine* 2015, 90(11 suppl), S63–S69.

11. Baghdady MT, Carnahan H, Lam E, Woods NN. Test-enhanced learning and its effect on comprehension and diagnostic accuracy. *Medical Education* 2014, 48, 181–188.

12. Bloom B, Krathwhol D, Masia C. Taxonomy of educational objectives, Vol. II. *The Affective Domain*. New York: David McKay Company, Inc., 1964.

13. Epstein RM, Dannefer EF, Nofziger AC, Hansen JT, Schultz SH, Jospe N, Connard LW, Meldrum SC, Henson LC. Comprehensive assessment of professional competence: The Rochester experiment. *Teaching and Learning in Medicine* 2004, 16(2), 186–196.

14. Lurie SJ, Nofziger AC, Meldrum S, Mooney C, Epstein RM. Effects of rater selection on peer assessment among medical students. *Medical Education* 2006, 40(11), 1088–1097.

15. Doherty EM, Nugent E. Personality factors and medical training: A review of the literature. *Medical Education* 2011, 45(2), 132–140.

16. Tyssen R, Dolatowski FC, Rovik JO, Thorkildsen RF, Ekeberg O, Hem E, Gude T, Gronvold NT, Vaglum P. Personality traits and types predict medical school stress: A six-year longitudinal and nationwide study. *Medical Education* 2007, 41(8), 781–787.

17. Dave RH. *Psychomotor Domain*. Berlin: International Conference of Educational Testing, 1967.

18. Jelovsek EJ, Kow N, Diwadkar GB. Tools for the direct observation and assessment of psychomotor skills in medical trainees: A systematic review. *Medical Education* 2013, 47, 650–673.

19. Miller GE. The assessment of clinical skills/competence/performance. *Academic Medicine* 1990, 65, s63–s67.

20. Ponton-Carss A, Hutchison C, Violato C. Assessment of communication, professionalism, and surgical skills in an objective structured performance-related examination (OSPRE): A psychometric study. *American Journal of Surgery* 2011, 202(4), 433–440.

11

Constructing
multiple-choice items

ADVANCED ORGANIZERS

- Multiple-choice items are objective tests, because they can be scored routinely according to a predetermined key, eliminating the judgments of the scorers.
- The first step to constructing valid tests is to develop a test blueprint as it serves as a tool to help ensure the content validity of an exam.
- The multiple-choice item consists of several parts: the stem, the keyed-response, and several distractors. The keyed-response is the "right" answer or the option indicated on the key. All of the possible alternative answers are called options.
- The stems should include verbs such as define, describe, identify (knowledge), defend, explain, interpret, explain (comprehension), and predict, operate, compute, discover, apply (application).
- In a review of 46 authoritative textbooks and other sources in educational measurement, Haladyna et al. developed a taxonomy of 43 multiple-choice item writing rules.
- In criterion-referenced testing, it is necessary to establish cutoff scores for pass/fail. One very common and simple way to do this is called a minimum performance level (MPL) in discussion among experts on the minimally competent candidate.
- For each distractor, experts identify the probability that they believe a hypothetical minimally competent examinee could rule out as incorrect. Quartile probabilities (e.g., 25%, 50%, etc.) are usually used though deciles (10%, 20%, etc.) could also be used. The probabilities for each expert (2–3) for each option are averaged. The total test score MPL (passing score) is the sum of each item MPL.

INTRODUCTION

The objectivity of a test refers to how it is scored. Tests are objectively scored to the extent that independent scorers can agree on the number of points answers should receive. If observers can agree on scoring criteria, subjective judgments, and opinions can be minimized, the test is said to be objective. Scoring procedures on some objective tests, such as multiple-choice questions (MCQs), have been so carefully planned that scoring can be automated on a computer.

Objectivity in scoring is necessary if measurements are to be useful. Multiple-choice items are objective tests because they can be scored routinely according to a predetermined key, eliminating the judgments of the scorers. Objective test items produce higher reliability assessments than do subjective test items (e.g., essays) and are therefore more desirable. MCQs are efficient and effective for assessing the first three levels of Bloom's taxonomy (*knowledge, comprehension, application*—Table 5.1) and, arguably, some higher levels (e.g., *analysis*). There is consensus among testing experts that MCQs can and should be used to measure the first three levels of Bloom's taxonomy because they are objective, efficient, and effective. Open-ended items (e.g., essays) should be used to assess learning outcomes at the higher levels (*analysis, synthesis, evaluation*) because this assessment requires originality, elaboration, and divergent thinking which cannot be done by MCQs. Open-ended or essay tests are discussed in Chapter 12.

BEFORE CONSTRUCTING ITEMS

The first step to constructing valid tests is to develop a TOS or test blueprint (see Table 5.2, Chapter 5). The test blueprint serves as a tool to help ensure the content validity of an exam. As you study the blueprint presented in Table 5.2, you will notice that the content of the course has been subdivided into a number of subtopics. Moreover, each section of the course has been given an overall percentage of emphasis for the test. For example, the subtopic *Preventive Cardiology* contains 20 items or 27% of the total test. By inference, the topic that receives the greatest emphasis on the test should also have received the greatest emphasis in the course learning activities. Very close to 27% of the course should have focused on *Preventive Cardiology*. If there is a discrepancy in this, alter the exam emphasis to reflect the course.

In addition to the appropriate emphasis, test construction benefits from considering the appropriate cognitive level of assessment. The accompanying test blueprint identifies the first four levels of Bloom's taxonomy (*i.e. knowledge, comprehension, application, higher*) as appropriate levels for the testing material related to the course (Table 5.1). The issue of cognitive levels for testing is elaborated below. In summary, using the test blueprint helps ensure that all required course topics are covered at an appropriate level of understanding thereby enhancing content validity.

CONSTRUCTING MULTIPLE-CHOICE TEST ITEMS

The multiple-choice item consists of several parts, the *stem*, the *keyed-response,* and several *distractors.* The keyed-response is the "right" answer or the *option* indicated on the *key.* All of the possible alternative answers are called *options.*

Stem

1. Widely spaced eyes, thin upper lip, and short eyelid openings in the preschool child are typical of

   Options

   A. Down's syndrome

   B. fetal alcohol syndrome*

   C. rubella during the child's prenatal development

   D. the effects of thalidomide

   * = *Keyed-response* (other options A, C, & D are distractors).

The stem presents the problem. It may be in two formats: (1) incomplete statement (as above) or (2) complete statement (such as a full interrogative). The stem may be quite brief as in the example above or may be lengthy and include numbers, formulae, charts, photographs, and other material. The point is to present a problem in the stem that is best solved or answered by one option (the keyed-response). The stem should be clear, well-written, and free from extraneous or irrelevant material.

Possibly the most difficult task in constructing multiple-choice items is to write *plausible* distractors. That is, distractors which may appear correct to the confused candidate or one with little or partial knowledge. "Schizophrenia," for example, would not be a plausible distractor in the above example, because even candidates with little or no knowledge could eliminate it as clearly incorrect. Following is an example of a more extensive MCQ:

2. A study of the etiology of breast cancer involves recruiting female volunteers to the study by their physicians. All participants are screened for previous cancer or pre-cancerous or chronic diseases. In other words, all patients are healthy at the beginning of the study. The study will last 25 years and women who become ill with breast cancer will be compared on social, psychological, biological, genetic, and familial factors to matched peers who have not become ill. This study design is best described as a

   A. direct, clinical observation study
   B. matched, cross-sectional/longitudinal study
   C. prospective, case-comparison study*
   D. retrospective, case-comparison study
   E. population-based panel study

The stem of this item is much longer than the previous item (#1) and therefore requires much more reading time although both receive an equal weight (1 point).

This is generally not a problem so long as the average reading time for each item is manageable for the allotted testing time.

Both of the items above (1 and 2) end with incomplete statements. Generally, the use of incomplete statement-type items should be minimized, because they do not define the problem adequately. This type of questions requires longer and more complex cognitive processing and therefore can add confusion to average or lower performing students. This then introduces unwanted error of measurement requiring "mental gymnastics" in addition to knowledge of the content area. The question, "Which of the following best describes this study design?" is better.

CONCEPTUAL DEPICTION OF MCQs

Diagrams representing an easy, moderate, and difficult MCQ are depicted in Figure 11.1. The first frame shows an easy item because the keyed-response

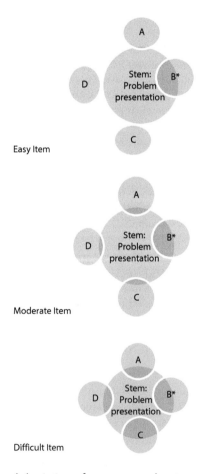

Figure 11.1 Conceptual depiction of an easy, moderate, and difficult MCQ item.

("correct answer") B clearly overlaps the problem presented in the stem, while options A, C, and D either do not (C, D) or only marginally (A) overlap with the stem or problem presented there. This type of item is typical of factual knowledge item—if the student knows the fact, the item is very easy.

The moderate difficult item in the second frame shows option B clearly overlapping with the stem but options A, C, and D also have some overlap and are therefore plausible alternatives. A student must know this concept quite well in order to select the keyed-response. Students with only superficial or partial knowledge will find this item somewhat challenging. Therefore, this item will "discriminate" (i.e., distinguish) between students who know the content and those that don't.

The difficult item frame indicates even more overlap between stem and distractors (options A, C, and D). Students will require superior knowledge in order to distinguish between the correct answer (B) and the distractors. High achievers will select the correct response, while moderate or low achievers will likely be confused by this item. This item, therefore, will discriminate between those that know the content very well and those that have only superficial or partial knowledge. Moderate and low-achieving students frequently refer to this type of item as "multiple guess"—putting the blame on the item rather than on the real source of the issue which is lack of knowledge. Any given test can consist of a mix of easy, moderate, and difficult items. A good distribution is 20% easy, 40% moderate, and 40% difficult items.

COGNITIVE LEVEL OF TEST ITEMS

The testing of simple recall has too frequently characterized the multiple-choice item format. This situation has been mistakenly attributed to some inherent weakness in the format itself, but this is not true. The multiple-choice format offers ample opportunity to construct items that are more complex than simple recall. Nevertheless, there are many situations where assessing the candidate's mastery of factual knowledge is a perfectly appropriate task (i.e., definition of a medical term). Criticism is warranted when a simple recall test item is used for material that should be assessed at the comprehension, application, and/or even analysis level. Therefore, an important step to constructing a test item is to consider the learning objective underlying the learning of the material. In doing so, the level of cognitive complexity that the item should reflect can be determined.

In constructing test items at various cognitive levels, refer to Bloom's Taxonomy (see Table 5.1). Remember from the table that there are six major cognitive categories, and the general objectives at each level provides the action verbs which are useful in constructing test items in each of these categories. While it is possible to construct items at the upper three levels of the taxonomy (i.e., analysis, synthesis, evaluation), this task is quite difficult. In general, items for high-stakes course exams and licensing exams are more likely to reflect the first three levels of the taxonomy (i.e., *knowledge, comprehension, application*). The actual distribution of cognitive categories for any particular exam will of course be influenced by the curriculum content being assessed. Consequently, it is not surprising that some exams are characterized primarily by knowledge and comprehension-type questions, while other exams may have a larger proportion of application-type questions.

The stems should include verbs such as define, describe, identify (*knowledge*), defend, interpret, explain (*comprehension*), and predict, operate, compute, discover, apply (*application*).

COMMON GUIDELINES FOR ITEM CONSTRUCTION

In a review of 46 authoritative textbooks and other sources in educational measurement, Haladyna et al. developed a taxonomy of 43 multiple-choice item writing rules.[1] The taxonomy, which is summarized here as Table 11.1, is exhaustive with a great deal of detail. We will focus on a subset of these rules with particular attention.

There are a variety of the multiple-choice test formats to consider when constructing these items. Table 11.2 contains six possible test item formats. In addition, format variation may also be found within the cognitive domains. For example, items developed at the knowledge level may be constructed to reflect different types of knowledge outcomes as indicated in Table 11.3.

Table 11.1 Item-writing guidelines

General item-writing (procedural)
1. Use either the best answer or the correct answer format.
2. Avoid the complex multiple-choice (Type K) format.
3. Format the item vertically, not horizontally.
4. Allow time for editing and other types of item revisions.
5. Use good grammar, punctuation, and spelling consistently.
6. Minimize examinee reading time in phrasing each item.
7. Avoid trick items, those that mislead or deceive examinees into answering.

General item-writing (content concerns)
8. Base each item on an educational or instructional objective.
9. Focus on a single problem.
10. Keep the vocabulary consistent with the examinees' level of understanding.
11. Avoid cuing one item with another; keep items independent of one another.
12. Use the author's examples as a basis for developing your items.
13. Avoid over specific knowledge when developing the item.
14. Avoid verbatim textbook phrasing when developing the item.

(Continued)

Table 11.1 (*Continued*) Item-writing guidelines

15. Avoid items based on opinions.
16. Use multiple-choice to measure higher-level thinking.
17. Test for important or significant material; avoid trivial material.

Stem construction

18. State the stem in either question form or completion form; use the question as much as possible
19. When using the completion format, don't leave a blank for completion in the beginning or middle of the stem.
20. Ensure that the directions in the stem are clear and that wording lets the examinee know exactly what is being asked.
21. Avoid window dressing (excessive verbiage) in the stem.
22. Word the stem positively; avoid negative phrasing.
23. Include the central idea and most of the phrasing in the stem.

General option development

24. Use as many options as are feasible; aim to use four options for all items.
25. Place options in logical or numerical order.
26. Keep options independent; options should not be overlapping.
27. Keep all options in an item homogeneous in content.
28. Keep the length of options fairly consistent.
29. Avoid, or use sparingly, the phrase "all of the above."
30. Avoid, or use sparingly, the phrase "none of the above."
31. Avoid the use of the phrase "I don't know."
32. Phrase options positively, not negatively.
33. Avoid distractors that can clue test-wise examinees; e.g., avoid associations, absurd options, formal prompts, or semantic (overly specific or overly general) clues.
34. Avoid giving clues through the use of faulty grammatical construction.
35. Avoid specific determiners, such as "never" and "always."

Correct option development

36. Position the correct option so that it appears about the same number of times in each possible position for a set of items.
37. Make sure there is one and only one correct option.

Distractor development

38. Use plausible distractor; avoid illogical distractors.
39. Incorporate common errors of students in distractors.
40. Avoid technically phrased distractors.
41. Use familiar yet incorrect phrases as distractors.
42. Use true statements that do no correctly answer the item.
43. Avoid the use of humor when developing options.

Source: Adapted from Haladyna et al.[1]

Table 11.2 Sample test item formats

1. Question format

Acute intermittent porphyria is the result of a defect in the biosynthetic pathway for which of the following?

A. Corticosteroid
B. Fatty acid
C. Glucose
D. Heme*

2. Completion format

An inherited metabolic disorder of carbohydrate metabolism is characterized by an abnormally increased concentration of hepatic glycogen with normal structure and no detectable increase in serum glucose concentration after oral administration of fructose. These two observations suggest that the disease is the result of the absence of

A. Fructokinase
B. Glucokinase
C. Glucose 6-phosphatase*
D. Phosphoglucomutase

3. Clinical association format

A 12-year-old girl with sickle cell disease has pain in her right arm. An x-ray of the right upper extremity shows bony lesions consistent with osteomyelitis. Which of the following is the most likely causal organism?

A. *Clostridium septicum*
B. *Enterococcus faecalis*
C. *Pseudomonas aeruginosa*
D. *Salmonella enteritidis**

4. Negative question format

Which of the following is **NOT** a continuous variable?

A. Height
B. Religion*
C. Temperature
D. Time to solve a problem

5. Statement format

Identify the 95% confidence interval for the population mean when a sample mean is 37 and the standard deviation of 5.

A. 37 ± 1.96 (15)
B. 37 ± 1.96 (5)*
C. 37 ± 0.95 (15)
D. 37 ± 0.95 (3)

(Continued)

Table 11.2 (*Continued*) Sample test item formats

6. Order/sequence format

The triad of the nephritic syndrome includes which of the following?

A. Hypotension, proteinuria, and haematuria

B. Hypertension, proteinuria, and edema*

C. Night sweats, edema, and haematuria

D. Urinary frequency, burning, and pain

Table 11.3 Measuring knowledge outcomes

Knowledge of terminology

Which one of the following statements best defines the word egress?

A. digress

B. enter

C. exit*

D. regress

Knowledge of specific facts

Who was the first US astronaut to orbit the earth in space?

A. Alan Shepard

B. John Glenn*

C. Scott Carpenter

D. Virgil Grissom

Knowledge of principles

Which of the following best describes the power of science?

A. Scientists are rational and apply logic in their thought processes

B. Science is public, self-correcting, and results are replicable*

C. Science provides an algorithm for solving problems

D. Scientists are well-educated in basic philosophical problems

Knowledge of methods and procedures

If you were conducting a scientific study of a problem, your first step should be to

A. Collect information about the problem*

B. Develop hypotheses to be tested

C. Design the experiment to be conducted

D. Select scientific equipment

CONSTRUCTING THE STEM

As we have seen, a multiple-choice item is composed of a stem and four or five options. One of the options is referred to as the keyed or correct response, while the remaining options serve as distractors. In a well-constructed multiple-choice item, the stem should present a self-contained question or problem. Moreover, there should be enough information in the stem to permit the test-taker to develop a possible answer without viewing the options. In the following example, Item 1 represents an incomplete stem, while Item 2 is a better format.

Item 1—**Poor** (Problem is not adequately specified in the stem).
  The bichrome test may fail for patients who have
  A. deuteranopia
  B. deuteranomaly
  C. protanopia
  D. tritanopia

Item 2—**Better** (Problem is more clearly specified in the stem).
  In which of the following patient conditions will the bichrome test, which is used to determine the spherical refractive error in clinical refraction, likely fail?
  A. Deuteranopia
  B. Deuteranomaly
  C. Protanopia
  D. Tritanopia

One of the most frequent but easily avoided errors in constructing the stem deals with the grammatical fit between the stem and all of the options. The item writer may have sometimes failed to proofread the item. To avoid such errors, it is useful to have a colleague read and edit the items. Someone, other than the item writer, can frequently spot errors in items more readily.

Negatively stated items

Negatively stated (i.e., not, except, least) items should be avoided but there are rare occasions when they are appropriate. In the case of treatment procedures, for example, there may be an action among several which should not be performed. It is quite reasonable to develop a negatively stated item to help determine if the candidate is aware of the danger of performing a particular action. As in the case of all negatively stated stems, capitalize and bold the negation component of the stem (i.e., which of the following is NOT an appropriate action when dealing with a head-injured patient?).

Example

You suspect placenta previa when a 26-year-old woman in her 23rd week of pregnancy comes to the emergency department with vaginal bleeding with bright red blood but is painless. Which of the following actions is **NOT** correct?

A. Conduct a digital pelvic exam*
B. Monitor the fetal heart rate
C. Order bed rest as a treatment
D. Order transvaginal ultrasonography as a diagnostic test
E. Order a complete blood count (CBC)

Constructing the options

How many options?

The four-option item is the most effective form to use (i.e., the stem and options a, b, c, d). The addition of a fifth option generally does not provide sufficient discrimination power and improvement in reliability to justify the effort required to construct it.[2] Given this evidence and the importance of a consistent format style throughout the exam, item writers are advised to construct all items in the four-option format.

The main reason for increasing the number of options in an item is to reduce the probability of selecting the keyed-response by chance alone. These probabilities are illustrated in Table 11.4.

Increasing the options beyond four does not decrease the probability of guessing very substantially. Increasing the options from two to three decreases the probability of guessing by 17% and three to four by an additional 8%. Going from four options to five only reduces the probability by 5% (Table 11.4). Given the difficulty in constructing four plausible distractors (a five-option item), it is advisable to use three plausible distractors (a four-option item) since the reduction of guessing is small (5%) compared to the effort in constructing an additional distractor. A number of empirical studies have found little or no improvement in the reliability or discrimination of tests by using five options versus four.[1]

Table 11.4 Probabilities of guessing with various options

Number of options	Probability of guessing (%)	Decrease in probability (%)
2	50	—
3	33	17
4	25	8
5	20	5
6	17	3

Option length

Frequently, the correct option is longer than the distractors. This is frequently because the longer option contains more information so as to make this option the best answer. Many test-wise candidates, however, are aware of this test construction error and will select the longest option. When a test-taker selects a correct option on the basis of some factor other than having the necessary knowledge, the value of the item is reduced.

The item below is typical of the length construction error. In general, try to keep the options approximately equal.

Option length error
   Neurotics are more likely than psychotics to
   A. be dangerous to society
   B. be dangerous to themselves
   C. have delusional symptoms
   D. have insight into their own inappropriate behavior but nevertheless feel
       rather helpless in terms of dealing with their difficulties*

Location of the correct answer

The location of the keyed-response should be randomized so that it appears at approximate equal frequency in each of the four options. Usually this is not the case, particularly for novice item writers. For reasons that are not fully understood, these writers favor "c" as the correct option. Indeed, the practice is so widespread that test-wise students have developed the dictum, "When in doubt pick 'c.'" Therefore, when reviewing your items, simply check to see that you have not favored "c" as the correct response. In a 100-item test, for example, the keyed-response should appear about 25 times in each of the four option positions.

In addition to determining the location of the correct response, consideration should be given to the order in which the options are presented. Whenever appropriate, the options should be placed in either ascending or descending order, usually in ascending order. When the options are comprised of numbers, for example, it is preferable to present the options in a serial order rather than put them in random order.

Example of numbers
   What proportion of a normal distribution falls between $z = -1.16$ and $z = +1.16$?
   A. 0.2460
   B. 0.3770
   C. 0.6230
   D. 0.7540*

Similarly, the options should be placed in either ascending or descending order alphabetically. As for numbers, it is usual to arrange the options in ascending order.

Example of alphabetical

A 22-year-old student comes in to the university health center with a mild fever (100F). On careful physical examination, you notice four small vesicular lesions, each on an erythematous base. The most likely diagnosis is primary infection with

A. Cytomegalovirus (CMV)
B. Herpes simplex virus type 2 (HSV-2)*
C. Human immunodeficiency virus type 1 (HIV-1)
D. Human papilloma virus type 6 (HPV-6)

All of the above or none of the above

These options should be avoided particularly when the item constructor plans to make them the correct response. It is very difficult to defend the position that a set of options are always the case or never the case. When "all of the above" or "none of the above" options serve as distractors, it is important for item constructors to recognize that many people will quickly eliminate these options. Test-wise candidates understand that the item constructor frequently uses these options as fillers due to the inability to create a third valid distractor.

Example: None of the Above

What effect would a thrombolytic drug administered to a heart attack patient arriving in the emergency department by ambulance have on the patient's systolic blood pressure?

A. Decrease it
B. Increase it
C. Neither increase nor decrease it*
D. None of the above

It is evident that option D as "none of the above" is nonsensical and was used only as a filler because it is very difficult to write a plausible distractor for that option. The problem in the stem should be re-worked to avoid this difficulty.

Example: All of the above (poor construction)

Which are characteristic of the nephritic syndrome?

A. Hypertension
B. Proteinuria
C. Edema
D. All of the above*

Example: All of the above (better construction)
  Which are characteristic of the nephritic syndrome?
  A. Hypertension, proteinuria, and edema*
  B. Hypotension, deuteranopia, and edema
  C. Hypertension, proteinuria, and deuteranopia
  D. Hypotension, proteinuria, and edema

For this "all of the above" option, even a student with partial knowledge could select D because the student might recognize two options (probably B and C) as correct so it follows that D must be the correct answer. Additionally, if "all of the above" rarely occurs, it probably is the correct answer. Finally, either of the two options (none/all of the above) frequently are not grammatically correct in relation to the stem. The best strategy is to never use either "all of the above" or "none of the above" or any other inclusive/exclusive options (e.g., A and B but not C).

Homogeneous distractors

It is important that all distractors be plausible and homogeneous. The rationale for this is simple. One of the major advantages of using the multiple-choice format is that it requires candidates to make discrimination among what should be a set of compelling options with only one representing the best choice. Any question that contains distractors that are easily eliminated reduces the overall value of the question. The following example represents this type of construction error.

Example: Poor
  Who is most closely associated with the theory of natural selection?
  A. Bell
  B. Darwin*
  C. Morse
  D. Pasteur

Example: Better
  Who is most closely associated with the theory of natural selection?
  A. Darwin*
  B. Fleming
  C. Pasteur
  D. Virchow

In the first example (poor), Darwin and Pasteur were both in the life sciences, while Bell and Morse were in the physical sciences. In the second example (better), the distractors are more homogeneous as all four are now in the life sciences.

Cueing the correct answer

There are ways in which a cue in the stem gives away the correct answer by repeating a key word from the stem in one of the options. The following represents an example of this type of error. In general, this particular error is found more frequently among items which involve technical language as in the case of science or medical-type items.

Providing obvious clues

Which of the following diseases is caused by a virus?

A. Gallstones
B. Scarlet fever
C. Typhoid fever
D. Viral pneumonia*

CONSTRUCTING THE CLINICAL VIGNETTE QUESTION

Questions can be written with a clinical vignette. The vignette allows testing at the comprehension or application level of knowledge and provides face validity for the item. The vignette commonly provides the patient's age, sex, chief complaint, and site of care, followed by personal history, family history (if relevant), then physical examination information, then laboratory data (if provided). Depending upon the purpose of the set, vignettes can be brief, prototypic presentations, or fuller descriptions that challenge examinees to identify key information. A good stem provides sufficient information but not irrelevant or distracting information such as patient's hair color if that is not relevant to the diagnosis. A good stem can be answered without referring to the options.

Dos and don'ts for effective writing of vignettes

- Each item should focus on an important concept, typically a common or potentially acute clinical problem.
  1. Don't assess knowledge of trivial facts
  2. Don't include trivial, "tricky," or overly complex questions
  3. Do focus on problems that would be encountered in real life

- Each item should assess comprehension or application of knowledge, not recall an isolated fact.
  1. Do use stems that may be relatively long
  2. Do use short options
  3. Do use the question format
  4. Do use a presenting problem of a patient for the clinical sciences
  5. Do follow with the history (including duration of signs and symptoms), physical findings, results of diagnostic studies, initial treatment, subsequent findings, etc.

6. Do use vignettes that may include only a subset of this information, but the information should be provided in this specified order
7. Don't use long patient vignettes for the basic sciences; keep them very brief
8. Do use laboratory vignettes for the basic sciences

- The stem of the item must pose a clear question, and it should be possible to arrive at an answer with the options covered.
    1. Do cover up the options to determine if the question is focused and clear; examinees should be able to pose an answer based only on the stem
    2. Do rewrite the stem and/or options if they could not
    3. Do write a vignette for each (or many) of the options in the list
    4. Do begin with the presenting problem of a patient, followed by the history (including duration of signs and symptoms), physical findings, results of diagnostic studies, initial treatment, subsequent findings, etc.
    5. Do pose a clear question in the lead-in of the stem so that the candidates can pose an answer without looking at the options
    6. Do satisfy the "cover-the-options" rule as an essential component of a good question

General vignette example*

A 22-year-old student comes in to the university health center with a mild fever (100F) and a "continuous tingling sensation running down the inside of her thighs" that has disturbed her sleep. On careful physical examination, you notice four small vesicular lesions, each on an erythematous base, adjacent to the vaginal opening. There are no other recognizable skin abnormalities but the inguinal (groin) lymph nodes are noticeably swollen and tender. Which primary infection is the most likely diagnosis that accounts for this young women's condition?

A. Cytomegalovirus (CMV)
B. Herpes simplex virus type 2 (HSV-2)*
C. Human immunodeficiency virus type 1 (HIV-1)
D. Human papilloma virus type 6 (HPV-6)
E. Varicella zoster virus (VZV)

---

* Many thanks to Dr. Peter Southern, Professor at the University of Minnesota Medical School who contributed this and several other items in this chapter.

Vignettes with x-rays example

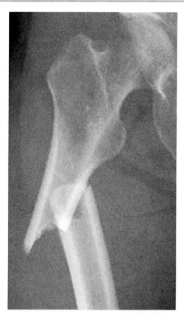

This X-ray is from a male patient with date of birth: May 20, 1975; side of extremity/body: right; and date of X-ray: May 01, 2018. What type of fracture is shown in the X-ray above?

A. Simple spiral
B. Simple oblique*
C. Simple transverse
D. Simple wedge
E. Simple fragmentary

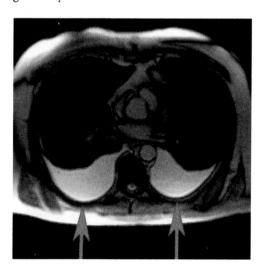

A 63-year-old man presents to the emergency department complaining of coughing that produces phlegm. He has fever, shortness of breath and difficulty breathing, chills, fatigue, sweating, and chest pain. You order a chest CT with the results below. What is the most likely differential diagnosis?

A. Cytomegalovirus of the lungs
B. Lung cancer
C. Pneumonia*
D. Tuberculosis
E. Emphysema

Vignettes with photographs example

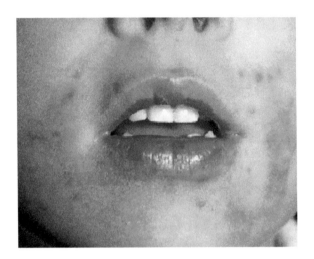

This 4-year-old child is generally happy and healthy although she does seem to have inherited a family susceptibility to atopic dermatitis. Shortly after beginning pre-school classes, she experiences an episode of skin disruption around her mouth and across her cheeks that progresses to fluid secretion and crusting, suggestive of secondary bacterial infection. What combination of bacteria is most likely to be causing the secondary skin infections when the Diagnostic Laboratory isolates a beta-hemolytic, gram-positive, coagulase positive organism and a lactose non-fermenting, non-spore-forming rod?

A. *Escherichia coli* and *Streptococcus pyogenes*
B. *Klebsiella pneumoniae* and *Streptococcus pyogenes*
C. *Pseudomonas aeruginosa* and *Staphylococcus aureus**
D. *Staphylococcus epidermidis* and *Pseudomonas aeruginosa*
E. *Streptococcus agalactiae* and *Pseudomonas aeruginosas*

Vignettes with lab data example

A 68-year-old woman's hospital discharge was delayed due to unavailability of a bed in a nursing home. She is bedridden and unable to attend to personal needs. During a 3-day period, her pulse increases from 79/min to 127/min, and blood pressure decreases from 128/76 mm Hg to 103/60 mm Hg. Laboratory values include:

	Day 1	Day 3
Hemoglobin	17.4 g/dL	18.8 g/dL
Serum		
Glucose	97 mg/dL	86 mg/dL
Urea nitrogen	20 mg/dL	58 mg/dL
Creatinine	1.1 mg/dL	1.2 mg/dL
Na+	133 mEq/L	148 mEq/L

Which of the following is the most likely diagnosis?

A. Hepatic globular disease
B. Dehydration*
C. Diabetic ketoacidosis
D. Duodenal hemorrhage
E. Renal failure

Table 11.5, which is adapted and modified based on Gronlund's and Cameron's text, is a very useful checklist to run through to check that you have avoided basic item writing errors that we have discussed throughout this chapter. Use this checklist frequently to review your item construction.

Table 11.5 Checklist for reviewing multiple-choice items[3]

	Yes	No
1. This is the most appropriate type of item for this assessment		
2. The amount or reading time is appropriate for each item		
3. As much as possible, the item stems are stated in positive terms		
4. The item stem is free of irrelevant material		
5. Negative wording (e.g., NOT) has been capitalized		
6. Each item stem presents a meaningful problem		
7. The alternatives are grammatically consistent with the item stem		

(Continued)

Table 11.5 (*Continued*) Checklist for reviewing multiple-choice items[3]

	Yes	No
8. You have avoided repetitive words or phrases in the alternatives		
9. There is only one correct or clearly BEST answer		
10. The distractors are plausible to non-achievers		
11. The alternative answers are brief without unnecessary words		
12. The alternatives are similar in length and form		
13. The items are free of verbal clues to the answers		
14. Verbal alternatives are in alphabetical order		
15. Numerical alternatives are in numerical order		
16. You have avoided "none of the above" and "all of the above"		
17. You have avoided inclusive/exclusive items (e.g., "A and B but NOT C")		
18. A colleague has reviewed your items		

SETTING PASS/FAIL SCORES FOR MCQs

The MPL method

In criterion-referenced testing, it is necessary to establish cutoff scores for pass/fail.[4] One very common and simple way to do this is called a minimum performance level (MPL) employing the Nedelsky method.

Here, we employ a modified version of the Nedelsky method. Experts (e.g., physicians, nurses, dentists, etc.) assign probabilities to multiple-choice test items based on the likelihood that a group of examinees should be able to rule out incorrect options.[5] These reference groups are hypothetical test-takers on the borderline between inadequate and adequate levels of performance. These are the minimally competent candidates (not failures, not stars, but those that just got their toes in the door). These also refer to the borderline between mastery and non-mastery of some domain of knowledge, ability, or skill.

A good way to proceed in setting the MPL is to have a discussion among experts on the minimally competent candidate. In this meeting, participants' discuss, describe, and clarify the hypothetical "borderline examinee." The participants can now leave the meeting and independently inspect each option in a MCQ of some of the items being calibrated. For each distractor, experts identify the probability that they believe a hypothetical minimally competent examinee could rule out as incorrect. Quartile probabilities (e.g., 25%, 50%, etc.) are usually used though deciles (10%, 20%, etc.) could also be used. We then average the probabilities for each expert (2–3) for each option.

The total test score MPL (passing score) is the sum of each item MPL. We must, therefore, establish an MPL for each item. The MPL is the value ranging between 0.25 and 1.0 which reflects the probability that even a minimally competent candidate can answer this item correctly. An MPL of 0.25 indicates a very difficult item with an MPL of 1.0 reflecting an easy one.

Once we have averaged the expert judgment for each option assigning a value (one of 0, 0.25, 0.50, 0.75, 1.0) to each distractor, the following formula is then applied to calculate the MPL of each item.

$$\text{MPL} = \frac{1}{O_p - \Sigma P_D}$$

where O_p = the number of options in the item

P_D = the probability that a minimally knowledgeable candidate can eliminate that option as clearly incorrect

MPL = minimum performance level for that item

Examples illustrate the procedure

1. When did World War II end?
   A. 1650
   B. 1859
   C. 1945*
   D. 1984

$$A = 1.0 \quad B = 1.0 \quad C = * \quad D = 1.0$$

In this example, each of the distractors, A, B, and D are assigned 1.0 because even a minimally competent candidate can almost certainly eliminate them as incorrect. The MPL, therefore, is

$$\frac{1}{O_p - \Sigma P_D} = \frac{1}{4 - (1.0 + 1.0 + 1.0)} = \frac{1}{4 - 3} = \frac{1}{1} = 1.0$$

The above item receives an MPL = 1.0, because it is very easy. We can increase the difficulty in item 2 by making the options overlap more closely with the stem.

2. When did World War II end?
   A. 1944
   B. 1945*
   C. 1948
   D. 1950

$$A = 0 \quad B = * \quad C = 0.50 \quad D = 0.75$$

"A." is assigned a value of 0 because a minimally competent candidate would be very unlikely to eliminate it, while "C." is easier to eliminate as is "D." The MPL is:

$$MPL = \frac{1}{4-(0+0.50+0.75)} = \frac{1}{2.75} = 0.36$$

This is a difficult item as reflected in the MPL = 0.36. We can increase the item difficulty even further by requiring even more fine-grained discrimination between the options and including more detail in the stem as in item 3.

3. When did World War II end in Europe?
   A. March 1945
   B. April 1945*
   C. May 1945
   D. June 1945

$$MPL = \frac{1}{4-0} = \frac{1}{4} = 0.25$$

This is a very difficult item as reflected in the MPL = 0.25, which is equivalent to chance guessing for this item.

All MCQs should then be referenced with their MPLs when stored in an item bank. As we indicated, the total test score MPL (passing score) is the sum of each item MPL. If we select 50 MCQs from an item bank, the passing score for that test is the sum of the 50 MPLs. Conceivably, the lowest MPL possible is 0.25 (25% to pass)—a very difficult test—to 1.00 (100% to pass). In practice, total test MPLs are usually in the range of 0.55–0.78. These are criterion-referenced tests because passing/failing is based on an absolute standard and not on the norm group performance.

SUMMARY AND MAIN POINTS

The objectivity of a test refers to how it is scored. Scoring procedures on some objective tests, such as multiple-choice questions (MCQs), have been so carefully planned that scoring can be automated on a computer. Multiple-choice items are objective tests because they can be scored routinely according to a predetermined key, eliminating the judgments of the scorers. Objective test items produce higher reliability assessments than do subjective test items (e.g., essays) and are therefore more desirable.

- The first step to constructing valid tests is to develop a test blueprint as it serves as a tool to help ensure the content validity of an exam.
- The multiple-choice item consists of several parts: the stem, the keyed-response, and several distractors. The keyed-response is the "right" answer or the option indicated on the key. All of the possible alternative answers are called options.

- The stems should include verbs such as define, describe, identify (knowledge), defend, explain, interpret, explain (comprehension), and predict, operate, compute, discover, apply (application).
- In a review of 46 authoritative textbooks and other sources in educational measurement, Haladyna et al developed a taxonomy of 43 multiple-choice item writing rules.
- In criterion-referenced testing, it is necessary to establish cutoff scores for pass/fail. One very common and simple way to do this is called a MPL in discussion among experts on the minimally competent candidate.
- For each distractor, experts identify the probability that they believe a hypothetical minimally competent examinee could rule out as incorrect. Quartile probabilities (e.g., 25%, 50%, etc.) are usually used though deciles (10%, 20%, etc.) could also be used. The probabilities for each expert (2–3) for each option are averaged. The total test score MPL (passing score) is the sum of each item MPL.

BOX 11.1: *Advocatus Diaboli*: Tricks for taking MCQ tests

Many students, particularly those who are anxious or suffer from test anxiety, may be compromised on MCQ tests. These candidates frequently report that such tests cause them to become very anxious, and as a result, their performance suffers significantly. Observations of unsuccessful test-takers have revealed at least two sources of difficulties. First, poor test-takers do not generally spend sufficient time reading the question component or stem of the MCQ. The stem frequently contains information that the test-taker can use to eliminate the incorrect options. Reading the stem too quickly results in missing such information and thereby, adds unnecessarily to the difficulty of the item. Second, racing through the stem in order to choose an option creates a frenzied pace for the student which adds to their already high anxiety.

The following strategy has been suggested[6] to help students in slowing their pace and thus read the stem more carefully and thoroughly. The strategy also gives the test-taker a greater feeling of control, and accordingly, reduces their anxiety somewhat.

Specific instructions to students
- Stop reading at the end of the stem and cover the options with your hand.
- Reflect on what information the stem provides and what you know about the specific content area of the question.

- Respond silently to the question with what you believe might be the correct answer. After completing this task, uncover the options.
- Confirm your tentative response with one of the options.

This is called the SRRC strategy. Many students, particularly those experiencing anxiety during an MCQ exam, have reported that this strategy has helped them to feel more in control during examinations and has helped to maximize their performance.

There are several additional strategies for approaching an MCQ test item.

- Turn the stem into a question. For some students, a stem such as "The field of epidemiology is concerned with" is more difficult to respond to than the question, "What is epidemiology?" While the reasons for this are not completely clear, there is evidence that converting open stems into complete questions does increase test scores.[7] One possibility is that converting the incomplete stem to a question more clearly focuses the problem and thus reduces the ambiguity of the question. Additionally, it probably increases the efficiency of cognitive processes such as decoding and memory searches.
- Try elimination. Students frequently perceive the task of selecting the correct answer in a four-option item as selecting one from four possibilities. Through the process of elimination, the choice can be reduced to one in two options. Even for questions which are very difficult, students usually have some knowledge about the item making the elimination of one or more options possible.
- Watch for qualifiers as *specific determiners*. Options that contain absolutes such as *never, only, always, certainly*, or *all* (specific determiners) are frequently incorrect responses. Test constructors sometimes use such options to easily render the option incorrect thus reducing the need to develop other plausible distractors. Therefore, they are rarely meant to be the correct responses and more often simply provide evidence of poor test construction. These are usually created as distractors. Conversely, options that equivocate with the use of words like *sometimes, frequently, in most cases, usually* (also specific determiners), and so on are generally correct options. Identifying these options and responding accordingly will allow students to capitalize on poorly constructed tests rather than be penalized by them.
- More words tend to be right. In any well-designed MCQ item, there is only one correct option. In order for this to be true, test writers construct the correct option to be complete and to account for all the possible information. On occasion, the need to construct a valid correct option results in too little attention to the construction of the distractors. Consequently, the distractors may be considerably shorter than the correct answer. Long complete options, therefore, frequently represent the correct answer.
- Look for cues from the stem to the options. These may be grammatical links (e.g., past tense), plural versus singular, repeated phrases or words, and so on.

PART A: EXAMPLE OF A TABLE OF SPECIFICATIONS FOR A CELLULAR PROCESSES TEST

Content area	Levels of understanding			
	Knowledge	Comprehension	Application	
1. Nucleus	2	5	1	8 (32%)
2. Chromosomes	2	4	2	8 (32%)
3. Active transport	2	3	4	9 (36%)
	6 (24%)	12 (48%)	7 (28%)	25

1. State the general purpose of the test, i.e., how will the test results be used? For example, are there diagnostic uses for the test? (**½ mark**)
2. State who will take the test. (**½ mark**)
3. The test should include a title, explicit instructions (i.e., where do students record their answers) and indicate the time allocated to write the exam. (**3 marks**)
4. Include a scoring key which includes a breakdown of the frequency of the correct answer (i.e., a = 7; b = 6; c = 6, d = 6). (**1 mark**)

PART B: WRITING THE TEST (25 MARKS—1 PER QUESTION)

According to your blueprint developed in Part A of this assignment, write a 25 item multiple-choice exam. Each item should have four options—a keyed-response and three distractors. Below is a list that will help you construct your test. First read through the criteria below and then, after your test is written, evaluate your questions using these criteria.

CRITERIA FOR MCQS: ONE MARK WILL BE DEDUCTED FOR EACH OF THE FOLLOWING NOT ATTENDED TO

1. Is the stem of the item meaningful *by itself* and does it present a definite problem? (Remember, the direct question (closed stem) tends to be easier for students to answer—who, what, where, when, why, how.)
2. Does the stem include as much of the item as possible and is it free of irrelevant material?
3. Have you used negatively stated stems only when significant learning outcomes require it? Have you clearly identified the negative qualifier (i.e., bold lettering, all capitals, underlining, etc.)?
4. Are all of the alternatives grammatically consistent with the stem?
5. Does each item contain only one correct or clearly best answer?

6. Are all the distractors plausible?
7. Have you avoided verbal associations between the stem and the correct answer?
8. Does the relative length of the alternatives provide a clue to the answer?
9. Does the correct answer appear in each of the alternative positions approximately an equal number of times, but in random order?
10. Have you used special alternatives such as "none of the above" or "all of the above" sparingly and only when significant learning outcomes require it?
11. Have you left *at least* one (1) blank line between the stem and the first alternative?
12. Are all maps/diagrams clearly labelled to indicate which questions correspond to them?
13. Have you provided references for materials taken from other sources?
14. Is the question and *all* of the options presented on the same page?
15. Questions with answers requiring mathematical calculations *must* have a rationale for each distractor.

PART C: REFLECTIONS

After you have completed this assignment, write a brief reflection (1-page type-written maximum) about your reactions to multiple-choice exams and the construction of a multiple-choice exam.

NOTE: the reflection is an important part of this assignment. Although the reflection is not marked, in order to receive a grade for the entire assignment, the reflection must be handed in.

TO SUBMIT TO THE INSTRUCTOR

1. Part A—Questions 1–4.
2. The multiple-choice exam (which includes Part A—Question 5).
3. The scoring key (which includes Part A—Question 6).
4. Your reflection.

All of the above should be typewritten.

REFERENCES

1. Haladyna TM, Downing SM, Rodriguez MC. (2002). A review of multiple-choice item-writing guidelines for classroom assessment. *Applied Measurement in Education*, 15, 309–334; Haladyna TM. (1994). *Developing and Validating Multiple-Choice Test Items*. Toronto, ON: Erlbaum; Downing SM, Haladyna TM. (2006). *Handbook of Test Development*. Mahwah, NJ: Lawrence Erlbaum.
2. Baghaei P, Amrahi N. (2011). The effects of the number of options on the psychometric characteristics of multiple choice items. *Psychological Test and Assessment Modelling*, 53(2), 192–211; Kilgour JM, Tayyaba S. (2016). An investigation into the

optimal number of distractors in single-best answer exams. *Advances in Health Science Education*, 21, 571–585.

3. Gronlund NE, Cameron IJ. (2005). *Assessment of Student Achievement*, Canadian Edition 1st Edition. Toronto, ON: Pearson.

4. Yousuf N, Violato C, Zuberi RW. (2015). Standard setting methods for pass/fail decisions on high stakes objective structured clinical examinations: A validity study. *Teaching and Learning in Medicine*, 27(3), 280–291.

5. Cizek GJ, Bunch MB. (2007). The Nedelsky method. In Cizek GJ, Bunch MB, eds., *Standard Setting* (pp. 68–74). Thousand Oaks, CA: SAGE Publications Ltd. doi:10.4135/9781412985918.

6. Violato C, McDougall D, Marini A. (1992). *Assessment of Classroom Learning*. Calgary, AB: Detselig.

7. Violato C, Marini AE. (1989). Effects of stem orientation and completeness of multiple choice items on item difficulty and discrimination. *Educational and Psychological Measurement*, 49(1), 287–296.

12

Constructed response items

- The constructed response or open-ended item is most commonly known as the essay test, but consists of any item format type where the examinee must construct a response rather than select one as in the multiple-choice format.
- These item types are sometimes also called subjective tests because scoring involves subjective judgments of the scorer. By contrast, the MCQ is referred to as objective, because no judgments are required to score the items.
- Constructed response questions are usually intended to assess students' ability at the higher levels of Bloom's taxonomy: application, analysis, synthesis, and evaluation.
- There are at least two types of essay questions, the restricted and extended response forms. This classification refers to the amount of freedom allowed to candidates in composing their responses. The restricted response question limits the character and breadth of the student's composition.
- There are two basic approaches to the scoring of constructed response test questions: analytic scoring and holistic scoring.
- Analytic scoring rubrics list specific elements of the response and specify the number of points to award each response.
- The holistic rubric contains statements of a typical response at each score level so that actual responses written by test-takers provide examples of a 10-point response, an 8-point response, a 5-point response, and so on.
- The total amount of effort in the use of either essay test or MCQs use is, in part, a function of the number of students to be tested. The greatest amount of effort for MCQ use is in the construction of the test items while for the essay it is the grading.

- The idea of grading essays by computer has been around since the mid-1960s. Researchers have recently made progress in using computers to score constructed item responses. Automated scoring reduces the time and cost of the scoring process.

INTRODUCTION

The constructed-response or open-ended item is most commonly known as the essay test but consists of any item format type where the examinee must construct a response rather than select one as in the multiple-choice format. In addition to a written answer, the constructed response may consist of other performance types such as presenting a case study, an interpretive dance, or performing a physical exam on a patient. Assessing clinical skills such as conducting a physical exam is usually done in an objective structured clinical exam (OSCE) and is the subject of Chapter 13.

Constructed-response items require students to apply knowledge, skills, and analytic thinking to authentic performance tasks. These are sometimes called open-response items, because there may be a number of ways to correctly answer the question; students are required to construct or develop their own answers without suggestions or choices. These item types are sometimes also called subjective tests, because scoring involves subjective judgments of the scorer. By contrast, the MCQ is referred to as objective because no judgments are required to score the items.

Constructed-response items can be simple, requiring a phrase or sentence or two as answers. Or they can be complex, requiring students to read a prompt or a paragraph and write an essay or analysis of the information. Based on Bloom's taxonomy of cognitive outcomes (Table 5.1), constructed-response questions are usually intended to assess students' ability at the higher levels of the taxonomy: application, analysis, synthesis, and evaluation. The constructed-response formant then is intended to require students to apply, analyze, synthesize, and evaluate knowledge, reasoning, and skills.

Illustrative verbs for the stems or questions for constructed-response items can include modify, operate, compute, discover, apply (*application*), identify, differentiate, discriminate, infer, relate, distinguish, detect, classify (*analysis*), combine, compose, design, plan, revise, deduce, produce (*synthesis*), and appraise, compare, contrast, criticize, support, justify (*evaluation*).

TABLE OF SPECIFICATIONS

Before writing the constructed-response test (or any other test), we begin with a table of specifications. Table 12.1 is an example of a TOS for an essay test with ten questions, three levels of understanding and three topics of evidence-based medicine. The numbers in the cells represent the number of essay question for that topic and level of understanding. For example, there are two essay questions for validity of empirical evidence at the *analysis* level of understanding.

Table 12.1 An example of a table of specifications for constructed response test

Content area	Levels of understanding			
Evidence-based medicine	Analysis	Synthesis	Evaluation	
1. Need for empirical evidence for clinical application	0	1	1	2 (20%)
2. Validity of empirical evidence	2	1	1	4 (40%)
3. Translation sciences and clinical practice	1	2	1	4 (40%)
	4 (40%)	4 (40%)	2 (20%)	10 (100%)

TYPES OF ESSAY ITEMS

There are at least two types of essay questions, the restricted and extended response forms. This classification refers to the amount of freedom allowed to candidates in composing their responses. The restricted response question limits the character and breadth of the student's composition. In this type of essay question, the following conditions are met: the student is directed toward a particular type of answer, the scope of the problem is limited, and the length of the essay is sometimes specified.

EXAMPLE 1

A restricted response essay: how might the principles of behaviorism help physicians to maintain motivation for their patients' adherence to treatment plans? In answering this question, at least complete the following tasks:

a. briefly describe the principles of behaviorism;
b. illustrate the use of these in maintaining motivation for their patients' adherence to treatment plans.

The answer should be between one and a half and two pages long.

The essay test outlined in Table 12.1 is a restricted-response essay. There are ten questions for a 4 h examination for approximately 24 min per question. The answers should be all of equal value (10 points), a maximum of one page long.

EXAMPLE 2

A restricted-response essay: a 30-year-old man is brought to the emergency department 30 min after being stung by several wasps. He is confused and has difficulty breathing. His temperature is 38°C (100.4°F), pulse is 122/min, respirations are 34/min, and blood pressure is 80/40 mm Hg. Physical examination shows dry skin and decreased capillary refill. There are multiple erythematous, inflamed marks on the back, and 1+ pitting edema of the ankles. The first treatment step is the administration of 0.9% saline solution.

a. What should be administered as the most appropriate next step in management?
b. Describe the pathophysiology in this patient that accounts for the clinical symptoms.
c. How does the treatment function to alleviate the symptoms?

The answer should be about two pages long.

These examples of restricted response essay questions aim the student at the desired answer. Moreover, the scope of the essay has been circumscribed. As compared to the extended essays, restricted-response questions promote greater reliability in scoring. They may also reduce the student's opportunity to apply, analyze, and synthesize disparate information into a coherent whole, however, thereby reducing divergent thinking, a major purpose of the constructed response.

The extended-response question places fewer limitations on discussion and the form of the answer. An example of the extended-response essay question is a follows:

EXAMPLE 3

An extended-response essay question: how might humanistic psychology be used to maintain motivation for their patients' adherence to treatment plans? Illustrate with appropriate examples the application of particular theoretical constructs from humanistic psychology in the maintenance of patients' motivation for adherence to treatment plans.

In answering this essay question, students may select the particular theoretical constructs from humanistic psychology which they deem to be most important and relevant in maintaining motivation in their patients'. This is in contrast to the previous example of a restricted-response question. In addition, the form of the extended-response essay remains the responsibility of the student and the length is unspecified, thus, allowing for more flexibility and creativity in responses.

EXAMPLE 4

An extended-response essay question: the main purpose of a clinical trial is to determine the efficacy and safety of a medical treatment such as a drug. Design a clinical trial to test the efficacy and safety of a medical treatment of your choice, adhering to the best practices and theory of clinical trials. Illustrate with appropriate discussion the application of particular theoretical and statistical principles of clinical trial design. Typical proposals of this sort are usually around 3,000 words of text. You may use tables, charts, appendices, etc. which are not included in the word count.

EXAMPLE 5

An extended-response essay question: a 25-year-old woman is brought to the emergency department 1 h after she fainted. She has had mild intermittent vaginal bleeding, sometimes associated with lower abdominal pain, during the past 3 days. She has had severe cramping pain in the right lower abdomen for 12 h. She has not had a menstrual period for 3 months; previously, menses occurred at regular 28-day intervals. Abdominal examination shows mild tenderness to palpation in the right lower quadrant. Bimanual pelvic examination shows a tender walnut-sized mass in the right parametrium. What is the most likely differential diagnosis? Based on this differential diagnosis, write a patient management plan, relevant treatments, prognosis, and follow-up plans.

GUIDELINES FOR PREPARING ESSAY ITEMS

- Allow adequate time to write, re-write, and edit the essay questions.
- Use restricted response questions whenever possible unless extended-response format is clearly required for higher level measurement of cognitive levels.
- State the problem in the form of a question or statement.
- Do not use optional questions. Optional questions will undermine the content validity of the test. If an essay topic is important enough for one student, it is important enough for all students. If it is not important enough for all students, it is not important enough for any student.
- When asking student's their opinions, require that they support them with knowledge and a rational argument.
- The essay examination should be given under standard conditions. The instructions, time, and place of writing should be uniform for all students.

- Clearly indicate the time allotted for the total test (e.g., 2 h, a week for take-home essays—give precise due dates).
- Teach your students how to write essay tests with the following guidelines:
  - Ensure that all understand the general instructions.
  - Teach your students to first read and understand the question.
  - Before students begin writing, they should spend about 10% of the total question time in understanding the question and developing an outline for the answer.
  - Teach them to answer the question: if the question asks to "compare and contrast", students should not simply describe. Teach students to use appropriate headings such as "How the two theories compare" and "How the two theories contrast".
  - Teach them to develop an outline with key ideas.
  - Each essay should have an introduction, the body of the essay, and a conclusion.
  - Teach students to use all of the allotted time.
- Create a scoring key for each question.

GUIDELINES FOR SCORING ESSAY QUESTIONS

- There are two basic approaches to the scoring of constructed-response test questions: analytic scoring and holistic scoring.
- In both cases, develop an answer key or rubric to aid the scoring of the essay. Even so, judgment about the quality will be subjectively determined at the time of scoring.
- The rubric tells the scorer what aspects of the response to identify and how many points to award.

Analytic scoring

- Analytic scoring rubrics list specific elements of the response and specify the number of points to award each. On a diagnostic question, the scorer awards 2 points for providing a correct clinical impression, 2 points explanation of the pathophysiology, and 1 point for the correct treatment (total points = 5).
- Each question with the same value (e.g., 5 points, 10 points, etc.).
- Set realistic performance standards.

Holistic scoring

- Holistic scoring is different from analytic scoring. The holistic rubric contains statements of a typical response at each score level so that actual responses written by test-takers provide examples of a 10-point response, an 8-point response, 5-point, and so on. The student examples may also include borderline cases such as a response that just is a minimal pass (e.g., a score of 5) or a response that fails (e.g., receive less than a score of 5).

- Holistic scoring is even less consistent that analytic scoring—the same response scored by two different scorers is less likely to receive the same score from both scorers than analytic scoring.
- For some types of constructed-response questions (e.g., measuring writing ability or moral reasoning), it may not be possible to identify specific elements of the essay. Responses to these can be scored holistically.
- The advantage of holistic scoring is that it allows for student creativity, divergent thinking, and novel responses.
- A good example of holistic scoring are the *Gold Foundation* annual essay contest that asks medical students to engage in a reflective writing exercise on a topical theme related to humanism in medicine (www. gold-foundation.org/2013-humanism-in-medicine-essay-contest-winners-announced/). First, second, and third place essays are chosen by a panel of physicians and noted writers. Winners receive a monetary award and their essays are published in *Academic Medicine*. Students write an essay or story of 1,000 words or less on themes such as: "Who is the 'good' doctor?" and "What do you think are the barriers to humanism in medicine today?"

General scoring guidelines

- Irrespective of analytical or holistic scoring, require proper grammatical responses with full sentence and paragraphs. Do not allow point form.
  - If there are multiple essay questions, grade one question at a time for all students.
  - Randomize the order of students and score all the answers to the first question.
  - Randomize again and score the second question, etc. until all are scored (this procedure will minimize item-to-item order effects as well as student-to-student order effects).
  - Score each test anonymously. Use numerical IDs only that mask student names. This will minimize the halo or horns effects.
  - Be wary of the dove and hawk effects, also called the generosity and severity effects. Some graders are doves and give easy marks, while others are hawks and mark very vigorously. Try to identify which one you are and guard against it.
  - Be wary of the central tendency effect or the average effect. That is, grading everyone as in the middle without extremes of good and bad.
  - Guard against unconscious bias, another common type of error. This refers to attitudes or stereotypes that are outside our awareness but nonetheless affect our judgments and grading. These are both positive and negative automatic associations about other people based on characteristics such as race, ethnicity, sex, age, social class, and appearance.
  - Write comments on each paper.

Computer scoring

The greatest problems in constructed-response testing are the time and expense involved in scoring. The scorers need to be highly trained as in the *Gold Foundation* essays and require elaborate systems for monitoring the consistency (reliability) and accuracy (validity) of the scores. Researchers have recently made progress in using computers to score constructed item responses. Automated scoring reduces the time and cost of the scoring process. For most testing situations, constructed response items requiring human scoring are impractical and prohibitively expensive. While a number of essay scoring programs have been developed, this approach remains very controversial and not very widely used.[1]

COMPARING TOTAL EFFORT FOR MCQ AND ESSAYS TESTS

The total amount of effort in the use of either MCQs or essay test use is, in part, a function of the number of students to be tested (Figure 12.1). The greatest amount of effort for MCQ use is in the construction of the test items. The effort in scoring is minimal, because these items can be scored by computers. The amount of effort in test construction for MCQs is large irrespective of the number of students to be tested, but the effort in scoring is relatively unaffected.

By contrast, the essay test is relatively easy to construct but most of the effort is in scoring the test—creating the scoring rubric and applying to the student responses. The effort in scoring increases rapidly as the number of students increases. Figure 12.1 shows the relationships between MCQs and essay test total effort as a function of the number of candidates tested.

Constructing a high-quality 100 MCQ test with clinical vignettes following the rules specified in Chapter 11 may take more than 33h (approximately 20min per

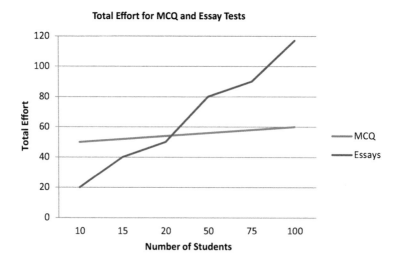

Figure 12.1 Comparison of total effort for MCQ and essays tests.

item). Once this is done, however, the effort for scoring is small and doesn't increase much even with a large number of candidates. Constructing a high-quality ten question essay test may take only about 2 h even strictly adhering to the rules as specified in this chapter. Scoring the results, however, may be quite effortful. For ten students, it may take about 5 h (30 min/student). For 20 students, it may take 10 h, for 50 students 25 h, for 100 students 50 h, and so on. Determining the testing format for any given situation is not dependent on the number of students but rather the levels of cognitive measurement. MCQs should be used for the first three levels of Bloom's taxonomy (*knowledge, comprehension, application*), and constructed response should be used for the next three (*analysis, synthesis, evaluation*).

BOX 12.1: *Advocatus Diaboli*: Automated essay scoring

Important skills such as critical thinking and problem solving are better assessed with constructed-response item formats, such as essays, than they are with MCQs and other selection items. Constructed-response assessments are very effortful to score (Figure 12.1), because they rely on human raters. The responses to constructed-response tasks are manually scored by content specialists who must be trained for the grading task, do the scoring, and monitored throughout to ensure that scores achieve adequate reliability.

Automated essay scoring (AES) technology involves the process of scoring and evaluating written text using a computer program that builds a scoring based on a rubric provided by humans. Then by using machine-learning algorithms, it compares features to the rubric so that the computer can classify, score, or grade new text material submitted by a new group of students. AES phase can assess many different types of written responses, such as patient case management and restricted response essays. The benefits of AES include improved reliability of scoring, reducing the time required for scoring, reducing scoring costs, and immediate feedback on the results.

The idea of grading essays by computer has been around since the mid-1960s; more than 50 years with the work of Ellis Page.[2] At that time, researchers worked with punch cards and mainframe computers. Notwithstanding advances in test theory and computer technology since then, AES still remains controversial and has not been widely implemented in education.

Some excitement was sparked in 2012 when the *Hewlett Foundation* sponsored a competition to determine if AES can be as reliable as human raters for scoring 22,029 essays. There were initial claims that the AES was as reliable as human scoring; this has since been criticized by a variety of commentators including the *Educational Testing Service*. The criticisms included[3] the following:

- five of the eight datasets analyzed consisted of paragraphs rather than essays

(Continued)

BOX 12.1 (*Continued*): *Advocatus Diaboli*: Automated essay scoring

- four of the eight datasets were graded by human readers for content only rather than for writing ability
- AES machines employed an artificial construct, the *resolved score*, rather than the true score thus giving AES an unfair advantage

Shermis and Hamner[4] in an evaluation of the result of the *Hewlett Foundation* competition concluded that AES has developed to the point where it can be reliably applied in both low-stakes assessment (e.g., instructional evaluation of essays) and for high-stakes testing as well. They suggested that Page's "fascinating inevitability," for the potential for AES in educational assessment has been realized. AES systems, however, cannot understand written text. Rather, AES uses approximate variables that correlate with the intrinsic variables of interest to classify written-response scores. AES is best used for well-defined, precise answers to questions.

In the field of medical education, Gierl et al.[1] conducted a study of clinical decision making (CDM) constructed response items used by the Medical Council of Canada (MCC) in Part I of its Qualifying Examination using an AES system. This test assesses the competence of candidates who have obtained their medical degree for entry into supervised clinical practice in postgraduate training programs. The CDM component consists of short-menu and short-answer write-in questions; candidates are allowed 4 h to complete. Gierl et al. utilized responses from six CDM write-in questions from the MCC database. Physicians scored the typed CDM open-ended responses using an established scoring rubric for grading the CDM-constructed responses. Each response was scored independently by two physician raters. Data from the 2013 administration served as the validation dataset. The computer program Light Summarization Integrated Development Environment (LightSIDE), open source software, was used to analyze the data as AES. Exact agreement between the computer classification and the human raters on the validation dataset ranged from 94.6% to 98.2%.

This confirmed, as Page predicted in 1966, that AES systems can classify scores at a rate as high as that of the agreement among human raters themselves. Notwithstanding, acceptance of AES has not been achieved among students, teachers, professors, and the public more generally. One criticism is that computers use a mechanistic process which is incapable of either understanding or appreciating written text. Because of this deficiency, scores are not considered valid. Another view is that the written responses of humans are best assessed using the knowledge, reasoning, and understanding of other humans. This is a criticism of machine learning and artificial intelligence generally. Page and Petersen[5] called this the humanist objection. The AES criteria, critics claim, are trivial (e.g., the use

(Continued)

BOX 12.1 (*Continued*): *Advocatus Diaboli*: Automated essay scoring

of the total number of words as for fluency, matching words for recognition, identified phrases for comprehension, etc.).

Geirl et al. asserted that AES provides a method for efficiently scoring constructed response tasks and could complement the widespread use of selected response items (e.g., MCQs) used in medical education. AES could serve medical education in two ways.

First, AES could be used to provide summative scores required for high-stakes testing. Human scoring would still be required for constructed response items on summative assessments but that AES could be the second scorer thus reducing costs and resources. Instead of using two human raters for each constructed response task, the initial score could be produced by one rater and the second score by the AES system.

Second, AES could assist medical educators by helping them to provide students with rich formative feedback. This would be particularly useful in large classrooms where providing this kind of feedback by human graders would be onerous. AES could not only evaluate students but also provide them with immediate, detailed feedback on their constructed responses. AES could provide the ability to measure, monitor, and improve writing skills in their students.

Current applications of AES require the judgments, expertise, and experiences of content specialists to produce the input and output required for machine learning. AES requires computer technology for the algorithmic task of extracting complex features from the essays scored by human raters. Although not yet widely accepted, AES still holds the promise of reliable and valid evaluations of written text thus automating the processing and evaluating written text. Page's 1966 prediction that AES systems can do better evaluations of written text than human raters may yet come true.

SUMMARY AND MAIN POINTS

Essay questions or constructed-response items can be used to measure at the higher levels of Bloom's taxonomy: application, analysis, synthesis, and evaluation. There are two basic types of essay questions, the restricted and the extended response. These can be scored by either the analytic method or the holistic method, both of which require the development of a rubric. There are well-established guidelines for scoring essays that help to reduce subjectivity of scoring and error of measurement. The total amount of effort in the use of either MCQs or essay test use is, in part, a function of the number of students to be tested. The greatest amount of effort for MCQ use is in the construction of the test items, while for the essay it is the grading time. The idea of grading essays by computer has been around since the mid-1960s. Notwithstanding advances in test theory and computer technology since then, AES still remains controversial and has not been widely implemented.

1. The constructed-response or open-ended item is most commonly known as the essay test but consists of any item format type where the examinee must construct a response rather than select one as in the multiple-choice format.
2. These item types are sometimes also called subjective tests because scoring involves subjective judgments of the scorer. By contrast, the MCQ is referred to as objective because no judgments are required to score the items.
3. Constructed-response questions are usually intended to assess students' ability at the higher levels of Bloom's taxonomy: application, analysis, synthesis, and evaluation.
4. There are at least two types of essay questions, the restricted and extended response forms. This classification refers to the amount of freedom allowed to candidates in composing their responses. The restricted response question limits the character and breadth of the student's composition
5. There are two basic approaches to the scoring of constructed-response test questions: analytic scoring and holistic scoring.
6. Analytic scoring rubrics list specific elements of the response and specify the number of points to award each response
7. The holistic rubric contains statements of a typical response at each score level so that actual responses written by test-takers provide examples of a 10-point response, an 8-point response, 5-point, and so on.
8. The total amount of effort in the use of either essay test or MCQs use is, in part, a function of the number of students to be tested. The greatest amount of effort for MCQ use is in the construction of the test items, while for the essay it is the grading.
9. The idea of grading essays by computer has been around since the mid-1960s. Researchers have recently made progress in using computers to score constructed item responses. Automated scoring reduces the time and cost of the scoring process.

REFLECTIONS AND EXERCISES

Essay test construction

30 marks
> **Purpose:** to practice and develop skills in writing an essay exam.
> **Directions:**

PART A: PLANNING THE TEST (6 MARKS)

Construct a four-item essay exam in a content/subject area in which you have some competence.

Table 12.2 An example of a table of specifications for organ transplantation

Content area	Levels of understanding		
Organ transplantation	Synthesis	Evaluation	
1. Need and quality of life	1	1	2 (50%)
2. Cost-benefit analysis	1	1	2 (50%)
	2 (50%)	2 (50%)	4

1. Outline the content area upon which the test is based. (**1 mark**)
2. Construct a two-way TOS with four cells (Two Levels of Understanding by two subsections of the Content Area). This table should include the following:
   a. two (2) levels of understanding: synthesis and evaluation. (**1 mark**)
   b. two (2) subsections of the content area. (**1 mark**)
   c. the number of test items for each cell. (**1 mark**)
   d. the total number of items. (**½ mark**)
   e. percentage weights for each level of understanding and for each content element. (**½ mark**)
3. State the general purpose of the test, i.e., how will the test results be used? (**½ mark**)
4. State who will take the test (Table 12.2). (**½ mark**)

PART B: WRITING THE TEST (22 MARKS)

According to your blueprint developed in Part A of this assignment:

1. Write a four-item, restricted response essay exam. (**2 marks each; 8 total**)
2. Write a sample answer for each essay question. Use full sentences and appropriate essay format (introduction, body, and conclusion). (**2 marks each; 8 total**)
3. Using an embedded scoring system within your sample answer, indicate how points are to be assigned for each answer. See the example below. (**1 mark each; 4 total**)
4. The test should include a title and explicit instructions (i.e., time for each question and value of each question). (**2 marks**)

EXAMPLE OF AN ESSAY QUESTION AND A RUBRIC WITH AN EMBEDDED SCORING SYSTEM VIGNETTE

A number of tests by the family doctor and specialists confirm the diagnosis of astrocytoma, grade 4, brain cancer (i.e., advance stage of development) for a 15-year-old girl.[6] There is no known cure for this type of cancer, but the doctors' suggest that they can slow the process if they begin ongoing chemotherapy immediately. After a few days, the mother and daughter decide to end the chemotherapy treatments to pursue a variety of alternative non-toxic therapies (e.g., herbology, nutritional modification, vitamin therapy). The girl's father, however, is in direct conflict with his wife and daughter and wants them to return to the original chemotherapy treatment plan.

QUESTION

In your opinion, what should the family doctor say to the family regarding their decision to pursue alternative therapies?

Support your answer with (3) reasons for your opinion. You will receive (1) mark for your opinion and (3) marks for each supporting reason for a total of 10 marks. You have 20 min to complete this essay.

SAMPLE ANSWER WITH EMBEDDED MARKS

In my opinion, it's always really up to the patient to determine what course they want to go on. The doctor is a kind of the moderator on these and that it's a horrible decision to have to make, especially for a 15-year-old girl (1).

If the doctor is confident that the 15-year-old girl and her mother have made a sound decision he/she would have to defend them in their decision. And the doctor would probably need to outline the conflict to the governing body because that seems to be of pretty big importance to this case. (3) So, the family doctor's obligations are to outline the options available, which are to be on chemotherapy or not be on chemotherapy. As a family doctor, I would try to work with the mother, father, and daughter to try and blend the two approaches and find a middle ground they might be comfortable with. (3) Also helping the father and mother realize that the social benefits to their daughter of good family relations are going to do way more for their daughter's health than either of the two treatment modalities. (3)

For these reasons, I feel that the doctor should be a moderator to help the whole family reach a decision on which they can be comfortable.

PART C: REFLECTION

After you have completed this assignment, write a brief reflection (one page typewritten maximum) about your reactions to essay exams and the construction of an essay exam.

NOTE: the reflection is an important part of this assignment. Although the reflection is not marked, in order to receive a grade for the entire assignment, the reflection must be handed in.

To submit to the instructor

1. Part A—Questions 1–4.
2. The essay exam which includes Part B—Question 4.
3. The sample answers with an embedded scoring system.
4. Your reflection about the construction of an essay exam.
5. Two (2) marks will be awarded for professional appearance of the exam (spelling and grammar).

All of the above should be type-written.

REFERENCES

1. Gierl MJ, Latifi S, Lai H, Boulais A, Champlain A. Automated essay scoring and the future of educational assessment in medical education. *Medical Education* 2014, 48:950–962.
2. Page EB. The imminence of grading essays by computers. *Phi Delta Kappan* 1966, 47:238–243.
3. Perelman L. When "the state of the art" is counting words. *Assessing Writing* 2014, 21:104–111; Bennett RE. The changing nature of educational assessment. *Review of Research in Education* 2015, 39(1):370–407.
4. Shermis MD, Hamner B. Contrasting state-of-the-art automated scoring of essays. In: Shermis MD, Burstein J, eds. *Handbook of Automated Essay Evaluation: Current Application and New Directions*. New York, NY: Routledge 2013:313–346.
5. Page EB, Petersen NS. The computer moves into essay grading: Updating the ancient test. *Phi Delta Kappan* 1995, 48:238–243.
6. Donnon T, Oddone-Paolucci E, Violato C. A predictive validity study of medical judgment vignettes to assess students' noncognitive attributes: A 3-year prospective longitudinal study. *Medical Teacher* 2009, 31(4):e148–e155. doi: 10.1080/01421590802512888.

13

Objective structured clinical exams

ADVANCED ORGANIZERS

- Due to the errors produced by traditional methods and the need to improve the reliability and validity of clinical competency measurement, the objective structured clinical examination (OSCE) has been introduced.
- The OSCE concentrates on skills, clinical reasoning, and attitudes—to a lesser degree basic knowledge. Content checklists and global rating scales are used to assess observed performance of specific tasks. Candidates circulate around a number of different stations containing various content areas from various health disciplines.
- Most OSCEs utilize standardized patients (SPs), who are typically actors trained to depict the clinical problems and presentations of real issues commonly taken from real patient cases.
- OSCE validity concerns are (1) content-based—defining the content to be assessed within the assessment; (2) concurrent-based—this requires evidence that OSCEs correlate with other competency tests that measure important areas of clinical ability; and (3) construct based—one of the ways of establishing construct validity with OSCEs is through differentiating the performance levels between groups of examinees at different points in their education.
- OSCE reliability concern is which reliability coefficient (inter-rater, ICC, Ep^2), how many raters are required, which people (e.g., SPs or MDs) make the best raters, and what is the appropriate number of stations in an OSCE?
- As OSCEs are used for both summative and formative purposes, it is important to determine the standards or the score cutoff (such as pass/fail) which define the level of expected performance for different groups of candidates.

- OSCEs are both time-consuming and resource-intensive. Administrative components, concerns such as test security and cost analysis play important roles ensuring the quality of the OSCEs.
- The OSCE has been adopted worldwide with very little scrutiny and study. There is not much systematic evidence of empirical validity for the OSCE.

INTRODUCTION

The traditional assessment of clinical competence since time immemorial consisted of bedside oral examinations, ward observations, casual conversations between clinical teachers and students, and chart audits. More recently, constructed response formats such as essays and selection formats such as MCQs have also been used. There are several major limitations of these assessment formats.

MCQs which provide objective measurements of biomedical knowledge primarily at the lower levels of Bloom's taxonomy are too superficial and lack ecological validity and are also disconnected from the real clinical context between patients and physicians. Bedside observations, oral exams, hallway conversations, and chart reviews contain nearly all possible sources of assessment error including (1) rater error (i.e., inconsistency due to subjectivity) such as the halo effect, hawk-dove effect, etc., (2) lack of standards for marking performance, (3) inadequate sampling of student interactions with patients and across content areas, (4) small numbers of real patients in which to observe student, resident, or physician performance, and (5) contrived situations and threatening environments in which to test student performance.

Due to the errors produced by these methods and the need to improve the psychometric aspects of clinical competency measurement, Harden and colleagues[1] pioneered a systematic and objective strategy for observing and evaluating clinical skills—the objective structured clinical examination (OSCE).

Clinical competence and OSCEs

As discussed in Chapter 2 and throughout this book, clinical competence is a multidimensional construct composed of several complex components: knowledge, skills, attitudes, professionalism, and so on. Miller described a four-tier pyramid of clinical ability, identifying the base of the pyramid as knowledge (measuring what someone knows), followed by competence (measuring how they know), performance (shows how they know), and lastly at the summit, action (behavior).[2] Clinical competence involves a complex interplay between attributes displayed within the physician–patient encounter which enable physicians to effectively deliver care. Before the introduction of the OSCE, however, the assessment of these basic clinical skills lacked reliability and validity.

The OSCE concentrates on skills, clinical reasoning, and attitudes; to a lesser degree, basic knowledge. The OSCE is not a test itself but rather a testing approach to which multiple testing activities, such as content checklists and global rating scales are used to assess observed performance of specific tasks.

The OSCE is a multiple station format. Candidates circulate around a number of different stations containing various content areas from various medical disciplines. The station lengths can range from between 5 min to 1 h, attempting to simulate a real-time medical encounter depending upon medical discipline. Family medicine physicians usually see patients for between 15 and 20 min, whereas palliative care physicians may spend 30–40 min with patients and their families. Content and principles from surgery, pediatrics, family medicine, orthopedics, and so forth are used within the OSCE.

Most OSCEs utilize standardized patients (SPs), who are typically actors trained to depict the clinical problems and presentations of real issues commonly taken from real patient cases. A specified and defined number of tasks are required to be performed by examinees and recorded on structured behavioral checklists and/or rating form by examiners (usually physician judges or SPs). The encounter can be video and audio recorded and assessed at a later time. This recording can also be used to provide specific formative feedback to the candidate.

Frequently, there are two components to the OSCE format, typically referred to as *couplet* stations where examinees first perform clinical tasks with an SP for a defined period of time (e.g., 10 min). Then they rotate to a post-encounter station containing x-ray or laboratory findings for the patient they have just seen. The post-encounter station offers a constructed-response format (i.e. various questions which require specific answers) related to the preceding patient encounter. The couplet stations are designed to measure both the application of practical skills as well as to measure the examinees ability to take and synthesize relevant patient information.

The major strengths of the OSCE are objectivity and structure for scoring of the examinees' performance, usually as a checklist or rating scale. Additionally, there is standardization of content, tasks, and processes accomplished through the training of SPs, who present the same information in a standard fashion across examinees.

The OSCE is a performance-based measure that satisfies two main assessment criteria: (1) reliability and validity can be determined and improved and (2) generalizations about the performance of examinees can be made. There can also be educational uses: (1) formative evaluation that provides feedback to clinical teachers and students and (2) summative evaluation that allows clinical teachers, regulatory bodies, and licensing bodies to make pass/fail decisions.

PSYCHOMETRIC ISSUES FOR OSCES

Traditional methods of clinical skill assessment were poor indicators of ability because they were confounded by unstandardized, uncontrolled, and subjective methods of evaluation. The major basic psychometric principles which underlie any measurement and evaluation are basic to OSCEs as well. These include aspects of validity, reliability, standard setting, and sources of measurement error.

Standardized patient accuracy

Does the simulated SP environment reflect the real-life context? Are these clinical environments such as SPs credible? How closely does it reflect the real context? Numerous studies have documented the accuracy of SP performance for real-life context including history taking, physical exam performance, communication, empathy, diagnoses, data collection and evaluation, prescribing, and so on.[3] This accuracy and consistency of SP performance depends on the effectiveness of SP training. Considerable error variance (e.g., 25%) can be introduced by SPs when they have not been effectively trained.

Tamblyn[4] has studied the standardized patient method extensively. She has identified three parameters that are central to portrayal by the SP.

1. Present the same information to every candidate. If the candidate asks about diet for example, all SPs should give the same response.
2. The information should be provided under the same conditions. Do some SPs but not others spontaneously volunteer information about their medications (e.g., "I'm taking Tylenol")? This type of variation is common and it has an impact on candidate performance.
3. The SP should not mention other problems that were not part of the official case or script (e.g., "I haven't been sleeping well"). Performance standards are designed to be case specific, so deviations in the content of the case bias performance measurement.

Other factors that contribute errors

- Sex differences
    1. Women SPs are more likely to receive a prescription for medication than men presenting with the same problem.
    2. A woman SP presenting with the precise same appendicitis symptoms as a man SP will receive irrelevant diagnoses of ectopic pregnancy and endometriosis.
- Body size: presenting a meningitis case, an overweight SP compared to an average weight one will attract investigations about diabetes and hypertension.
- Consistency of portrayal: an SP portraying high fever with DVT sprays water on forehead to simulate sweating. When the spray bottle runs dry, candidates receive a different portrayal than did the earlier ones.
- SPs that prompt a candidate that is faltering (e.g., "my pain level is 7/10").
- SPs that make evaluative comments (e.g., good, or that's wrong) during the exam.

Employing well-trained SPs with accuracy of case presentation reduces error. When properly trained, SPs can and do uniformly present the case in a way that reduces measurement errors arising from content presentation.

OSCE validity concerns

CONTENT-BASED

Defining the content to be assessed within the evaluation is one of the most important priorities of measurement design. Content validity is concerned with comprehensiveness and relies on the adequacy and representativeness of the items sampled within the domain of interest. As with any assessment, developing a table of specifications, or TOS (Chapter 5) that incorporates the sample of items and level of measurement is central to content validity. Many studies have documented the high-content validity of the OSCE approach. Table 13.1 represents a TOS for a 12-station family medicine OSCE.

Table 13.1 Table of specifications of OSCE stations utilized to evaluate residents

Patient and condition	Assessments	Differential diagnoses and/or management
1. Stuart Kim 62-year-old male complaining of problems urinating	• History taking • Physical assessment • Counselling	Benign prostatic hypertrophy
2. Pat Soffer 39-year-old male arrives at rural emergency room after vomiting bright red blood	• Immediate assessment and treatment • History taking • Physical assessment and emergency management dealing with ABCs	Peptic ulcer disease, Mallory Weiss tear, esophageal varices, gastritis, and malignancy
3. Daisy Long 75-year-old female presenting with fatigue	• History taking with preliminary psychiatric assessment • Communication skills	Diuretic induced-hypokalemia, hypertension
4. Andrew Voight 45-year-old male admitted 5 days previously with chest pain	• History taking • Counselling • Risk assessment and management for non Q-wave myocardial infarction	Advise on use of medication and warning signs for seeking healthcare
5. Nancy Posture 58-year-old female presenting with difficulty sleeping, headaches, loss of appetite, and feeling as though "on an emotional roller coaster"	• History taking • Counselling with special risk management for suicidal tendencies	Depression and excessive alcohol intake

(Continued)

Table 13.1 (*Continued*) Table of specifications of OSCE stations utilized to evaluate residents

Patient and condition	Assessments	Differential diagnoses and/or management
6. Terry Spencer 64-year-old female complaining of severe right leg pain	• History taking • Physical assessment • Promptness of management and information Sharing	Necrotizing fasciitis, Gangrene
7. Terry Heinsen 48-year-old male complaining of fever 3 days after an open cholecystectomy	• History taking • Physical assessment of abdomen post-operatively	Deep vein thrombosis
8. Katherine Jones 35-year-old female who wants to discuss her risk of getting breast cancer after her younger sister was just diagnosed	• History taking • Risk assessment • Counselling	Addressing concerns of breast cancer in the family
9. Laura Zhang 21-year-old female complaining of a severe headache	• History taking • Physical assessment of the central nervous system	Meningitis
10. Jaden Bogart 17-year-old male complaining of 'shortness of breath'	• History taking • Physical assessment • Information sharing	Asthma, aggravating factors such as pets, grass, and perfumes, inhaler use, Ventolin, smoking
11. Sandy Monteiro 15-year-old female presenting with "excessive weight loss"	• History taking (weight loss) • History taking (family, past) • Interpersonal skills	Anorexia nervosa, anxiety, depression, obsessive compulsive disorder
12. Jason Browne 23-year-old male wanting a note that he is 'sick' to avoid an exam	• History taking • Ethical issue • Counselling	Discuss ethics Non-judgemental and empathic Counselling/ Actions

CONCURRENT-BASED

This requires evidence that OSCEs correlate with other competency tests that measure important areas of clinical ability (Chapter 6). OSCEs in pediatrics can explore the degree to which OSCE scores on various sub-components of skills correlated with final MCQ examinations. There might be correlations between patient management skills and final MCQs testing of knowledge. Other correlations could be between OSCE practical skills and clinical teacher's evaluation of performance on hospital wards. Other concurrent validity study may involve determining correlations between OSCE total test scores and clerkship and residency ratings and also performance on USMLE exams. Correlations between OSCEs and other objective measurements of clinical ability, specifically testing skills and knowledge domains can provide evidence of concurrent validity.

CONSTRUCT-BASED

A construct is a hypothetical entity which cannot be directly observed but must be inferred from observable behaviors and responses to test items (Chapter 6). One of the ways of establishing construct validity with OSCEs is through differentiating the performance levels between groups of examinees at different points in their education. Evidence of construct validity, for example, is provided when performance differences are exhibited between medical students, clerks, and, residents (Years 1, 2, 3, 4, or 5) on some performance as these groups have increasing level of knowledge and expertise. This is the "known group difference effect."

In a study of 27 second-year surgery residents in a 19-station OSCE covering history taking and physical exam skills, management skills, problem-solving skills, and technical skills revealed significant between-group differences ($p < 0.05$). These results were corroborated by Stillman et al. who compared performance between three groups of residents (i.e. PGY1 ($n = 63$) vs. PGY 2 ($n = 98$) vs. PGY3 and 4 ($n = 80$) across 19 residency programs in the United States.[5]

The researchers were interested in examining differences in performance on cases related to content, communication, physical findings, and differential diagnosis by residency level.

Using the mean scores attained for each of the four OSCE cases, results revealed significant between group differences ($p < 0.05$) for the content and differential diagnosis cases between all years, as scores increased as a function of increased year in residency. There were only significant differences observed for the communication and physical findings cases, however, among first-, third-, and fourth-year residents.

The two studies provided as examples are stable findings observed in studies comparing various levels of undergraduate and post-graduate for differences in proficiency levels across skills (i.e. history-taking, communication and interpersonal skills, problem-solving skills, technical skills) and across medical disciplines. These results taken together provide some evidence of construct validity for the use of OSCEs.

Sources of measurement error in validity

There are several types of factors that contribute errors:

- Order effects (two types are typical): fatigue and practice effects. Examiner, candidate, and/or SP fatigue is a factor contributing to sources of measurement error in the assessment of clinical competence using OSCEs. Similarly practice effects of examiner, candidate, and/or SP can introduce error of measurement
- Anxiety and motivation: increased performance for OSCE order may be due to decreased student anxiety as they move through the stations, higher motivation, and increase in comfort level as a result of increased experience with the OSCE format
- SP factors. The SP's understanding of the clinical problem to be presented, SPs previous experience with the simulation context and prior acting experience, SPs with similar health-related problems as the cases portrayed
- The best solution in reducing these types of errors is controlling the testing environment, particularly by ensuring that SPs are well trained

RELIABILITY

In performance-based assessments, variance can be decomposed into several components: between raters (inter-rater reliability), between stations (inter-station reliability), between items (internal consistency), and between observed performance and an estimate of future performance (test reliability). Examinees' scores are typically decomposed into two main components: raters and stations (or cases), which refer to inter-rater and inter-station reliability. Generalizability theory can be applied to this type of problem (Chapter 9).

Multiple sources of measurement error

Generally, the standard reliability coefficient (inter-rater, ICC) is set at 0.80. How many raters are required to achieve this standard of 0.80? What people (e.g., SPs or MDs) make the best raters? What is the appropriate test length or number of stations in an OSCE?

In their review, van der Vleuten and Swanson[6] found that (1) one rater provides as good an estimate of reliability for station scores and rater consistency as two or more raters, as increasing the number of stations is more important than increasing the number of raters; (2) there are comparable inter-rater reliabilities between SPs and physician raters; (3) inter-station reliability is the most variable among the sources of reliability estimates, as an examinee's performance on one station does not predict well with performance on another station; and (4) an average of between 7 and 15 plus stations over a minimum of 3–6 h of testing time is typically required to achieve a $Ep^2 \geq 0.80$. Inter-rater reliability is generally higher than reliabilities for inter-station reliability.

Inter-station reliability

Many studies have consistently shown that performance on one station is a poor predictor of performance on another station. Newble and Swanson[7] indicated that inter-station reliability is a complex issue because it deals with two types of error: (1) the inconsistency of performance across stations and (2) inconsistency in rater agreement, both affecting the score. Other factors that have been shown to produce error in examinee scores are (1) heterogeneity of examinee group, (2) SP performance, (3) examiners, (4) scoring, and (5) integrity of the data. Another source of error in testing clinical competence involves the use of checklists versus global rating scales.

CHECKLIST VS. GLOBAL RATING SCALE

Checklists contain many items, and itemize examinee performance into small units compared to global ratings, which are broader and less exhaustive than checklists. Items in a checklist can range from a few items to many items about the expected tasks to be performed within a station. Conversely, items in global rating forms are broader, and range from a single overall item to fewer than a dozen items relating to more broad-based tasks or behaviors that are observed.

The differences in reliability between checklists and global rating scales are marginal. Regehr et al. have found that although there are differences between these two rating form types, they are different by chance fluctuation not by statistical difference.[8] Global rating scales, though, have better validity than checklists as they correlate better with end of course written examinations (concurrent validity) and are better at discriminating levels of performance (construct validity) than checklists.

GENERALIZABILITY THEORY

Generalizability theory, though underemployed, has an important place in performance-based measurement particularly when OSCEs are employed. G theory permits the calculation of a dependability estimate and attempts to determine how accurate one can be about generalizing a candidate's observed score to the range of behaviors estimated. The goal is to ascertain how much within and between variability is accounted for by each facet (Chapter 9).

Three variance components and Ep^2 are usually calculated: (1) between raters (inter-rater), (2) from the same rater across performance on different stations (inter-station), and (3) all of the test across for all raters. In one study,[9] the Ep^2 for the two-facet nested design (SP nested into case) based on the two assessment formats was 0.84 and 0.74 (checklist and global rating, respectively—Table 13.2).

The Ep^2 indicated that higher reliability was achieved by checklist scores than global scores. The latter may provide better assessment of coherence of clinical competency than checklists.

Sources of error arise in the percent variance components for the SP and the examiner facets due to SP and examiner variability (approximately 20% of the

Table 13.2 The variance, percentage variance, and generalizability coefficients for the two-facet nested design (SP nested into case)

Assessment	Facets	Variance	Variance (%)	Ep^2
Checklist	Candidates (p)	30.9609	20.0	0.84
	Cases (c)	11.6028	7.5	
	SPs nested in case	27.0727	17.5	
	p x c, res[a]	85.0487	55.0	
	Total	154.6851	100	
Global	Candidates (p)	0.1474	12.6	0.74
	Cases (c)	0.0162	1.4	
	SPs nested in case	0.2698	23.1	
	p x c, res[a]	0.7323	62.8	
	Total	1.1657	100	

[a] The variability as a result of the interaction effect (p x c) also includes random error (res) which cannot be separated and are combined and labelled as the residual.

variance). Generally, examiner inconsistency is the largest threat to the reliability of an assessment. It is therefore important to train the examiners on how to use the assessment instruments. Similarly, SP measurement error can be introduced via the inconsistent and inaccurate SP performance, choice of SP to portray the case, and/or the SP's portrayal of the case. Therefore, careful selection and training of SPs is important.

STANDARD SETTING

As OSCEs are used for both summative and formative purposes, it is important then to determine the standards or the score cut-point (such as pass/fail) which define the level of expected performance for different groups of candidates. The absolute standard-setting method based on judgments about items in a station test using the Ebel method is generally preferred in OSCE standard setting because it takes into account two dimensions of each item: relevance and difficulty.

The Ebel method is a good approach in high-stakes exams. This method focuses on content items on the checklists and rates items based on their difficulty and relevance, thus placing more emphasis on ensuring content validity of the checklist or rating scale itself (Table 13.3). Judges establish standards through reviewing each potential item and rating the item by its difficulty concerning the level of ability of examinees and to its relative importance related to the necessary skills to be executed for proper fulfillment of the case. The advantage of this method is that it is thorough and strengthens the content validity of the scoring method used within the station, however the process of determining the specifics are time consuming.

Employing the nine-category grid in Table 13.3, each OSCE[10] item is classified into one of the cells based on its difficulty and relevance. This method for setting

Table 13.3 Ebel procedure for setting MPLs of clinical skills, tasks, and procedures

		Difficulty		
Relevancy		Easy	Medium	Hard
	Essential	EE	ME	HE
	Important	EI	MI	HI
	Marginal	EM	MM	HM

MPLs has been shown to have empirical evidence of validity.[11] For relevancy, three levels are used: essential, important, and marginal. Similarly, three levels are used for difficulty: easy, medium, and hard.

Judges independently classify each task or clinical skill into one of the nine cells on the difficulty by relevancy table above. A clinical skill may be judged as easy and essential (EE), for example, although another may be judged as medium difficulty and important (MI). Through this process, an Ebel rating is given to each clinical skill, procedure, or task. The overall cutoff score for the station is the sum of the MPLs.

EXAMPLES

- Asking the patient about the intensity of pain ("On a scale of 1–10, how much does it hurt?"), for example, may be judged easy to do and important (EI) to the assessment.
- In some instances, listening to heart sounds may be judged as hard to do and marginal to the presenting problem (HM)

Judges are instructed to independently classify each item into one of the nine cells in Table 13.3. They are given the following instructions: *do not agonize over each but provide your BEST clinical intuition of the difficulty and relevance of each skill relevant to the particular case. Write your classification (e.g. EM) in pencil on the left-hand side of each item on the checklist.*

The items are circulated to the judges electronically such as Excel worksheets and the judges provide their ratings on the spread sheet. At least two judges rate each item independently. Subsequently, these are averaged to determine a weight for the item MPL.

OSCE LOGISTICS

OSCEs are both time-consuming and resource-intensive. There are several theoretical and psychometric issues that arise from the use of OSCEs: test length, sample size, training time of SP's, and establishing inter-rater reliability. Additionally, administrative components, concerns such as test security, and cost analysis play important roles ensuring the quality of the OSCEs. Test security becomes an issue particularly when dealing with large groups of candidates, such as those tested by national licensing bodies for entering practice at various stages of the educational spectrum (e.g., end of undergraduate medical education or post-graduate medical education). To manage the volume of candidates tested whether at a local school or at a national level (i.e., MCC, NBME, *National Council Licensure Examination*-RN), parallel forms of tests are used to minimize the potential confounds influencing candidate performance. The major concern to repeatedly testing candidates with the same station content is that sharing of information between candidates may compromise the validity of the exams.

OSCEs can be very costly, as SPs, examiners, and other personnel and administrative staff must be paid. Cost consideration can compromise psychometric criteria such as attaining high validity and reproducibility of scores. About 12 stations are required to achieve adequate reliability, particularly for total test reliability. If the stations are very well-designed and executed, Ep^2 coefficients > 0.70 can be achieved with as few as seven stations. These and other logistical concerns are important to consider when designing the TOS for the OSCE. Disadvantages include the extensive time commitment required to create the cases, the expense of resources needed (e.g., testing rooms), personnel costs (e.g., SPs and their trainers and physician examiners), and candidate testing time frequently compromise psychometric results.

STATISTICAL RESULTS OF THE FAMILY MEDICINE OSCE DESCRIBED IN TABLE 13.1

There were 51 family medicine residents that took the 12-station OSCE described in Table 13.1. The results of the exam are summarized in Table 13.4 that contains the overall results and the pass/fail for each of the OSCE stations. The mean number of stations passed overall was 9.45.

Table 13.4 Descriptive statistics and psychometric results of OSCE assessments

Station	Min	Max	Mean	SD	α
Station 1	11	18	14.06	2.32	0.63
Station 2	8	15	12.03	2.24	0.67
Station 3	14	24	20.68	3.07	0.60
Station 4	20	29	23.90	3.13	0.74
Station 5	15	29	23.87	4.75	0.78
Station 6	18	28	21.45	2.51	0.70
Station 7	13	16	14.84	1.21	0.73
Station 8	17	26	21.84	2.22	0.81
Station 9	19	30	23.13	3.24	0.70
Station 10	11	21	15.65	3.71	0.75
Station 11	16	24	20.26	3.26	0.68
Station 12	10	18	13.52	2.74	0.71
Overall ratings and communication					
Overall examiner ratings	1.8	3.9	3.49	0.46	—
Communication	3.1	4.0	3.60	0.32	0.86

SD, Standard Deviation; α, Cronbach's alpha of internal consistency reliability.

The internal consistency reliabilities (Cronbach's alpha) are also summarized in Table 13.4. They range from 0.60 (Station 3) to 0.86 (Communication). The overall ratings on the stations and the communication scale are also summarized in Table 13.4. G-theory analyses for this OSCE was a two-facet nested design (SP nested into case) based on the two assessment formats $Ep^2 = 0.84$, a value acceptable for high-stakes assessments.

SUMMARY AND CONCLUSION

Harden et al. developed the OSCE in response to the highly error-laden techniques such as chart audits, MCQs, unstructured hallway conversations, infrequent student observations, and lack of structured protocols in which to establish rater consistency among clinical teachers. This work helped renew interest in the focus and application of basic psychometric principals which underlie all measurement. Through standardization and proper training, SPs can accurately and reliably present case material with high ecological validity (indistinguishable between real and simulated performance). As well, SPs are comparable to physician examiners to reliably assess the skills of examinees and provide feedback that is useful and helpful for examines.

Like all assessment tasks, OSCE development should begin with a TOS. This will allow control over various testing components such as (1) that test items are specific to the objectives of real clinical tasks and are appropriate for different educational levels of examinees, (2) ensuring an adequate number of stations, content areas, and objectivity in rating performance, and (3) choosing the Ebel method of setting standards.

Major limitations to designing and implementing OSCEs are practical issues such as SP training, test security and costs. Confounding variables such as order effects and error due to inadequate sampling of stations due to lack of resources can compromise reliability and validity. Although these are practical (as opposed to theoretical) aspects of the testing design, they can have a profound impact on the outcomes of the testing approach if not properly controlled and are incongruent to the goals and objectives of the OSCEs.

The challenges to using OSCEs include threats to basic measurement criteria such as inter-rater and inter-station reliability and aspects of validity. OSCEs can measure clinical skills, such as physical exams, history taking, communication, and technical procedures in a uniform and systematic manner. With careful construction, training of both assessors and SPs, and controlled application, OSCEs can adequately and accurately capture important elements of clinical competence that is fundamental disciplines of medical and healthcare practice.

- The OSCE concentrates on skills, clinical reasoning, and attitudes; to a lesser degree basic knowledge. Content checklists and global rating scales are used to assess observed performance of specific tasks.
- Most OSCEs utilize SPs.
- OSCE validity concerns are (1) content based; (2) concurrent based; and (3) construct based—differentiating the performance levels between groups of examinees at different points in their education.

- OSCE reliability concerns how many raters, which people make the best raters and what is the appropriate number of stations?
- Cutoff scores (such as pass/fail) can be set with the Ebel method.
- OSCEs are both time-consuming and resource-intensive.
- The OSCE has been adopted worldwide notwithstanding the paucity of empirical validity evidence for the OSCE.

BOX 13.1: *Advocatus Diaboli*: The trouble with OSCEs

Most assessments in medical and health sciences education lack evidence of construct validity. This includes the OSCE, a performance-based assessment. It is second in popularity and use only to the MCQ formats. There has been a rapid increase in medical, nursing, dental and other health education worldwide in the use of OSCE assessment methods.

The major advantages of the OSCE format include controlling the complexity of the station based on the skill level of the candidates, the ability to sample a wide range of knowledge and skills, and clearly defining the knowledge, skills, and attitudes to be assessed. The disadvantages include the extensive time commitment required to create the cases, the expense in resources needed (e.g., testing rooms), and personnel costs (e.g., SPs and their trainers; physician examiners). Notwithstanding the widespread use, there is a need for further construct validity evidence for the use of the OSCE assessment format for assessing professionalism and competence, particularly for high-stakes outcomes (e.g., licensing or certification).

Construct validity focuses on whether a test successfully measures the characteristics it is designed to assess and whether the interpretation of the test score is meaningful. In order for an assessment to be valid, it must be reliable. For measurements of performance to produce evidence of reliability, there must be a sufficient sample of observations, and these observations should be gathered with a degree of structure and standardization.

Few studies have investigated the empirical evidence of validity of OSCEs. Construct validity of an assessment method includes all other forms of validity and even more extensive research such as the known group difference group method, the MTMM approach, as well as exploratory and confirmatory factor analyses. Although rare, some studies have directly investigated construct validity of OSCEs. Blaskiewicz et al.[12] utilized multiple regression analysis to study the relationship between psychiatry OSCE scores from the clinical skills examination, an obstetrics/gynecology OSCE, and the NBME psychiatry subject examination. They found that the pattern and magnitude of convergence and discrimination of scores were indicative of inadequate construct validity for both the psychiatry checklist scores and global scores.

(Continued)

BOX 13.1 (Continued): Advocatus Diaboli: The trouble with OSCEs

Baig et al.[13] employed a MTMM to study the construct validity of clinical competence—including aspects assessed by an OSCE—and identified both method and trait variance. With few exceptions, however, there is a scarcity of studies directly investigating the construct validity of measurements of clinical competence, particularly OSCEs.[14] In a predictive validity of a high-stakes OSCE used to select candidates for a 3-month clinical rotation to assess practice-readiness status, Vallevand and Violato[9] provided evidence of predictive validity with a 100% correct classification rate in the pass/fail rotation results.

Notwithstanding these examples, insufficient systematic research has been conducted to investigate the predictive and construct validity of OSCEs. The principal function of any assessment protocol is to provide inferences about the competency, abilities, or traits of the candidates—inferences that extend beyond the sample of cases or stations included in the examination. Regardless of an assessment's intention (e.g., formative vs. summative examination) the assessment process must be reliable, valid, defensible, and feasible.

The OSCE has been adopted worldwide with very little scrutiny and study. It is so popular that it has even made an appearance on the television show *Seinfeld*, even though it is not a good model to conduct this exam.[15] There is insufficient systematic evidence of empirical validity for the OSCE. The sample sizes are frequently too small for running complex statistical procedures such as generalizability, factor, or discriminant analyses required to establish evidence of construct validity. It is also typical to only have one rater per station which compromises the determination of inter-rater reliability. Future research should be designed for Ep^2 analyses with fully crossed designs. More work needs to be done on the empirical evidence (e.g., criterion-related and construct) for the OSCE, since this aspects has been neglected. The focus in past research has been primarily on face and content validity, and the OSCE has been accepted more-or-less uncritically.

REFLECTIONS AND EXERCISES

Reflections

1. Notwithstanding the scant validity evidence, the OSCE has gained worldwide acceptance and use. Critically evaluate the reasons for the ascendancy of the OSCE. (Maximum 500 word answer)

2. Compare and contrast the efficacy of various assessors in the OSCE (e.g., SPs, physicians, undergraduate students, etc.). What are the important characteristics of the assessors for improving the reliability and validity of the OSCE? (Maximum 500 word answer)
3. Design an ideal study to investigate the construct validity of the OSCE. (Maximum 500 word answer)

Exercises

1. Using the template in Table 13.1, develop a table of specifications for an eight-station OSCE in any area of your interest.
2. What major psychometric analyses would you conduct in an OSCE? (*hint*: descriptive statistics, reliability, validity, item analyses, etc.)
3. For a ten-station OSCE to assess 150 students, how would you design a generalizability (Ep^2) study to address variance due to students, assessors, stations, etc.? Consider maximum efficiency and cost constraints.
4. Develop a point-by-point plan for adequately training SPs in an OSCE.

REFERENCES

1. Harden R, Gleeson F. Assessment of clinical competence using an objective structured clinical examination (OSCE). *Medical Education*, 1979; 13: 41–54.
2. Miller GE. The assessment of clinical skills/competence/performance. *Academic Medicine*, 1990; 65: s63–s67.
3. Harden RM. Twelve tips for organizing an objective structured clinical examination (OSCE). *Medical Teacher*, 1990; 12: 259–264.
4. Tamblyn RM. Use of standardized patients in the assessment of medical practice. *Canadian Medical Association Journal*, 1998; 158: 205–207.
5. Stillman P, Swanson D, Regan MB, Philbin MM, Nelson V, Ebert T, Ley B, Parrino T, Shorey J, Stillman A, Hatem C, Kizirian J, Kopelman R, Levenson D, Levinson G, McCue J, Pohl H, Schiffman F, Schwartz J, Thane M, Wolf M. Assessment of clinical skills of residents utilizing standardized patients. *Annals of Internal Medicine*, 1991; 114: 393–401.
6. van der Vleuten CPM, Swanson DB. Assessment of clinical skills with standardized patients: state of the art. *Teaching and Learning in Medicine*, 1990; 2: 58–76.
7. Newble DI, Swanson DB. Psychometric characteristics of the objective structured clinical examination. *Medical Education*, 1988; 22: 325–334.
8. Regehr G, MacRae H, Reznick RK, Szalay D. Comparing the psychometric properties of checklists and global rating scales for assessing performance on an OSCE-format examination. *Academic Medicine*, 1998; 73: 993–997.

9. Vallevand A, Violato C. A predictive and construct validity study of a high-stakes objective clinical examination for assessing the clinical competence of international medical graduates. *Teaching and Learning in Medicine*, 2012; 24: 168–176.

10. Ebel RL, Frisbee DA. *Essentials of Educational Measurement* (4th ed). Toronto, ON: Prentice Hall, 1986.

11. Violato C, Marini A, Lee C. A validity study of expert judgment procedures for setting cutoff scores on high-stakes credentialing examinations using cluster analysis. *Evaluation & the Health Professions*, 2003; 26: 59–72.

12. Blaskiewicz RJ, Park RS, Chibnall JT, Powell JK. The influence of testing context and clinical rotation order on students' OSCE performance. *Academic Medicine*, 2004; 79(6): 597–601.

13. Baig L, Violato C, Crutcher R. A construct validity study of clinical competence: A multitrait multimethod matrix approach. *Journal of Continuing Education in the Health Professions*, 2010; 30(1): 19–25.

14. Patricio M, Juliao M, Fareleira F, Young M, Norman G, Vaz Carneiro A. A comprehensive checklist for reporting the use of OSCEs. *Medical Teacher*, 2009; 31(2): 112–124.

15. www.youtube.com/watch?v=wLRlbsBJhio

14

Checklists, rating scales, rubrics, and questionnaires

ADVANCED ORGANIZERS

- Checklists, rating scales, rubrics, and questionnaires are instruments that state specific criteria to gather information and to make judgments about what students, trainees, and instructors know and can do in outcomes. They offer systematic ways of collecting data about specific behaviors, knowledge, skills, and attitudes and can be used at higher levels of Miller's Pyramid.
- A checklist is an instrument for identifying the presence or absence of knowledge, skills, behaviors, or attitudes used for identifying whether tasks in a procedure, process, or activity have been done.
- Surgery has made extensive use of checklists as have many other disciplines such as oncology and cardiology.
- A rating scale is an instrument used for assessing the performance of tasks, skill levels, procedures, processes, and products, but they indicate the degree of behavior rather than dichotomous judgment as in checklists.
- Rating scales allow the degree or frequency of the behaviors, skills, and strategies to be rated. Rating scales state the criteria and provide selections to describe the quality or frequency of the performance. A five-point scale is preferred because it provides the best all-around psychometrics.
- There are four basic types of rating scales: (1) numeric rating scale, (2) graphic rating scale, (3) descriptive graphic rating scale, and (4) visual analogue scale.
- A rubric is a scoring guide used to evaluate the quality of constructed responses. Rubrics employ specific criteria to evaluate performance. They consist of a fixed measurement scale and detailed description, which focus on the quality of performance with the intention of including the result in a grade.

- Questionnaires are instrument consisting of a series of questions (or prompts) for the purpose of gathering information from respondents. A main advantage of questionnaires is that a great deal of information can be gathered effectively and with little cost. Unlike telephone surveys, they require much less effort and often have standardized answers that make it simple to compile data. A disadvantage of the standardized answer is that they don't permit alternative responses.

INTRODUCTION

Checklists, rating scales, rubrics, and questionnaires are instruments that state specific criteria to gather information and to make judgments about what students, trainees, and instructors know and can do in outcomes. They offer systematic ways of collecting data about specific behaviors, knowledge, skills, and attitudes and can be used at higher levels of Miller's Pyramid.

The purpose of checklists, rating scales, rubrics, and questionnaires is to devise instruments for:

- systematic recording of observations
- self-assessment
- determine criteria for learners prior to collecting and evaluating data on their work
- record the development of specific skills, strategies, attitudes, and behaviors that demonstrate learning
- clarify learners' instructional by recording current accomplishments

WHAT IS A CHECKLIST?

A checklist is an instrument for identifying the presence or absence of knowledge, skills, behaviors, or attitudes. They are used for identifying whether tasks in a procedure, process, or activity have been done. The activity may be a sequence of steps and include items to verify that the correct sequence was followed. The assessor usually observes the activity because it cannot be judged from the end product. Some attitudes, like showing respect for patients, can only be observed indirectly. A checklist itemizes task descriptions and provides a space beside each item to check off the completion of the task.

CHARACTERISTICS OF GOOD CHECKLISTS

Checklists should have the following characteristics:

- space for other information such as the trainees' name, date, case, assessor
- clear criteria for success based on outcomes
- tasks organized into logical sections or flow from start to finish
- highlight critical tasks
- clear with detailed wording to avoid confusion
- brief and practical (e.g., one sheet of paper)

Table 14.1 is a checklist to be used for an OSCE station with an SP portraying a patient with lung cancer. The assessor observes the trainee and checks-off the behaviors as "attempted" or "done satisfactorily." If the performance was not attempted, the checks are left blank. The assessor will check item 2 "What patient

Table 14.1 Checklist for a station of a patient with lung cancer

Candidate_____ Assessor_____ Date_____Time: ___begin ____end

History of presenting complaint—enquires about	Attempted	Done satisfactorily
1. Other symptoms (nausea, headache)	O	O
2. What patient has been taking for pain	O	O
3. Further treatment after surgery	O	O
4. Relationship status	O	O
5. Nature of relationships with wife and children	O	O
6. Employment status	O	O
7. Asks about patient's feelings, displays empathy	O	O
8. Asks about coping mechanisms after initial diagnosis	O	O
Information sharing		
9. Informs patient of results of CT scan	O	O
10. Indicates that tumors are metastases from lung cancer	O	O
11. Indicates that there is no cure	O	O
12. Reassures patient that failing to stop smoking did NOT cause cancer to spread	O	O
13. Indicates will make appointment with a specialist to discuss palliative treatment options	O	O
14. Inquires how patient will be getting home	O	O
15. Arranges follow-up with family members	O	O
Questions to be asked by examiner (at 10 min)		
16. What sort of follow-up would you arrange for this patient?		
17. Would follow-up regularly	O	O
18. Demonstrates knowledge of other community resources	O	O
19. How would you respond if the patient asks about alternative (non-conventional) treatments?		
20. Ask which treatment in particular the patient was thinking of using and why	O	O
21. Reflect back patient's seeking alternative treatment as a reflection of patient's desperation and offer to work with patient to explore all options	O	O

has been taking for pain" and item 9 "Informs patient of results of CT scan", for example, as "attempted" or "done satisfactorily" or left blank.

Table 14.1 has all of the characteristics of a good checklist: clear criteria for performance, one page, organized into logical sections and flow, clear with detailed wording, and has spaces to record trainees' names, assessor, date, etc.

Surgery has made extensive use of checklists as they have been promoted in an attempt to prevent mistakes related to surgery. Checklists have been widely adopted, not only in Western countries but throughout the world for increasing patient safety.[1] They have been associated with improved health outcomes, including decreased surgical complications and surgical site infections. Surgical complications represent a significant cause of morbidity and mortality with the rate of major complications after in-patient surgery estimated at 3–17% in industrialized countries.

The World Health Organization (WHO) has developed a surgical safety checklist (Table 14.2) that has been widely disseminated and adopted. This checklist

Table 14.2 World Health Organization surgical safety checklist[2]

---

1. Has the patient confirmed his/her identity, site, procedure, and consent?

2. Is the site marked?

3. Is the anesthesia machine and medication checked completely?

4. Is the pulse oximeter on the patient functioning?

5. Does the patient have a:
   - Known allergy?
   - Difficult airway or aspiration risk?
   - Yes, and equipment/assistance available

6. Risk of >500 ml blood loss (7 ml/kg in children)? Yes, and two IVs/central access and fluids planned

7. Confirm all team members have introduced themselves by name and role

8. Confirm the patient's name, procedure, and where the incision will be made

9. Has antibiotic prophylaxis been given within the last 60 min?

10. Anticipated critical events

11. To Surgeon:
    - What are the critical or non-routine steps?
    - How long will the case take?
    - What is the anticipated blood loss?

12. To Anesthetist:
    - Are there any patient-specific concerns?

13. To Nursing Team:
    - Has sterility (including indicator results) been confirmed?

(Continued)

Table 14.2 (*Continued*) World Health Organization surgical safety checklist[2]

 • Are there equipment issues or any concerns?

 • Is essential imaging displayed?

14. Nurse Verbally Confirms:

 • The name of the procedure

 • Completion of instrument, sponge, and needle counts

 • Specimen labelling (read specimen labels aloud, including patient name)

 • Whether there are any equipment problems to be addressed

15. To Surgeon, Anesthetist, and Nurse:

 • What are the key concerns for recovery and management of this patient?

Source: http://apps.who.int/iris/bitstream/10665/44186/2/9789241598590_eng_
    Checklist.pdf.

was explicitly designed for varying cultural and geographic contexts with a very clear and simple presentation. It contains most of the elements of good checklists: clear criteria for performance, one page, organized into logical sections and flow, clear with detailed wording. The statements are primarily framed in the interrogative as questions to which the answer must be either "yes" or "no." Some of the important questions, for example, are: "3. Is the anesthesia machine and medication checked completely?" and "9. Has antibiotic prophylaxis been given within the last 60 min?"

Surgical checklists are a simple and promising way for addressing surgical patient safety worldwide. Further research may be able to determine to what degree checklists improve clinical outcomes and whether improvements may be more pronounced in some settings over others.

Another area which checklists have been applied is for scoring an electrocardiogram (ECG) examination protocol (Table 14.3). Cardiologist candidates that are applying for board certification are given a number of ECG examples and are asked to read them and record their answers on a 50-item answer sheet. The checklist in Table 14.3 is used by the assessor to check each item that the candidate recorded on their answer sheet.

Scoring and candidates' score

Table 14.4 summarizes the protocol for scoring each item together with the pertinent Ebel score, item value, the score for each examiner (for an example candidate), and the average score for each item. The total score for each candidate is the sum of the average score and the overall MPL is the sum of the Ebel scores for each item. If a candidate's score is equal to or greater to the MPL, it is a "pass"; if less, it is a "fail." A total of 150 candidates wrote this test.

Three examiners independently scored each protocol and the results were averaged over the three examiners (Table 14.4). A generalizability analysis (fully

Table 14.3 Checklist for scoring ECG protocol (Check each item that was written by the candidates on the answer sheet)

1	Sinus/Atrial/Supraventricular
	PVC (± unifocal)
	Arrythmia—sinus/otheratrial
2	Sinus
	Bradycardia
	Anterior/Anteroseptal/Anterolateral
	Recent/Acute
3	Sinus
	1° AV Block
	LBBB
4	Junctional (supraventricular)
	Atrial (sinus) Bradycardia
	Occasional atrial capture of ventricles
	Anterior ischema or definite repolarization changes
5	Pacemaker LBBB (not required)
	Dual Chamber (DDD)
	Sinus/Atrial Beats
	1° AV Block
6	Sinus
	PACs
	LAH/LAD
	Possible ant MI/Poor R wave prog
	Repolarization changes
7	Sinus
	1° AV Block
	RBBB
	Long QT
	Antero....MI
8	Sinus
	Inferior MI
	Left atrial abnormality
9	Atrial fibrillation
	Rapid ventricular response
	Nonspecific ST/T changes
10	Atrial Flutter
	Atrial Fib-Flutter
	2:1 AV conduction
	Inferior MI
11	Sinus
	Long QT
	Anterior or lateral T-wave changes

(Continued)

Table 14.3 (*Continued*) Checklist for scoring ECG protocol (Check each item that was written by the candidates on the answer sheet)

12	Pacemaker
	VVI (ventricular)
	3° AV Block
	Sinus
13	Atrial fibrillation
	3° AV Block
	Junctional rhythm
	ST&T changes/repolarization changes
14	Sinus
	(Consider) Pericarditis
	Inferior Infract
15	(probable, possible, etc.) Ventricular rhythm
	Tachycardia
16	Sinus
	RBBB
	Left Anterior Hemiblock/Left Axis Deviation
	1° AV Block
	Long QT
	Anterior MI
17	Sinus
	RBBB
	LAH/LAD
	Anterior MI
	PAC
18	Sinus
	Supraventricular tachycardia
19	Junctional rhythm
	Accelerated
	Inferior MI
	Posterior MI
20	Sinus
	Second-degree AV Block
	Mobitz II
	RBBB
	Acute Ant MI
	Left anterior hemiblock/LAD
21	Sinus
	Inferior MI
	Posterior MI
	Lateral MI
	Non-acute MI (or equivalent words)

(Continued)

Table 14.3 (*Continued*) Checklist for scoring ECG protocol (Check each item that was written by the candidates on the answer sheet)

22	Sinus tachycardia
	Inferior MI
	Acute MI
	Posterior MI
23	Sinus
	Non-specific T-wave changes
	Limb lead reversal (malposition)
24	Non-sinus supraventricular rhythm (or equivalent words)
	Right ventric. conduction delay (or IRBBB or RV hypertrophy)
25	Sinus
	WPW
26	Sinus
	Pericarditis (±consider)
27	DELETED
28	Sinus
	Left bundle branch block
	Septal MI
29	Sinus
	2° AV Block (high grade AV Block) (2:1 AV Block)
	RAD
	RBBB
30	Atrial fibrillation
	Actual or controlled: ventricular rate
	Non-specific ST&T changes/repolarization changes
31	Sinus
	Inferior MI
	Acute or recent or indeterminate
32	Sinus
	Left ventricular hypertrophy
	Left atrial abnormality
33	Sinus
	Lead reversal (malposition)
	Left atrial abnormality
34	Atrial fibrillation
	Fast (uncontrolled) ventricular rate
	RBBB
35	Sinus tachycardia
	Left bundle branch block
	(possible) Anterior MI
	Left atrial abnormality

(*Continued*)

Table 14.3 (*Continued*) Checklist for scoring ECG protocol (Check each item that was written by the candidates on the answer sheet)

36	Normal (or no abnormality mentioned)
	Sinus (or just normal)
	i.e., Normal, sinus rhythm, or both
37	Atrial rhythm
	Sinus bradycardia
38	Sinus
	3° or complete AV block
	"Idioventricular rhythm" or "junctional rhythm with LBBB"
39	Sinus
	2° AV block
	Mobitz I
	Acute or recent inferior MI
	Acute or recent posterior MI
40	Atrial tachycardia or atrial flutter
	2:1 AV block
	Anteroseptal MI (or anterior or septal)
	Non-diagnostic ST&T changes
41	Sinus bradycardia
	1° AV Block
	Blocked PACs
	Non-specific ST-T changes
42	Supraventricular tachycardia (or PAT)
	Non-specific ST-T changes
43	Sinus or sinus tachycardia
	High grade / (2:1) / 2° AV Block
	RBBB
	Non-acute anteroseptal or anterior MI
	Non-acute inferior MI
44	DELETE
45	Sinus arrhythmia or PACs or sinus exit block
	Acute inferior MI
	Posterior MI
46	Atrial flutter
	Inferior MI
	Posterior MI
	Possible acute/Recent MI
47	Sinus
	Artifact
	Acute anterior MI
	Left atrial abnormality

(*Continued*)

Table 14.3 (*Continued*) Checklist for scoring ECG protocol (Check each item that was written by the candidates on the answer sheet)

48	Sinus
	Lead reversal (malposition)
	Acute anterior MI
49	Sinus
	Right bundle branch block
	Acute anteroseptal MI
	Non-acute inferior MI
	LAD/LAH
50	Sinus
	WPW

Table 14.4 Selected results (items 1 and 2) of the scoring ECG protocol

				Candidate #2			
Item #	Item	Ebel score	Item value	Examiner 1	Examiner 2	Examiner 3	Average score
1	Sinus/Atrial/ Supraventricular	0.9	1	0	0	0	0
	PVC C (± unifocal)	0.9	1	1	1	1	1
	Arrythmia—sinus/ otheratrial	0.7	1	0	0	0	0
2	Sinus	0.9	1	1	1	1	1
	Bradycardia	0.5	1	1	1	0	0.67
	Anterior/ Anteroseptal/ Anterolateral	0.9	1	1	1	1	1
	Recent/Acute	0.9	1	1	1	1	1

Ep^2 (examiners) = 0.97.

crossed, one facet design) for the results showed that the scores had very high dependability across the three examiners: variance component (rater) = 4340.642; variance component (residual) = 96.154; and $Ep^2 = 4340.642/(4340.642 + 96.154) = 4340.642/4436.796 = 0.97 - Ep^2 = 0.97$.

WHAT IS A RATING SCALE?

A rating scale is an instrument used for assessing the performance of tasks, skill levels, procedures, processes, and products. Rating scales are similar to checklists except that they indicate the *degree* of behavior rather than dichotomous judgment such as "yes" or "no" (Table 14.2). They are composed of a list of performance statements and behavior in descriptive words usually with numbers. Two items from a rating scale of teacher effectiveness, for example, are:

1. Encourages students to participate in discussion

   $1 =$ never $2 =$ rarely $3 =$ sometimes $4 =$ frequently $5 =$ consistently

All rating scales can be classified into one of three types.

Numeric rating scale (examples are Items #1 above and #2 below)

1. Stimulates students to bring up problems

   $1 =$ never $2 =$ rarely $3 =$ sometimes $4 =$ frequently $5 =$ consistently

Graphic-rating scale (an example is below)

Rate your colleague based on the quality of work, neatness, and accuracy.

1. Poor: careless worker that repeats similar mistakes
2. Average: work is sometimes unsatisfactory due to messiness
3. Good: work is acceptable without many errors
4. Very Good: reliable worker producing good quality work
5. Excellent: work is of high quality; errors are rare and there is little wasted effort

Descriptive graphic-rating scale

This scale is intended to be simple and self-explanatory. It can be easily used with children and impaired respondents (Figure 14.1).

Visual analogue scale (VAS)

This scale is continuous (or analogue) and different from discrete scales such as the Likert scale. The visual analogue scales may give more precise values and superior metrics than discrete scales, thus they produce a true continuous ration

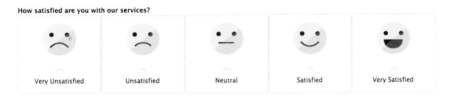

How satisfied are you with our services?

Very Unsatisfied   Unsatisfied   Neutral   Satisfied   Very Satisfied

Figure 14.1 A common example of a descriptive graphic-rating scale.

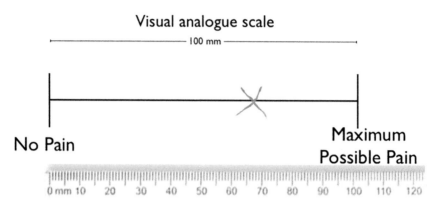

Figure 14.2 An example of a visual analogue scale.

scale (Figure 14.2). When this scale is electronically linked on modern computers, the respondent moves the indicator up and down the scale by dragging it with the mouse and a value (e.g., 3.65) is automatically calculated. The low-tech version above shows how the value can be calculated from pencil-and-paper application.

These ratings form the scale and can indicate a range of feeling (no pain to maximum possible pain) or performance such as from poor to excellent, never to always, beginning to exemplary, never to consistently, or strongly disagree (SD) to strongly agree (SA). The last scale, SD to SA (Item #1 above), is a Likert scale. Any scale that is not dichotomous (i.e., two options such as yes or no) is generally referred to as a multi-point scale. A common error that is made is to refer to all five-point scales as Likert scales but this only refers to the SD to SA scales.

How many points should a scale have? It is common to see scales range from 3 to 12 points. Considerable research has demonstrated that generally, the five-point scale is preferred because it provides the best all-around psychometrics. McKelvie in some experiments found that the five-point scale was most reliable, and confidence judgments using continuous scales indicated that respondents were operating with five categories. Other evidence suggested that while there is no psychometric advantage in a large number of scale categories (greater than 9–12), there may be a loss of discriminant power and validity with fewer than five.[3] The default, therefore, is five points.

Characteristics of rating scales

Rating scales should have clearly defined, operationalized, detailed statements to be rated. On the teacher effectiveness rating scale (Table 14.5), for example, #7 is "Listens attentively to students." This is a clearly defined statement.

The range of numbers should always increase or always decrease. If the statements are positive (e.g., #8 is respectful toward students), then the highest

Table 14.5 A rating scale for teacher effectiveness in a clinical environment

	Factor					
	Stud center	Teach skills	Feed-back	Learn object	Evaluation	Motivation
1. Encourages students to participate in discussions	0.416	0.674				
2. Stimulates students to bring up problems		0.654				
3. Keeps to teaching goals; avoids digressions		0.653				
4. Prepares well for teaching presentations		0.600		0.447		
5. Teaches on ward rounds, at clinics, and OR		0.569				
6. Cover all the topics which are in the curriculum		0.494		0.523		
7. Listens attentively to students	0.713					
8. Is respectful toward students	0.790					
9. Is available regularly for the students	0.699					
10. Is easily approachable for discussions	0.771					
11. States learning goals clearly				0.697		
12. Prioritizes learning goals and topics				0.675		
13. Debriefing the learning goals periodically				0.689		
14. Evaluates student's specialized knowledge					0.653	
15. Evaluates student's analytical abilities					0.676	

(Continued)

Table 14.5 (*Continued*) A rating scale for teacher effectiveness in a clinical environment

	Factor					
	Stud center	Teach skills	Feed-back	Learn object	Evaluation	Motivation
16. Evaluates student's application of knowledge to specific patient					0.657	
17. Evaluates student's medical skills regularly			0.500		0.554	
18. Evaluates student's communication and professionalism skills			0.536		0.497	
19. Regularly gives constructive feedback			0.648			
20. Explains why students are incorrect			0.609			
21. Offers suggestions for improvement			0.663			
22. Gives students chance to reflect on feedback			0.650			
23. Motivates students to study more						0.671
24. Stimulates students to keep up with the literature						0.651
25. Motivates students to learn independently						0.699

1, strongly disagree; 2,disagree; 3, neutral; 4, agree; 5, strongly agree.

number (5) should be the positive term ("strongly agree" or "always") with the lowest number (1) the negative term ("strongly disagree" or "never"). The characteristics and descriptors listed should clear, specific, and observable.

Table 14.6 contains an adapted version of the mini-CEX to directly assess clerkship students' medical competence. The current version of mini-CEX is an eight-item, global-rating scale (1–5) that is designed to evaluate residents' patient

Table 14.6 Rating scale (modified mini-CEX assessment form)

Assessor _____   Student _____

Date _____   Patient Problem/Dx(s) _____

Patient Age ___   Patient Sex: M   F   Setting (I/O)_____

ENCOUNTER COMPLEXITY: ___ Low ___ Moderate ___ High

	Not yet meets criteria	Meets criteria	Exceeds criteria	Not observed
1. Communication skills	N1 N2	M3 E4	E5	NO
2. Medical interviewing skills				
3. Physical examination skills				
4. Professionalism/humanistic qualities				
5. Clinical reasoning				
6. Management planning				
7. Organization/efficacy of encounter				
8. Oral presentation				
9. Overall clinical competence				

Mini-CEX time: Observing ___ min

Assessor providing feedback to student ___ min

Comments on Student's Performance

Areas of Strength:

Areas for Improvement

_____   _____

Student Signature   Assessor Signature

encounters, followed by open-ended comments. After a 15–20 min observation, an attending physician provides scale ratings on nine dimensions.

This mini-CEX has been programmed to be used on mobile devices (e.g., phones, iPad, laptop, etc.) with voice-activated input. The data can be automatically downloaded to a website by activating the "submit" button. Assessors can also record the patient problems, age, sex, setting (inpatient/outpatient), and encounter complexity (low, moderate, high). Ratings range from 1–5, where 1 = not close to meeting criterion; 2 = not yet meets criterion; 3 = meets criterion; 4 = just exceeds criterion; 5 = well exceeds criterion.

Rating scales allow instructors or students to indicate the degree or frequency of the behaviors, skills, and strategies displayed by the person rated. Rating scales state the criteria and provide selections to describe the quality or frequency of the performance. The descriptive word is very important; the more precise are the words for each scale point, the more reliable the scale.

Effective rating scales use descriptors with clearly understood measures, such as frequency (e.g., never to always). Subjective descriptors of quality (e.g., fair, good or excellent) introduce ambiguity because the adjective requires some subjective judgment.

The 25-item clinical-teacher-effectiveness scale (Table 14.5) was completed by clerkship students for 585 clinical rotations. The data were factor analyzed with principal components extraction and varimax rotation resulting in six factors (student-centered, teaching skills, feedback, learning objectives, evaluation, and motivation). These six factors accounted for nearly 90% (89.3%) of the variance. In the clinical environment, it is evident that students can distinguish teaching effectiveness into its components. These factors are cohesive and theoretically meaningful.

WHAT IS A RUBRIC?

A rubric is a scoring guide used to evaluate the quality of constructed responses. They usually are in table format and can be used by assessors when grading and by students when planning work.

Rubrics employ specific criteria to evaluate performance. They may be used to assess individuals or groups and, as with rating scales, results may be compared over time. They consist of a fixed measurement scale and detailed description of the characteristics for each level of performance. These descriptions focus on the *quality* of performance with the intention of including the result in a grade. Rubrics can increase the consistency and reliability of scoring.

Developing rubrics

The scoring criteria for a rubric communicate expectations of level of performance. The scoring criteria are frequently used to delineate consistent standards for grading. Scoring criteria allow assessors and trainee alike to evaluate criteria, which can be intricate and subjective. A rubric can also provide self-assessment, reflection, and peer review. This integration of performance and feedback provides formative as well as summative assessment.

Rubrics are increasingly recognized as a way to both effectively assess learning and communicate expectations directly, clearly, and concisely to students. The inclusion of rubrics provides opportunities to consider what demonstrations of learning look like and to describe stages in the development and growth of knowledge, comprehension, and application. To be most effective, rubrics should allow students to see the progression of mastery in the development of comprehension and skills. Table 14.7 contains a rubric to assess participation and discussion performance in case of based small group learning.

Table 14.7 Rubric to assess participation and discussion performance in case based small group learning

Component	Proficient	Competent	Not yet competent	Unacceptable
Conduct	Shows respect for members of the group. Does not dominate discussion; challenges ideas respectfully	Shows respect for members of the group. Sometimes has difficulty accepting challenges to ideas or maintain respect	Shows little respect for the group. Sometimes resorts to ad hominem attacks when disagrees	Shows lack of respect for members of the group. Argues or dismissive; resorts to ad hominem attacks
Leadership	Takes responsibility for maintaining the discussion whenever needed. Gives constructive feedback	Will take on responsibility for maintaining the discussion. Sometimes encourages others to participate	Rarely takes an active role in maintaining the discussion. Constrains or biases the discussion	Does not play an active role in maintaining the discussion or undermines effort to facilitate discussion
Reasoning	Arguments are reasonable, supported with evidence. Provides analysis of complex ideas for the inquiry and further the conversation	Arguments are reasonable and mostly supported by evidence. Comments and ideas contribute to understanding of the material and concepts	Contributions are often based on opinion or unclear views. Comments suggest a difficulty in following complex lines of argument	Comments are frequently so illogical or without substantiation. Resorts to ad hominem attacks on the author instead
Listening	Always actively attends to what others say as evidenced by regularly building on others' comments	Usually listens well and takes steps to check comprehension by asking clarifying and probing questions	Does not regularly listen well as indicated by the repetition of comments or questions; frequent non sequiturs	Fails to listen or attend discussion as indicated by repetition of comments or questions; non sequiturs, off-task
Preparation	Has carefully read and understood the readings. Comes prepared with questions and critiques of the readings	Has read and understood the readings. Sometimes interpretations are questionable. Comes prepared with questions	Has read the material; didn't read or think carefully about it. Inconsistent commitment to preparation	Doesn't understand and interpret the material; comes unprepared; can't answer basic questions or discussion

To develop a rubric, the quality of performance based on the learning outcomes needs to be defined. Examples of high and low performance need to be used to demonstrate what excellent or acceptable achievement is. This provides a model of high-quality work for learners. Once the standard is established, exemplary levels and less-than-satisfactory levels of performance can be articulated. Like rating scales, rubrics should have four to five-point descriptive levels to allow for discrimination in the evaluation of the task or performance.

Table 14.7 contains several components or traits of performance: conduct, leadership, reasoning, listening, and preparation. Each participant is rated on one of four categories on each component: proficient, competent, not yet competent, and unacceptable. There are descriptions of participant behavior that exemplifies that rating in each of the cells. For a *proficient* rating on conduct, for example, the student "Shows respect for members of the group; does not dominate discussion; challenges ideas respectfully" but for an unacceptable rating, "Shows lack of respect for members of the group. Argues or dismissive; resorts to *ad hominem* attacks." Similarly, a *not yet competence* rating for reasoning is "Contributions are often based on opinion or unclear views. Comments suggest a difficulty in following complex lines of argument."

QUESTIONNAIRES

Questionnaires are instrument consisting of a series of questions (or prompts) for the purpose of gathering information from respondents. A main advantage of questionnaires is that a great deal of information can be gathered effectively and with little cost. Unlike telephone surveys, they require much less effort and often have standardized answers that make it simple to compile data. A disadvantage of the standardized answer is that they don't permit alternative responses. Respondents must be able to read to answer the questions and therefore may not be suitable for some groups (e.g., children, impaired patients, foreign-language speakers). The questionnaire survey is possibly the most popularly used research method in the social, health, and educational sciences.

A patient questionnaire for encounters with medical radiation technologists is summarized in Table 14.8. This brief 12-item questionnaire is intended to be completed by the patient immediately after the treatment or procedure. It employs Likert-type items.

Questionnaires are commonly employed to conduct surveys, as they are very flexible in the content and formats employed. The information collected from individual questions or items become data that can be analyzed statistically. These analyses can range from descriptive statistics to factor analysis, multiple regression, and latent variable path analyses. A single survey may focus on various topics such as opinions (e.g., should assisted suicide be legal?), preferences (e.g., car vs. public transportation), behavior (e.g., eating and exercise), or factual information (e.g., illnesses), depending on its purpose. The success of survey research depends on the quality of the questionnaire and the representativeness of the sample from target populations of interest.

Table 14.8 Patient questionnaire

Medical Radiation Technologist (MRT's) Name: _____

Specialty: _____

Patient age _____   Sex (circle): Man   Woman

Treatment or Procedure_____

Respond to the statement about this MRT using the following:				
	Strongly agree	**Agree**	**Neutral**	**Disagree**	**Strongly disagree**
1. Adequately explained my treatment or procedures	1	2	3	4	5
2. Explained if and when to return for follow-up care	1	2	3	4	5
3. Shows interest in me as a patient	1	2	3	4	5
4. Treats me with respect	1	2	3	4	5
5. Helps me with my fears and worries	1	2	3	4	5
6. Provides adequate privacy	1	2	3	4	5
7. Prevents other patients from hearing confidential information about me	1	2	3	4	5
8. I would go back to this MRT	1	2	3	4	5
9. Answers my questions well	1	2	3	4	5
10. I would send a friend to this MRT	1	2	3	4	5
11. Shows concern for my comfort	1	2	3	4	5
12. Shows concern for my safety	1	2	3	4	5

An example of questionnaire survey research: Leadership

Leadership is a complex, multifaceted phenomenon that is widely observed but poorly understood. Empirical work in leadership—particularly in medical education—is required as it is associated with student achievement and successful team functioning. A recent study employed a survey questionnaire that was sent to medical education leaders to identify the primary competencies of medical education leadership.[4] Survey participants were from medical schools

Table 14.9 Descriptive statistics for 20 of the 63 items from the leadership questionnaire

Items	Min	Max	Mean	SD
1. Maintain quality	1	5	4.16	0.77
2. Succession planning/recruiting	1	5	4.31	0.82
3. Personnel decision quality	1	5	4.54	0.69
4. Maintaining safety	1	5	4.13	0.87
5. Enhancing task knowledge	2	5	4.24	0.70
6. Eliminating barriers to performance	1	5	4.26	0.72
7. Strategic task management	1	5	4.43	0.70
8. Communication with community	1	5	3.85	0.90
9. Providing a good example	2	5	4.58	0.67
10. Knowledge of organizational justice	2	5	4.44	0.72
11. Legal regulations	1	5	4.29	0.75
12. Open-door policy	2	5	4.41	0.78
13. Explaining decisions respect	1	5	4.55	0.66
14. Servant leadership	1	5	4.30	0.77
15. Distributing rewards fairly	1	5	4.28	0.85
16. Responsibility for others	1	5	4.24	0.81
17. Financial ethics	1	5	4.17	0.93
18. Honesty and integrity	1	5	4.76	0.59
19. Being accountable	1	5	4.71	0.61
20. Time management	1	5	4.24	0.71

in several countries—Austria, Canada, Germany, Switzerland, United Kingdom, and the USA—provided demographic data.

A five-point survey of 63 competencies (1 = not required, 2 = of very little importance, 3 = somewhat important, 4 = important, 5 = very important) was sent by email to professors, associate professors, and assistant professors. Most of the participants rated each item as important (4) or very important (5) but for many items the entire scale (1–5) was utilized. As examples of the items and responses, the first 20 competencies are summarized in Table 14.9. The means of the items ranged from 3.85 (#8. Communication with Community) to 4.76 (#18: Honesty and Integrity). The standard deviations are typical (<1.0) for five-point items, indicating that data points are clustered closely around the mean.

Factor analyses of the data indicated that core competencies in medical education leadership can be empirically identified and categorized into five factors: (1) social responsibility, (2) innovation, (3) self-management, (4) task management, and (5) justice orientation. The majority of respondents were physicians, nurses, followed by physiotherapists, midwives, and educators. Accordingly, the competencies appear to be stable and coherent across health professions. This study explicitly defined and provided empirical evidence for the most important leadership competencies in health sciences education.

SUMMARY AND MAIN POINTS

Checklists, rating scales, rubrics, and questionnaires are instruments that state specific criteria to gather information and to make judgments about what students, trainees, and instructors know and can do on outcomes. They offer systematic ways of collecting data about specific behaviors, knowledge, skills, and attitudes and can be used at higher levels of Miller's Pyramid.

The purpose of using checklists, rating scales, rubrics, and questionnaires is to devise instruments for systematic recording of observations, self-assessment, determine criteria for learners prior to collecting and evaluating data on their work. Another purpose is to record the development of specific skills, strategies, attitudes, and behaviors that demonstrate learning and clarify learners' instructional by recording current accomplishments.

- A checklist is an instrument for identifying the presence or absence of knowledge, skills, behaviors, or attitudes used for identifying whether tasks in a procedure, process, or activity have been done.
- Surgery has made extensive use of checklists as have many other disciplines such as oncology and cardiology.
- A rating scale is an instrument used for assessing the performance of tasks, skill levels, procedures, processes, and products, but they indicate the degree of behavior rather than dichotomous judgment as in checklists.
- Rating scales allow the degree or frequency of the behaviors, skills, and strategies to be rated. Rating scales state the criteria and provide selections to describe the quality or frequency of the performance. The five-point scale is preferred because it provides the best all-around psychometrics.
- There are four basic types of rating scales: (1) numeric-rating scale, (2) graphic-rating scale, (3) descriptive graphic-rating scale, and (4) visual analogue scale.
- A rubric is a scoring guide used to evaluate the quality of constructed responses. Rubrics employ specific criteria to evaluate performance. They consist of a fixed measurement scale and detailed description, which focus on the quality of performance with the intention of including the result in a grade.
- Questionnaires are instruments consisting of a series of questions (or prompts) for the purpose of gathering information from respondents. A main advantage of questionnaires is that a great deal of information can be gathered effectively and with little cost. Unlike telephone surveys, they require much less effort and often have standardized answers that make it simple to compile data. A disadvantage of the standardized answer is that they don't permit alternative responses.

REFLECTIONS AND EXERCISES

Reflections

1. Critically evaluate the use of checklists and rating scales in health sciences education. (Maximum 500 words)
2. Describe the application of rating scales based on the Miller's Pyramid of assessment. (Maximum 500 words)
3. Describe the application of rating scales based on Bloom's taxonomies of assessment. (Maximum 500 words)
4. Compare and contrast Miller's Pyramid and Bloom's taxonomies for the use of rating scale and checklists. Describe the application of rating scales based on Miller's Pyramid of assessment. (Maximum 500 words)
5. Discuss the leadership characteristics for health professions education identified in the leadership study (Table 14.9). (Maximum 500 words)

Exercises

1. Checklists have been considered very successful in surgery for reducing errors and improving patient safety. Propose an application of a checklist in any area of health professions that interests you. Develop a table of specifications and some examples items for your checklist. (Maximum 250 words)
2. Discuss the six factors identified on the "Clinical Effectiveness Rating Scale" in Table 14.5. Do the results of the factor analysis provide evidence for construct validity? (Maximum 250 words)
3. Apply the rubric in Table 14.7 to an assessment situation in any area of your interest. How would you modify it? (Maximum 250 words)
4. Propose a survey study in any area of health professions that interests you. Develop a table of specifications and some examples items for your questionnaire. (Maximum 250 words)

REFERENCES

1. Treadwell JR, Lucas S, Tsou AY. Surgical checklists: a systematic review of impacts and implementation. *BMJ Quality&Safety* 2014; 23(4): 299–318.
2. WHO 2009. http://apps.who.int/iris/bitstream/10665/44186/2/9789241598590_eng_Checklist.pdf.
3. McKelvie SJ. Graphic rating scales—How many categories? *British Journal of Psychology*, 1987; 69: 185–202.
4. Citaku F, Violato C, Beran T, Donnon T, Hecker K, Cawthorpe D. Leadership competencies for medical education and healthcare professions: population-based study. *BMJ Open*. 2012; 2(2): e000812.

15

Evaluating tests and assessments: Item analyses

ADVANCED ORGANIZERS

- A complete analysis of a test requires an item analysis together with descriptive statistics and reliability.
- There are three essential features for an item analysis for multiple-choice questions (MCQs): (1) difficulty of the item, (2) item discrimination, and (3) distractor effectiveness. All of these criteria apply to every other test or assessment form (e.g., OSCE, restricted essay, extended essay, survey) except for distractor effectiveness since there are no distractors in these test formats.
- The difficulty of the item is the percentage or proportion of people who got the item correct. If everyone gets the item correct, it is an easy item; if very few test-takers get the item correct, it is a very difficult item. Item difficulty (P) is usually expressed as a proportion such as $P = 0.72$ (72% got it correct).
- Item discrimination has to do with the extent to which an item distinguishes or "discriminates" between high test scorers and low test scorers. Positive D indicates discrimination in the correct direction. The point-biserial is commonly used for item discrimination D. Distractor effectiveness refers to the ability of distractors in attracting responses.
- The other important criteria of evaluating a test are descriptive statistics.
- The internal consistency reliability, Cronbach's α and the mean discrimination index are also helpful in evaluating test quality. The item analysis, pass/fail rate, MPL, and reliability all help interpret the value of a test.

ITEM ANALYSIS

A complete analysis of a test requires an item analysis together with descriptive statistics and reliability. There are three essential features for an item analysis for MCQs: (1) difficulty of the item, (2) item discrimination, and (3) distractor effectiveness.

The difficulty of the item is the percentage or proportion of people who got the item correct. If everyone gets the item correct, it is an easy item. Conversely, if very few test-takers (10%–20%) get the item correct, it is a very difficult item. An item of average difficulty has approximately 40%–50% correct response rate. Item difficulty (P) is usually expressed as a proportion such as $P = 0.72$ (72% got it correct).

Item discrimination has to do with the extent to which an item distinguishes or "discriminates" between high-test scorers and low-test scorers. Suppose that an item has a difficulty of $P = 0.50$ (50% of the test-takers got it correct). Which half got it correct? Was it the high achievers or was it the low achievers? Depending on which half got it correct, the item discriminates between them. This is item discrimination D. Distractor effectiveness refers to the ability of distractors in attracting responses. A distractor that attracts no responses is not effective; it begins to become effective when it attracts some responses.

To conduct an item analysis, you must identify a high-scoring group or an upper group (U) and a low-scoring group (L). To do this, sort the papers into rank-order. Split the group into half and designate the highest as U and the lowest as L.

The following formulae are used to compute the difficulty and discrimination.

Difficulty

$$P = \frac{R \times 100}{T}$$

where
P = percent who got the item correct
R = number who got the item correct
T = number who tried it

Discrimination

$$D = \frac{RU - RL}{1/2T}$$

where
D = discrimination
RU = number who got it right in the upper group
RL = number who got it right in the lower group
T = number who tried the item

Distractor effectiveness

Determine the number and percentage of test-takers that selected that particular distractor. If 80% selected a distractor, then it is too attractive and may overlap with the correct answer. If no one selected it, then it is not attractive enough. Generally, *some* (perhaps 10%–20%) test-takers should select a distractor to indicate that it is effective.

EXAMPLE MCQ TEST WITH ITEM ANALYSIS

Table 15.1 contains four MCQs from a test of biomedical knowledge administered to second-year medical students (Items 3 and 4 are vignette type items as found on Step 1 of the USMLE board exam). Table 15.2 contains a portion of an item analysis that was conducted on a computer using the MicroCAT software. Several item characteristics are summarized in the item analysis (Proportion Correct = Difficulty; Disc. Index = Discrimination; Point-Biserial = correlation between item performance and

Table 15.1 Examples of multiple-choice questions

1. Widely spaced eyes, thin upper lip, and short eyelid openings in the preschool child are typical of
   A. the effects of thalidomide
   B. Down's syndrome
   C. rubella during prenatal development
   D. fetal alcohol syndrome

2. The bichrome test may fail for patients who have
   A. deuteranopia
   B. protanopia
   C. deuteranomaly
   D. tritanopia

3. A 25-year-old woman is brought to the emergency department 1 h after she fainted. She has had mild intermittent vaginal bleeding, sometimes associated with lower abdominal pain, during the past 3 days. She has had severe cramping pain in the right lower abdomen for 12 h. She has not had a menstrual period for 3 months; previously, menses occurred at regular 28-day intervals. Abdominal examination shows mild tenderness to palpation in the right lower quadrant. Bimanual pelvic examination shows a tender walnut-sized mass in the right parametrium. Which of the following is the most likely diagnosis?
   A. Appendicitis
   B. Cancer of the ovary
   C. Ectopic pregnancy
   D. Endometriosis

4. A 55-year-old man with a history of drug and alcohol abuse undergoes operative placement of a portosystemic shunt to relieve portal hypertension. During this procedure, it is most appropriate for the physician to anastomose a major tributary of the portal vein to which of the following vessels?
   A. Left renal vein
   B. Left gastric vein
   C. Splenic vein
   D. Superior mesenteric vein

Table 15.2 Example item analysis

MicroCAT (tm) Testing System

Item analysis for data from file A:\Exam_M2017.DAT

Date: 06-26-17   Time: 10:24 am

Type of Correlations: Point-Biserial

Number of test-takers: 190

Ability Grouping: YES

Subgroup Analysis: NO

Express Endorsements as: PROPORTIONS

Seq. No.	Scale-Item	Item Statistics			Alt.	Alternative Statistics				
		Prop. Correct	Disc. Index	Point-Biser.		Prop. Total	Endorsing		Point- Biser.	Key
							Low	High		
1	0–1	0.69	0.27	0.24	A	0.09	0.13	0.03	−0.13	
					B	0.13	0.17	0.13	−0.11	
					C	0.09	0.14	0.03	−0.11	
					D	0.69	0.54	0.81	0.24	*
					Other	0.00	0.00	0.00	0.00	
2	0–4	0.28	0.40	0.44	A	0.22	0.46	0.09	−0.27	
					B	0.42	0.46	0.38	−0.18	
					C	0.28	0.04	0.44	0.44	*
					D	0.08	0.04	0.09	0.01	
					Other	0.00	0.00	0.00	0.00	

(Continued)

Table 15.2 (Continued) Example item analysis

| | Item Statistics | | | | | Alternative Statistics | | | | |
Seq. No.	Scale-Item	Prop. Correct	Disc. Index	Point-Biser.	Alt.	Prop. Total	Endorsing Low	Endorsing High	Point- Biser.	Key
3	0–5	0.86	0.30	0.42	A	0.01	0.04	0.00	−0.14	
					B	0.01	0.04	0.00	−0.24	
					C	0.86	0.67	0.97	0.42	*
					D	0.12	0.25	0.03	−0.33	
					Other	0.00	0.00	0.00		
4	0–2	0.63	0.25	0.18	A	0.63	0.50	0.75	0.18	*
					B	0.21	0.29	0.16	−0.15	
					C	0.01	0.00	0.00	−0.04	
					D	0.14	0.21	0.09	−0.06	
					Other	0.00	0.00	0.00		
5	0–3	0.69	0.23	0.23	A	0.18	0.25	0.16	−0.11	
					B	0.08	0.08	0.00	−0.10	
					C	0.69	0.58	0.81	0.23	*
					D	0.06	0.08	0.03	−0.16	
					Other	0.00	0.00	0.00		

Table 15.3 Summary of statistics from the test

There were 190 students in the data file.						
Scale:	1	2	3	4	5	6
Number of Items	16	16	20	20	12	16
Number of Students	190	190	190	190	190	190
Mean	10.756	11.033	13.911	15.356	7.344	13.478
Variance	4.385	4.543	4.103	3.474	1.937	3.694
Std. Dev.	2.094	2.132	2.026	1.864	1.392	1.922
Skew	0.115	−0.491	−0.232	−0.566	0.013	−0.947
Kurtosis	−0.280	0.757	0.011	0.516	−0.704	0.756
Minimum	6.000	4.000	8.000	9.000	4.000	7.000
Maximum	16.000	16.000	18.000	19.000	10.000	16.000
Median	11.000	11.000	14.000	15.000	7.000	14.000
Mean P	0.672	0.690	0.696	0.768	0.612	0.842
Mean Item-Tot.	0.297	0.319	0.248	0.253	0.313	0.347
Mean Biserial	0.402	0.455	0.366	0.390	0.488	0.554
Max Score (Low)	9	10	12	14	6	13
N (Low Group)	24	33	25	28	26	39
Min Score (High)	12	12	15	17	8	15
N (High Group)	32	38	35	29	39	31

Reliability: Total Scale Alpha = 0.83.

total test score—this is another type of discrimination index). Several statistics are summarized in Table 15.3 that provide other data about how this test performed (these are described in Chapter 3).

INTERPRETING THE ITEM ANALYSIS AND OTHER STATISTICS FOR THE EXAMPLE MCQS

A total of 190 second-year medical students wrote this test. The results in Table 15.2 show the details of the four items in Table 15.1. The P for Item 1 was 0.69 and the D (point-biserial) was 0.24. This item is moderately easy (nearly 70% correct) with a small discrimination. Each of distractors A, B, and C were selected by some test-takers (9%, 13%, 9%, respectively). The overall results of this item indicate that it is quite good; moderate difficulty with some discrimination and all of the distractors are effective. This item does not need revision.

Item 2 has a serious problem; only 28% ($P = 0.28$) selected the right answer, C. Nearly half of the students selected option B as correct (42%). Although this item has very good discrimination ($D = 0.44$), it needs revision before further use. Option B may need rewriting to make it less attractive to the mid-performing students. As it now stands, it appears to students as a "trick question." Items 3 and 4 are working somewhat with some discrimination though Item 3 may be slightly too easy, while Item 4 may be slightly too difficult (interpret the item analysis of Item 5).

The overall 100 MCQ test contained six subscales ranging from 12 to 20 items each (Table 15.3). The reliability was high—Cronbach's $\alpha = 0.83$. The overall test difficulty was $P = 0.71$ (71%) but the subscales difficulty (Table 15.3—mean P) varied with subscale six the easiest, $P = 0.84$. The mean discrimination indices (D) for each subscale are summarized in Table 15.3. The overall results of the item analysis (Table 15.2) and test statistics (Table 15.3) indicate that this exam is working well psychometrically. Nonetheless, it requires some improvement and re-writing (e.g., Item 2).

CONDUCTING AN ITEM ANALYSIS FOR OBJECTIVE-STRUCTURED CLINICAL EXAMS (OSCES)

OSCEs are intended to measure clinical skills, professionalism, communications, clinical reasoning, interprofessional collaboration, etc. which cannot be measured by MCQs or written exams. OSCEs usually contain several stations (typically, 4–15) that measure several aspects of candidate performance. Tables 15.4 and 15.5 contain stations with cases that are intended for 15 min each.

A complete analysis of an OSCE requires an item analysis together with descriptive statistics and reliability. The OSCE, unlike MCQs, have only two essential features that constitute an item analysis: (1) difficulty of the item and (2) item discrimination. Of course, there is no distractor effectiveness as there are no distractors.

Station 1: Coronary artery disease

In this station, a patient comes to your clinic complaining of "tightness in his chest". The checklist in Table 15.4 describes this case, coronary artery disease or stable angina. As you can see, Table 15.4 has several subscales for assessments: history of presenting complaint, past history, family history, social history, physical exam, and a differential diagnosis. A total of 188 candidates (residents) took this OSCE station. The item analysis is summarized in Table 15.5. From these results, it can be seen that most poorly performed items were (#1) Asking for patient's age ($P = 0.17$; $D = 0.12$) and (#12) Aggravating factors (anxiety) ($P = 0.29$; $D = 0.10$) with low P values and poor D values. The items on which performance was best were (#18) Asking about job ($P = 0.63$; $D = 0.38$) and (#24) Checking peripheral pulse ($P = 0.48$; $D = 0.48$).

The descriptive statistics of this 31-item station are a minimum score of 13 (43.3%) and a maximum of 30 (96.8%), with the mean score = 22.06 (73.5%), SD = 3.04 (10.1%), and a negative skew (−0.12). The minimum performance level (MPL) = 21 (67.7%). A total of 122 candidates passed (64.9%) this station. The internal consistency reliability, Cronbach's $\alpha = 0.76$. The mean difficulty $P = 0.74$ and discrimination $D = 0.23$. The item analysis, pass/fail rate, MPL, and reliability indicate that this is a good station for candidates at this level (residents). Nearly everyone got the diagnosis correct (90%) even though they may not have done well on some components of the checklist.

Table 15.4 Coronary artery disease (stable angina)

Checklist	
History of presenting complaint	**Done**
1. Age of patient	○
2. Pain described as dull ache in center of chest	○
3. Severity 6–7/10	○
4. Radiates to neck and jaw (toothache)	○
5. Began 3 months ago	○
6. Frequency of pain has increased (now every 2–3 days)	○
7. Pain associated with exercise (climbing stairs)	○
8. Pain relieved by rest	○
9. No shortness of breath	○
10. No nausea and vomiting	○
11. Occasionally feels weak & sweaty with pain	○
12. Aggravated by anxiety	○
Past history	
13. Cholesterol levels (unknown)	○
14. History of hypertension (negative)	○
15. History of diabetes (negative)	○
Family history	
16. Adopted and does not know biological parents; sons are healthy	○
Social history	
17. Happily married with two sons ages 21 & 19 years	○
18. Stressful job (firefighter)	○
19. Smokes ½ a pack a day X 15 years	○
20. Exercise: Walks dog four blocks three times a week	○
Physical examination	
21. Looks for evidence of shortness of breath, color, etc.	○
22. Measures blood pressure (told it is 160/90)	○
23. Palpates radial pulse	○
24. Palpates peripheral pulses	○
25. Checks capillary refill	○
26. Determines jugular venous pressure	○
27. Palpates Apex beat	○
28. Auscultates heart for abnormal sounds or murmurs	○
29. Auscultates lung fields	○
30. Check for leg edema	○
31. **QUESTION: What is the diagnosis? Answer:** Coronary Artery Disease (Stable angina)	○

Table 15.5 Coronary artery disease (stable angina)—item analysis (n = 188)

Item		Number, proportion correct response, & discrimination		
		n	P^β	D^γ
1.	Age of patient	32	0.17	0.12
2.	Pain described as dull ache in center of chest	176	0.94	0.22
3.	Severity 6–7/10	151	0.80	0.27
4.	Radiates to neck and jaw (toothache)	175	0.93	0.16
5.	Began 3 months ago	177	0.94	0.15
6.	Frequency of pain has increased (now every 2–3 days)	131	0.70	0.31
7.	Pain associated with exercise (climbing stairs)	177	0.94	0.25
8.	Pain relieved by rest	172	0.92	0.19
9.	No shortness of breath	123	0.65	0.19
10.	No nausea and vomiting	93	0.50	0.27
11.	Occasionally feels weak & sweaty with pain	102	0.54	0.19
12.	Aggravated by anxiety	55	0.29	0.10
13.	Cholesterol levels unknown	135	0.72	0.23
14.	History of hypertension (negative)	167	0.89	0.21
15.	History of diabetes (negative)	156	0.83	0.18
16.	Adopted; doesn't know biological parents; sons are healthy	165	0.88	0.28
17.	Happily married with two sons ages 21 & 19 years	60	0.32	0.30
18.	Stressful job (firefighter)	118	0.63	0.38
19.	Smokes ½ a pack a day X 15 years	181	0.96	0.26
20.	Exercise: Walks dog four blocks three times a week	83	0.44	0.27
21.	Looks for evidence of shortness of breath, color, etc.	142	0.76	0.31
22.	Measures blood pressure (told it is 160/90)	120	0.64	0.23
23.	Palpates radial pulse	131	0.70	0.20
24.	Checks peripheral pulses	90	0.48	0.48
25.	Checks capillary refill	67	0.36	0.28
26.	Determines jugular venous pressure	130	0.69	0.32
27.	Palpates apex beat	143	0.76	0.24
28.	Auscultates heart for abnormal sounds or murmurs	164	0.87	0.17
29.	Auscultates lung fields	99	0.53	0.11
30.	Check for leg edema	76	0.40	0.26
31.	What is your diagnosis? Answer: Coronary heart disease and/or angina	169	0.90	0.16

P^β = Proportion correct; D^γ = Discrimination (point-biserial correlation).

Station 2: Knife wound to the hand

In this station, a patient comes to the emergency department with a knife wound in the hand sustained in a fight (Table 15.6). You can see from Table 15.6 there are several subscales for assessments: history, examination, diagnosis, and management. The same 188 candidates (residents) took this OSCE station. The item analysis is in Table 15.6.

From these results, you can see that most poorly performed items were (#17) Anesthetize area ($P = 0.19$; $D = 0.16$), (#18) Hemastasis ($P = 0.21$; $D = 0.26$), and (#22) Splint hand in position of safety (explains) ($P = 0.08$; $D = 0.23$). The best performing

Table 15.6 Knife wound to the hand ($n = 188$)

		P^{β}	D^{γ}
History			
1.	Wound was the result of a knife fight	0.98	0.16
2.	Happened 2 h ago	0.91	0.21
3.	No significant past medical problems	0.74	0.41
4.	Have you ever had a Tetanus shot (no history)	0.84	0.29
5.	Are you taking any medications (no)	0.55	0.34
6.	Allergies (none)	0.55	0.35
Examination			
7.	Notice position of hand at rest with middle finger pulled out of line	0.58	0.43
8.	Examine wound and note it is in Zone 2	0.28	0.25
9.	Observe color of hand	0.30	0.31
10.	Demonstrates artery test	0.40	0.15
11.	Tests deep flexor tendons of middle finger	0.46	0.66
12.	Tests superficial flexor tendons of middle finger	0.45	0.62
13.	Tests deep superficial flexor tendons on index and ring finger	0.36	0.61
14.	Test median nerves—sensation (pinprick)	0.82	0.34
15.	Asks patient to pinch thumb against little finger	0.37	0.30
Diagnosis and management			
16.	Diagnosis of injured superficial and deep flexor tendons of the left middle fingers	0.50	0.60
17.	Anesthetize area	0.19	0.16
18.	Hemastasis	0.21	0.26
19.	Clean wound	0.77	0.13
20.	Explore wound	0.45	0.50
21.	Suture the tendons	0.45	0.46
22.	Splint hand in position of safety (explains)	0.08	0.23
23.	Tetanus toxoid	0.78	0.24

P^{β} = Proportion correct; D^{γ} = Discrimination (point-biserial correlation).

items were (#11) Tests deep flexor tendons middle finger ($P = 0.46$; $D = 0.66$), (#12) Tests superficial flexor tendons middle finger ($P = 0.45$; $D = 0.62$), and (#13) Tests deep superficial flexor tendons on index and ring finger ($P = 0.36$; $D = 0.61$). The pattern of P and D for these items indicates that the top performing candidates got these items correct.

The descriptive statistics of this 23-item station were a minimum score of 3 (13%), maximum = 21 (91%), mean = 14.09 (61.26%), SD = 3.59 (15.6%), and normally distributed (skew = 0.006). The minimum performance level (MPL) = 14.5 (63.0%). A total of 104 candidates passed (55.3%) this station. The internal consistency reliability, Cronbach's $\alpha = 0.71$ with a mean discrimination index $D = 0.35$. The item analysis, pass/fail rate, MPL, and reliability indicate that this is an adequate but difficult station for candidates at this level (residents). The failure rate was nearly half (44.7%) and many did poorly on some components of the checklist such as Diagnosis and Management (mean $P = 0.43$; mean $D = 0.32$). It is likely that residents are not getting enough experience and training in this type of hand injury.

ASSESSING COMMUNICATION IN OSCES

It is common practice in OSCEs to have the standardized patients assess the candidates' communication skills. Table 15.7 contains an 11-item scale used on the OSCE stations above together with the means and standard deviations of the items. The highest rated item was (#5) the doctor explained things to me so that I know what may be the matter with me (mean = 4.10; SD = 0.49). The lowest rated was (#7) the doctor gave me the opportunity to express my feelings or ideas in

Table 15.7 Communication scale completed by standardized patients ($n = 188$)

Item five-point scale (1 = strongly disagree to 5 = strongly agree)	Mean	SD
1. The doctor wanted to understand how I saw things	3.50	0.37
2. The doctor usually sensed or realized what I was feeling	4.00	0.34
3. The doctor treated me with respect & courtesy	3.20	0.42
4. I was able to explain my problem to the doctor as fully as needed	3.30	0.49
5. The doctor explained things to me so that I know what may be the matter with me	4.10	0.49
6. The doctor explained what treatment, tests or other follow-up is going to be	3.20	0.31
7. The doctor gave me the opportunity to express my feelings or ideas in planning treatment, tests, or follow-up	2.90	0.46
8. The doctor gave me the opportunity to ask questions	3.40	0.43
9. The doctor used understandable and non-technical language	3.00	0.52
10. The doctor was careful and thorough	3.20	0.54
11. I am satisfied with the medical care that I received	3.50	0.48

Cronbach's $\alpha = 0.96$.

planning treatment, tests, or follow-up (mean = 2.90; SD = 0.46). Interestingly, while the SPs tended to agree that the doctor explained things to them (#5), they disagreed that the doctor involved them in treatment planning or follow-up (#7). The overall scale reliability was very high, Cronbach's $\alpha = 0.96$.

From these results, it is evident that communication skills need improvement for several items but in particular for Items 3, 6, 7, 9, and 10.

ESSAY TEST ANALYSES

The essay examination challenges the examinee to construct a written response to a question. A great deal of freedom is permitted and the responses usually vary in merit with no given answer is considered entirely correct. Although an answer key in the form of a rubric may aid the scoring of the essay, judgment about the quality is subjectively determined at the time of scoring. The essay examination is given under standard conditions. The instructions, time, and place of writing are uniform for all students. Essay examinations are tests in which students are asked to compose written statements, discussions, summaries or descriptions that are to be used as measures of knowledge, understanding, clinical reasoning, or writing proficiency. Important aspect of the essay is that it can assess organization of material, logic, flow and coherence of an argument, synthesis of information, originality of responses, and evaluation of theories, content, data, and technique. The rubric for scoring the essay need not contain all of these but usually contains some of them. For instance, the essay instructions may require the writer to synthesize and evaluate competing theories so the scoring rubric will focus on these but not on originality of response.

TYPES OF ESSAY ITEMS

There are at least two types of essay questions, the restricted and extended response forms. This classification refers to the amount of freedom allowed to students in composing their responses. The restricted response question limits the character and breadth of the student's composition. In this type of essay question, the following conditions are met: the student is directed toward a particular type of answer, the scope of the problem is limited, and the length of the essay is sometimes specified. Restricted response essay questions are sometimes called short answers.

A restricted response essay

A total of 106 third-year medical students wrote a restricted response essay test that contains three sections: diagnosis-type case, investigation-type case, and a treatment-type case.[1]

Diagnosis-type case

Clinical scenario: a 75-year-old woman is admitted to the ward for dyspnea, which has been progressively getting worse over the past 3 months. She also has cough for 2 months and bilateral pedal edema for 1 month. She has bilateral crepitations on auscultation. Past history includes hypertension and diabetes mellitus.

a. Briefly describe the pathophysiology causing these signs and symptoms
b. What are your diagnoses?
c. Rate each of your diagnoses: 1 = possible, 2 = likely, 3 = very likely or almost certain

Investigation-type case

Clinical scenario: a 27-year-old woman is mechanically ventilated for severe acute pneumonia, hypoxemia, and septic shock. She has persistent fever with frothy blood-stained secretions after 7 days of IV Augmentin. Blood cultures grew *Streptococcus pneumoniae* sensitive to augmentin. FIO_2 requirements exceed 70%. She was previously healthy.

a. Briefly describe investigations that you would do
b. Provide justification for each investigation
c. Rate each of your investigation: 1 = somewhat useful, 2 = highly useful, 3 = completely or almost completely necessary

Treatment-type case

Clinical scenario: an 82-year-old man is admitted for left-sided pneumothorax and is treated with tube thoracostomy. He has chronic obstructive pulmonary disease, ischemic heart disease, chronic heart failure, diabetes mellitus, and chronic renal failure. The chest drain is still bubbling after 7 days.

a. What is causing the chest drain bubbling?
b. What are your treatments?
c. Rate the value of your treatments: 1 = somewhat useful, 2 = highly useful, 3 = completely or almost completely necessary

---

These examples of restricted response essay questions aim the student at the desired answer. Moreover, the scope of the essay response is circumscribed. As compared to the extended essays, restricted response questions promote greater reliability in scoring. They may also reduce the student's opportunity to synthesize disparate information into a coherent whole, however, thereby restricting divergent thinking—also characteristics of short-answer questions (Table 15.8).

The overall item analysis for this exam is good. The mean difficulty of this test is $P = 0.74$ and a mean $D = 0.35$ with internal consistency reliability Cronbach's $\alpha = 0.79$. The MPL = 0.63 resulting in a pass rate of 92.6%.

Table 15.8 Scoring results of restricted response essay, pulmonary, and critical care medicine

	P^β	D^γ
DIAGNOSIS-TYPE CASE: a 75-year-old woman		
a. briefly describe the pathophysiology causing these signs and symptoms	0.84	0.21
b. what are your diagnoses?	0.62	0.32
c. rate each of your diagnoses: 1 = possible, 2 = likely, 3 = very likely or almost certain	0.71	0.45
Possible diagnosis: lung cancer, heart failure, pulmonary embolism		
INVESTIGATION-TYPE CASE: a 27-year-old woman		
a. briefly describe investigations that you would do	0.61	0.41
b. provide justification for each investigation	0.73	0.22
c. rate each of your investigation: 1 = somewhat useful, 2 = highly useful, 3 = completely useful	0.70	0.46
Possible investigations: echocardiogram, bronchoscopy, CT thorax		
TREATMENT-TYPE CASE: an 82-year-old man		
a. what is causing the chest drain bubbling?	0.75	0.35
b. what are your treatments?	0.82	0.30
c. rate the value of your treatments: 1 = somewhat useful, 2 = highly useful, 3 = completely or almost completely necessary	0.86	0.44
Possible treatments: blood pleurodesis, watch/wait, surgical pleurectomy, and pleurodesis		

P^β = proportion correct; D^γ = point-biserial.

The extended response question places fewer limitations on discussion and the form of the answer. Example of the extended response essay question follows.

1. Is waist size related to risk of diabetes and heart attack?
2. What is the best way to keep your brain healthy for life?
3. How dangerous is a concussion? What is the best way to treat a concussion?
4. How can polio be eliminated?
5. What is inflammatory bowel disease? What are the best treatments? Can the food you eat help you avoid this chronic illness?
6. Identify some microorganisms that live inside and on humans. How do they help and hurt us?
7. Can the odors of our bodily fluids give us clue about our health?
8. Based on a cost-benefit analysis, is organ transplantation a viable medical treatment?
9. What are the most effective means to help cut death rates in heart attack patients?

10. Are eating disorders fatal? Can they be prevented?
11. Is there a best and healthiest diet for humans? Is there such a thing as a healthy heart diet?
12. Does waist size increase heart attack risk?

An extended response essay question: how might humanistic psychology be used to maintain engagement in the medical classroom? Illustrate with appropriate classroom examples the application of particular theoretical constructs from humanistic psychology in the maintenance of classroom engagement. A total of 176 second-year medical students responded to this essay question.

In answering this essay question, students may select the particular theoretical constructs from humanistic psychology, which they deem to be most important and relevant in maintaining discipline in the classroom. This is in contrast to the previous example of a restricted response question. In addition, the form of the extended response essay remains the responsibility of the student, and the length is unspecified, thus allowing for more flexibility and creativity in responses.

GUIDELINES FOR PREPARING ESSAY ITEMS

- Give yourself adequate time to write, re-write, and edit the questions
- Use restricted response questions whenever possible
- State the problem in the form of a question
- Do not provide optional questions
- When asking student's their opinions, it is required that they support them with knowledge and a rational argument
- Create a scoring key for each question

GUIDELINES FOR SCORING ESSAY QUESTIONS

- Set realistic performance standards
- Grade one question at a time for all students
- Preserve anonymity when grading
- Write comments on each paper
- Create a rubric for the scoring

The overall item analysis for this extended essay test is good. The mean difficulty of this test is $P = 0.67$ and a mean $D = 0.33$. Inter-rater reliability based on agreement of scoring for a random subset of the essays ($n = 20$) resulted in an initial 92% agreement. With subsequent review and discussion, the raters achieved 100% agreement. The MPL $= 0.60$, resulting in a pass rate of 82.6%. Students who did not pass had to remediate and write a subsequent parallel essay exam (Tables 15.9 and 15.10).

Table 15.9 Example rubric for scoring the humanistic psychology extend response essay

Category	4 = Excellent	3 = Good	2 = Adequate	1 = Poor
1. Summarizes theoretical constructs from humanistic psychology				
2. Problem identification and issues of humanistic psychology				
3. Classroom examples				
4. Logic and reasoning				
5. Evidence (e.g., empirical studies)				
6. Writing quality				
7. Flexibility and creativity				

Total Possible marks = 28.

Table 15.10 Item analyses of extended response essay

Category	P	D
1. Summarizes theoretical constructs from humanistic psychology	0.81	0.21
2. Problem identification and issues of humanistic psychology	0.74	0.27
3. Classroom examples	0.60	0.46
4. Logic and reasoning	0.71	0.41
5. Evidence (e.g., empirical studies)	0.53	0.22
6. Writing quality	0.67	0.32
7. Flexibility and creativity	0.61	0.41

SURVEY ANALYSES

A needs-assessment for faculty development of 241 professors at a medical school (MD program) was conducted recently. The professors responded on a five-point scale to 11 statements and provided demographic information.

ITEM ANALYSIS FOR FACULTY DEVELOPMENT SCALE

The aim of the faculty development survey was to develop and psychometrically assess the dimension of perceived needs assessment for faculty development for medicine. A total of 241 professors (representing 18 departments) teaching in the Faculty of Medicine at a major university (84% MD, 16% PhDs) participated. Nearly half (44%) held an academic position for more than 10 years. The 11-item scale (Tables 15.11 and 15.12) was developed through expert panel discussion and a literature review on needs assessments to establish face and content validity. Each item was rated on a five-point scale on the importance of each method of teaching.

The results of the item analyses are summarized in Table 15.12. The highest rated needs for faculty development were (4) giving feedback, (1) teaching in clinical environment, and (2) small group teaching. For the total scale, Cronbach's $\alpha = 0.85$.

The results provide an example of how a psychometrically sound teaching needs assessment scale can be developed to be used in determining professors' perceptions of the importance of various aspects of teaching. These types of needs assessments are critical in developing and improving medical education programs.

Table 15.11 Faculty development survey

Indicate how important you rate each item below for your teaching work (scale for items below).

1, Not important; 2, Somewhat important; 3, Neutral; 4, Important; 5, Very important.

Check the box for your choice:	1	2	3	4	5
1. Teaching in clinical environment					
2. Small group teaching					
3. Large group teaching					
4. Giving feedback					
5. Designing & teaching for web-based or distance learning					
6. Teaching medical skills or procedure					
7. Organizing medical knowledge					
8. Course or curriculum planning					
9. Assessment in the clinical environment					
10. Course or program planning					
11. Evaluating medical skills or procedures					

Demographics

1. I am MD (or equivalent): Yes   No
2. I am PhD (or equivalent): Yes   No
3. I am Other (indicate, e.g., MSc, etc.):
4. Other: i am other
5. I have held an academic appointment at a university for
6. My department is:

Table 15.12 Item analysis for faculty development survey

Item	Degree	n	Mean	SD	Min	Max
1. Teaching in clinical environment	PhD	33	2.61	1.69	1	5
	MD	199	3.87	1.19	1	5
	Total	232	3.69	1.35	1	5
2. Small group teaching	PhD	35	3.40	1.22	1	5
	MD	199	3.70	1.03	1	5
	Total	234	3.66	1.06	1	5
3. Large group teaching	PhD	34	2.91	1.11	1	5
	MD	199	3.14	1.07	1	5
	Total	233	3.10	1.07	1	5
4. Giving feedback	PhD	34	3.32	1.25	1	5
	MD	194	3.85	1.02	1	5
	Total	228	3.77	1.07	1	5
5. Designing & teaching for web-based or distance learning	PhD	33	2.85	1.48	1	5
	MD	196	2.93	1.25	1	5
	Total	229	2.92	1.28	1	5
6. Teaching medical skills or procedure	PhD	33	2.58	1.60	1	5
	MD	198	3.65	1.15	1	5
	Total	231	3.50	1.28	1	5
7. Organizing medical knowledge	PhD	34	2.59	1.35	1	5
	MD	200	3.55	1.10	1	5
	Total	234	3.41	1.19	1	5
8. Course or curriculum planning	PhD	35	2.94	1.37	1	5
	MD	197	3.03	1.22	1	5
	Total	232	3.01	1.24	1	5
9. Assessment in the clinical environment	PhD	33	2.64	1.69	1	5
	MD	196	3.80	1.06	1	5
	Total	229	3.63	1.23	1	5
10. Course or program planning	PhD	34	2.97	1.31	1	5
	MD	199	3.28	1.09	1	5
	Total	233	3.24	1.13	1	5
11. Evaluating medical skills or procedures	PhD	35	2.57	1.54	1	5
	MD	198	3.72	1.00	1	5
	Total	233	3.55	1.17	1	5

SUMMARY AND CONCLUSIONS

This chapter dealt with test and item analysis. A complete analysis of a test requires an item analysis together with descriptive statistics and reliability. There are three essential features for an item analysis for MCQs: (1) difficulty of the item, (2) item discrimination, and (3) distractor effectiveness. All of these criteria apply to every other test or assessment form (e.g., OSCE, restricted essay, extended essay, survey) except for distractor effectiveness since there are no distractors in these test formats.

The difficulty of the item is the percentage or proportion of people who got the item correct. If everyone gets the item correct, it is an easy item; if very few test-takers get the item correct, it is a very difficult item. Item difficulty (P) is usually expressed as a proportion such as $P = 0.68$ (68% got it correct).

Item discrimination has to do with the extent to which an item distinguishes or "discriminates" between high-test scorers and low-test scorers. Depending on which half got it correct, the item discriminates between them. The point-biserial is commonly used for item discrimination, D. Distractor effectiveness refers to the ability of distractors in attracting responses. A distractor that attracts no responses is not effective; it begins to become effective when it attracts some responses.

The other important criteria of evaluating a test are descriptive statistics (minimum/maximum score, mean, mode, median, skewness, minimum performance level (MPL) and number of candidates that passed the assessment. The internal consistency reliability, Cronbach's $\alpha = 0.71$, and the mean discrimination index are also helpful in evaluating test quality. The item analysis, pass/fail rate, MPL, and reliability all help interpret the value of a test.

EXERCISES AND REFLECTIONS 15.1

Item analysis

Purpose: to conduct an item analysis of multiple-choice items.
15 marks
The following are the responses to five MCQs by 20 students. (U = upper 10 students; L = lower 10 students.)

		Option		
Item	**A**	**B**	**C**	**D**
1. U10	0	2	0	8[a]
L10	3	3	0	4
2. U10	0	9[a]	1	0
L10	0	7	1	2
3. U10	7[a]	1	1	1
L10	7	1	1	1
4. U10	0	10[a]	0	0
L10	2	2	3	3
5. U10	0	3	4[a]	3
L10	2	1	6	1

[a] indicates the keyed-response.

Directions

1. Using the following formulas, calculate the Difficulty (*P*) and discrimination (*D*) value for each item. Write these in a table similar to the sample one found below (**5 marks**).

$$\text{Difficulty} = P = \frac{R \times 100}{T}$$

$$\text{Discrimination} = D = \frac{RU - RL}{1/2T}$$

An example of an item analysis table

Item	Difficulty (%)	Comment	Discrimination	Comment
11	35	Too difficult	0.35	Very good
12	75	Good	−0.25	Mis-keyed
13	85	Fair	0.55	Ideal
14	55	Ideal	0.15	Fair
15	95	Too easy	0.05	Poor

Note: your answers will be different.

2. For each item in the above table, analyze and describe the difficulty, discrimination, and distractor effectiveness. (**5 marks**)
3. For each item, indicate what option (if any) you would change (including the keyed-response) and explain your rationale for doing so (1–2 sentences each). (**5 marks**).

15 marks

TO SUBMIT TO THE INSTRUCTOR

1. A table indicating item number (1–5), difficulty and discrimination values and relevant comments.
2. A brief description of the distractor effectiveness for each item.
3. A description of what option (if any) you would change and why for each item (1–5).

EXERCISES AND REFLECTIONS 15.2

Essay test construction

30 marks
  Purpose: to practice and develop skills in writing an essay exam.

Directions

PART A: PLANNING THE TEST (6 MARKS)

Construct a 4-item essay exam in a content/subject area in which you have some competence.

1. Outline the content area upon which the test is based. (**1 mark**)
2. Construct a two-way table of specifications with four cells (2 Levels of Understanding by 2 subsections of the Content Area). This table should include:
   a. two (2) levels of understanding: synthesis and evaluation. (**1 mark**)
   b. two (2) subsections of the content area. (**1 mark**)
   c. the number of test items for each cell. (**1 mark**)
   d. the total number of items. (**½ mark**)
   e. percentage weights for each level of understanding and for each content element. (**½ mark**)

   An example of a table of specifications

Content area	Levels of understanding		
Anatomy of the heart	Synthesis	Evaluation	
1. Physical characteristics	1	1	2 (50%)
2. Functional characteristics	1	1	2 (50%)
	2 (50%)	2 (50%)	4

3. State the general purpose of the test, i.e., how will the test results be used? (**½ mark**)
4. State who will take the test. (**½ mark**)

PART B: WRITING THE TEST (22 MARKS)

According to your blueprint developed in Part A of this assignment:

1. Write a 4-item, restricted response essay exam. (**2 marks each; 8 total**)
2. Write a sample answer for each essay question. Use full sentences and appropriate essay format (introduction, body, and conclusion). (**2 marks each; 8 total**)
3. Using an embedded scoring system within your sample answer, indicate how points are to be assigned for each answer. See the example below. (**1 mark each; 4 total**)
4. The test should include a title and explicit instructions (i.e., time for each question and value of each question). (**2 marks**)

EXAMPLE OF AN ESSAY QUESTION AND EMBEDDED SCORING SYSTEM

Vignette

A 15-year-old teenage girl is suffering from swollen glands and complains of being lethargic.[2] After a number of tests, the family doctor and specialists confirm the diagnosis of astrocytoma, grade 4, brain cancer (i.e., advance stage of development). The family is informed that there is no known cure for this type of cancer, but the doctors suggest that they can slow the process if they begin to address the disease immediately through ongoing chemotherapy. After a few days, the mother and daughter decide to end the chemotherapy treatments, which they say are leaving the girl feeling constantly sick and disorientated. Instead, the mother and daughter decide to pursue a variety of alternative non-toxic therapies outside of the recognized medical system of practice (e.g., herbology, nutritional modification, vitamin therapy). The girl's father, however, is in direct conflict with his wife and daughter and wants them to return to the original chemotherapy treatment plan. After a frustrating week of family discussions, the father has decided to take legal action against his wife for sole custody of his daughter in support of his decision to get her back into chemotherapy.

Probing questions

- What should the family doctor say to the mother and daughter about the medical system's ability to provide care at the cancer treatment center?
- What should the family doctor say to the mother and daughter regarding their decision to pursue alternative therapies?
- What should the family doctor say to the father when he comes to ask for assistance in pursuing support from the doctor in convincing his wife and daughter to continue chemotherapy treatment?

You will receive (1) mark for your opinion and (2) for each supporting reason for each probing question, for a total of 12 marks. You have 20 min to complete this essay.

Sample answer

I don't think it's the doctor's role to suggest to people that they go elsewhere. (1) He/she should stick to what they know best, mainly medicine, and that includes describing the limitations of medicine. (2) I think that as far as I know, it's always really up to the patient to determine what course they want to go on (1). If they want to pursue an alternative treatment, then I think that the doctor needs to explain everything that he can do for them (1). I think you have to pursue both sides of this … that it's a horrible decision to have to make (1). Especially for a 15-year-old girl … I think the family doctor could play a role in somehow moderating this (1). If they are confident that the 15-year-old girl and her mother have made sound decisions in their practices and he/she would have to defend them in their decisions (2). The family doctor's obligations are to outline the options available, which are to be on chemotherapy or not to be on chemotherapy (1). As a family doctor, I would try to work with the mother and daughter to try and blend the two approaches and find a middle ground they might be comfortable with (1).

PART C: REFLECTION

After you have completed this assignment, write a brief reflection (1-page type-written maximum) about your reactions to essay exams and the construction of an essay exam.

NOTE: the reflection is an important part of this assignment. Although the reflection is not marked, in order to receive a grade for the entire assignment, the reflection must be handed in.

TO SUBMIT TO THE INSTRUCTOR

1. Part A — questions 1–4.
2. The essay exam, which includes Part B — question 4.
3. The sample answers with an embedded scoring system.
4. Your reflection about the construction of an essay exam.
5. Two (2) marks will be awarded for professional appearance of the exam (spelling and grammar).

   – All of the above should be typewritten.

REFERENCES

1. See KC, Tan KL, Lim K. (2014) The script concordance test for clinical reasoning: re-examining its utility and potential weakness. *Med. Educ.* 48: 1069–1077.
2. Donnon T, Oddone-Paolucci E, Violato C. (2009) A predictive validity study of medical judgment vignettes to assess students' noncognitive attributes: a 3-year prospective longitudinal study. *Med Teach.* 31(4):148–55. doi:10.1080/01421590802512888.

Grading, reporting, and standard setting

ADVANCED ORGANIZERS

- The main purposes of grading and reporting is to provide feedback to the learner, act as a source of accountability, and to reward and motivate learner efforts. The main problem with grades is that they lack universal meaning across instructors, courses, and schools.
- Grading systems can be based on norm-referenced (grading on the curve) or on criterion-referenced bases. All of these systems have some problems associated with them.
- The main and historically oldest symbols for grading are the letter grade, usually ranging from A to F. Substitutes have been attempted but have achieved little success because these usually involve reducing the number of categories (e.g., good, satisfactory, unsatisfactory).
- Numerical grades (% or 1–10) have also met with limited success, as have pass/fail systems and checklists of objectives.
- Norm-referenced grading is frequently called grading on the curve based on peer group performance. Criterion-referenced or absolute methods identify passing scores based on a predetermined level or standard of performance.
- The anecdotal record, the narrative report, or the portfolio is gaining popularity. Because of the various problems associated with this system, it is likely to find only restricted and specialized use.
- In order to determine final grades, various components must be combined in some fashion. Measurements that produce the highest variance in the scores will tend to influence the final grade disproportionately unless some weighting system is employed.
- Assignments are primarily intended as learning devices and are not intended as measurement instruments. Their reliability and validity are

likely to be low. Therefore, they should figure as little as possible and not exceed a value of 25% of the total course grade.

- The Dean's Letter or *Medical Student Performance Evaluation* should employ multiple reporting systems dealing with the cognitive, affective, and skills domains. There should be provisions for reporting learner achievement, effort, attitudes, interest, social and personal development, and other noteworthy outcomes. The wealth of information on the MSPE, however, should be balanced against the need for brevity and simplicity so that it can be readily understood.
- The instructor–student conference has a number of advantages, in that it allows for enhanced communication between students and instructors and may engage the student further in their education.
- Instructors are frequently called on to interpret standardized test score results to learners. When standardized test scores are used (e.g., z-scores; T-scores), they should always be interpreted in conjunction with another system such as percentile ranks.

INTRODUCTION: GRADING AND REPORTING

Grading and reporting is a necessary function of all educational enterprises for them to be most effective. The chapter begins with a discussion of the functions of grading and reporting and then several grading systems are described. Each grading system has advantages and disadvantages. A number of symbols including letter grades and numeric systems are commonly used to assign grades. Each of these has strengths and weaknesses.

Procedures for determining grades by weighting components differentially are necessary so as to control the effect of different variances of each component. Grading assignments present special problems for grading. Problems of reporting systems and examples of several are presented in this chapter and some guidelines for developing sound reporting systems are summarized. The chapter concludes with some guidelines for conducting the information and feedback conference with learners and explaining the meaning of test scores, assessments, and evaluations.

Purposes of grading and reporting

Some form of grading and reporting is part of every educational enterprise from nursery school to medical school to graduate school. Grading and reporting provide several functions including feedback, accountability, directing learner effort, as well as rewarding and motivating effort.

Grades (also called marks) provide feedback on performance to the learners, future teachers, and prospective employers and residency directors. This information is usually provided via transcripts, summative reports—i.e., Dean's Letter—and feedback conferences. Grades and other data communicated in this manner can be used by the learners and instructors to monitor the educational progress of the students and thereby facilitate decisions about educational plans.

Such information can indicate areas of strength, weakness, or deficit that require attention. Based on this feedback, appropriate action may be suggested and taken to improve the teaching and learning that the learner is engaged in. Instructors, professors, and school administrators are thereby also kept informed and involved in the educational process.

Grading and reporting also provides a form of accountability. Since periodic reporting is done, this holds the instructor, educational institution, and learner accountable for their educational activity. These reports provide analogous functions in education that financial statements play in business. Without such formal reporting systems, there would be no mechanism to hold all those involved in the educational enterprise accountable for their actions. Such accountability ultimately helps to improve education, as it requires planning, thought, and review of the outcomes of education.

Weaknesses, deficits, and strengths are identified by grades and are communicated by reporting. This helps to direct future efforts and interests. Efforts may be directed to correct deficits, and strengths may be further developed and interests shaped accordingly. Exceptional achievement in surgery rotations, for example, may be identified by grading and therefore affect decisions about future efforts in a surgical career. Deficits in professionalism may also be identified by grading, and the reporting to the learner may help them direct their efforts to overcome the problem.

GRADES AND MOTIVATION

Grades can motivate learners to work harder. Receiving high grades can motivate further effort by learners and may stimulate keen interest in the subject. High grades also serve to reward hard work and effort. Conversely, poor grades can motivate effort to improve performance.

PROBLEMS WITH GRADES

There are, however, a number of real or perceived problems with grades. The main problem lies in the meaning of grades. Marks may have different meanings across instructors, courses, and schools. Performance that received an A in one nursing school may produce only a B in another nursing school. Even within the same school, one professor may assign a C to a learner, while another professor might give the same learner a D for the same work. This lack of universal meaning for grades is a problem that can be at least partially solved by more valid assessment procedures.

The discrepancy of grading among instructors, courses, and schools is directly due to the lack of universal objective evidence for assigning grades. While it is common for most schools to have adjective descriptors associated with letter grades such as "excellent" for A, "good" for B, "fair" for C, "poor" for D, and "fail" for F, the objective evidence for assigning these letters and thus the adjective descriptors for individual learners is lacking. There is no universal scale to which instructors or course directors can refer to assign these letter grades. Thus, course and clerkship directors are left to their own judgment to what is the meaning and the evidence for assigning the marks. Recent studies have identified universal problems with medical and other health professions student evaluations, particularly during clerkships and other clinical experiences.

CLERKSHIP GRADES

There are serious concerns about the variability and lack of precision of student evaluation despite standardized curricula and mandated accreditation. A study of clerkship evaluations in American medical schools found huge discrepancies in clerkship evaluation. Alexander et al.[1] obtained clerkship evaluation data for AAMC-affiliated medical schools. Reports were analyzed to define the grading system and the percentage of each class within each grading tier. Inter- and intra-medical school grading variation was assessed by comparing the proportion of students receiving top grade.

Alexander et al.[1] found dramatic variation among the medical schools. They documented eight different grading systems using 27 unique sets of descriptive terminology. The eight different grading tiers ranged from 2 (pass/fail), 4 (Honors/Satisfactory/Low Satisfactory/Fail), to 9 (Honors/A/A–/B+/B/B–/C+/C/C–), and to 11 categories (A/A–/B+/B/B–/C+/C/C–/D+/D/D–/F).

Lack of precision of grading was obvious. Schools frequently used the same wording (e.g., "honors") with different meanings. The percentage of students awarded the top grade in any clerkship showed extreme variability (range 2%–93%) from school to school, as well as from clerkship to clerkship within the same school (range 18%–81%). Ninety-seven percent of all U.S. clerkship students were awarded one of the top-three grades regardless of the number of grading tiers. In the whole country, less than 1% of students failed any required clerkship.

There exists great heterogeneity of grading systems and imprecision of grade meaning throughout the U.S. medical education system. It is very likely worse in the rest of the world. Systematic changes to increase consistency, transparency, and reliability of grade meaning are needed to improve the student evaluation process at the national and global level. While this problem is difficult to solve completely, it can be mitigated by using as reliable and valid measuring instruments as possible.

GRADES AND IMPORTANT LEARNING

A major criticism of grades is that learners are motivated to work for grades rather than for significant educational outcomes or important learning. This is more a perceived problem than a real problem with grades. It is really a criticism of the validity of the use of grades than of the inherent nature of them. If grades do not reflect important learning it is because they have not been adequately tied to important educational outcomes. The solution to this problem is to make the use of grades more valid and thus reflect important learning outcomes. Accordingly, the learner will work for both grades and important learning.

Teacher-assigned grades have been shown to be notoriously unreliable.[2] When the grade or score is assigned largely or wholly on subjective grounds, as is frequently the case in the assessment of clinical rotations, numerous irrelevant factors influence the result. These include learner appearance, politeness, sex, attractiveness, height, and so on. This problem, of course, is not that grades are inherently flawed but rather that the data used to compute the grades are too subjective and therefore unreliable. The solution to the problem is to use data that are objective and reliable.

A final problem that is frequently identified with grades is that they are responsible for a variety of detrimental side effects like anxiety, self-concept problems, hostility, cheating, and produce negative attitudes toward learning and education when low grades are received. That some learners have low self-concepts, are anxious, cheat, and are hostile to learning is undeniable. These problems, however, are not caused by grades. They are a result of more fundamental factors. Most students readily know how well (or poorly) they can understand biostatistics, whether or not they are competent learners, how attractive they are, and how competent they are in athletics. All of these factors are far more important in learner anxiety, self-concept problems, hostility, and so on than are instructor assigned grades.

Recently, there has been concern in health sciences education of student burnout and wellbeing. Burnout of medical students in the United States is assessed each year with *Oldenburg Burnout Inventory* (OBI) that assesses two dimensions: (1) Disengagement and (2) Exhaustion, by the AAMC annual graduation questionnaire (GQ). There is considerable concern about the "burnout" rates in medical students but these are likely due to poor teaching, an overburdened curriculum, and excessive amounts of information to be learned, some of which is of questionable value. Grades are not the problems that lead to burnout; only when they are used without consideration for their validity.

GRADING AND MARKING SYSTEMS

There are a number of systems that can be used to assign grades and marks. These together with their strengths and weaknesses are discussed in turn.

Norm-referenced grading

This system is frequently called grading on the curve. Here, it is assumed that final achievement of a class is normally distributed and that marks can be derived based on the standard deviation and the mean of the distribution. The most commonly used technique for this is the Cajori method which sets +1.5 standard deviations and above for As (7% of the class), +0.5 to +1.5 for Bs (24%), −0.5 to +0.5 for Cs (38%), −0.5 to −1.5 for Ds (24%), and below −1.5 for Fs (7%). Essentially, grading on the curve amounts to determining a priori the numbers of As, Bs, Cs, Ds, and Fs that there will be in any given class.

There are some assumptions underlying this method, which are rarely met in practice. First, it is assumed that the underlying distribution is normal. This is rarely the case because typical classes are not large enough to produce data that even approaches a normal distribution. Moreover, few classroom tests are sufficiently reliable and valid to result in a normal distribution even with large classes. Second, it is assumed that educational performances of less than 1.5 standard deviations below the mean represent a failure. There are no good pedagogical or measurement reasons to make this assumption, which is quite arbitrary. Third, there is little reason to assume that any given class is "normal" and thus assumptions of the normal distribution cannot be applied. If the distribution is highly skewed either way, it may result in failure to assign any of the extreme grades (i.e., A or F). If the scores are positively skewed, none may fall below −1.5 standard deviations and thus no Fs would be assigned.

It is rarely advisable to apply grading on the curve strictly to any situation. Perhaps, it may be most defensibly used with very large enrollment classes of 300 or more students. Few health sciences classes are this large. Even here, however, it is assumed that the measurements were sufficiently reliable and valid to result in a normal distribution. Norm-referenced methods are based on the performance/ability of the students groups taking the examination and are neither based on the level of the student nor on the content of the examination. As a result, a fixed number of candidates may fail irrespective of their competence. In relative standard setting methods, the examinees' ability influences the standard so the passing score may be low when less competent students are taking the test resulting in false positive decisions and high when more competent students are taking the test resulting in false negative decisions. These relative methods are most suitable for selection or admission purposes, where a defined number of students have to be selected, and the top scorers are admitted.

Criterion-referenced grading

This method is an attempt to overcome the relativistic nature of norm-referenced grading by setting absolute standards called criteria or cutoff scores. Using a criterion for evaluating learner performance is an attempt to address the concern that students should be graded against an absolute standard of performance and not against each other. On the surface of it, this seems like a very sensible idea. In practice, however, this method requires considerable effort and expertise to implement.

In the past, it was common practice to use percentage cutoffs as though they were meaningful evaluation criteria. It is still common, for example, to consider 50% as the cutoff for pass–fail but there is no good pedagogical, measurement, or theoretical reasons to use this value. Some medical schools set equally arbitrary 70% cutoff scores for passing particularly in the pre-clinical or basic sciences courses. Nor are there defensible reasons to use 90% as a cutoff for an A, 80% for a B, and so on. Even if such a universal system was employed, it is obviously rather arbitrary. It is possible to establish absolute standards by systematic methods that are defensible.

STANDARD SETTING METHODS

There are several criterion-referenced standard-setting methods. Criterion-based or absolute methods identify passing scores based on a predetermined level of expected competency of students in that phase or stage of learning and the content of the examination, irrespective of group or class performance. Hence, absolute standard setting methods are preferred for competence-based assessments, for example, OSCEs as we saw in Chapter 13.

Angoff method

The Angoff method is one of the oldest and most widely used standard setting methods, which has been successfully used for both MCQs and OSCEs in medicine and health sciences education. The passing scores using the Angoff method are identified by a group of judges prior to the administration of the examination. The judges review each question or item independently and estimate the probability of a borderline student to answer correctly or perform the item skill. A borderline student is defined as a student who has 50:50 chance of failing or passing the examination or a student who may pass on good days and fail on bad days. These probabilities are added across items to identify the passing score for that station.

The average of the passing scores of all questions or items represents the standard for the whole examination. The Angoff method is supported by large amount of research but a few concerns still remain for this method.

- Judges may set standards that are unrealistically high or low. Accordingly, it is usually recommended that after the first round when judges have set their initial standards, they are provided with an opportunity to review the actual students' performance scores on these items and revise their standards as needed. This step is known as *reality check*. It can also be applied after the items have been administered for the first time on the examination.
- Another limitation of the Angoff method is the number of judges (as many as 5–6) required in identifying a reliable passing score and the amount of time required to set the standards.
- The judges and the examiners may be different with different understanding of performance expectations from the level of the student on the content being assessed.

Ebel method

The Ebel procedure[3] for setting MPLs that has been shown to have empirical evidence of validity.[4] An expert evaluates each clinical skill or task to be performed as identified on the checklist on two dimensions: difficulty and relevancy. For relevancy, three levels are used: essential, important, and marginal. Similarly, three levels are used for difficulty: easy, medium, and hard.

Each task or clinical skill is classified into one of the nine cells on the difficulty by relevancy table (Table 13.3). A clinical skill may be judged as easy and essential (EE), for example, although another may be judged as medium difficulty and important (MI). Through this process, an Ebel rating is given to each clinical skill, procedure, or task. The Ebel for setting pass/fail cutoff scores, particularly for OSCEs, is documented in detail in Chapter 13.

Nedelsky method

Another common and simple way to set cutoff scores in criterion-referenced testing is the Nedelsky method employing MPLs. Experts (e.g., physicians, nurses, dentists, etc.) assign probabilities to multiple-choice test items based on the likelihood that a group of examinees should be able to rule out incorrect options. These reference groups are hypothetical test-takers on the borderline between inadequate and adequate levels of performance. These are the minimally competent candidates (not failures, not stars, but those that just got their toes in the door). These also refer to the borderline between mastery and non-mastery of some domain of knowledge, ability, or skill. The procedure for employing the Nedelsky method for setting pass/fail cutoff scores for MCQ tests is explained in detail in Chapter 11.

Borderline group method

To determine the passing score using the borderline group method, the scores of all students rated as borderline on the test are considered. The mean or median scores of the identified borderline students is calculated and used as the passing score for the exam.

This procedure can also be used on a global-rating scale with borderline students further categorized into borderline unsatisfactory or fail and borderline satisfactory or pass. The passing score is then identified as the mean or median of the complete borderline group including both borderline fail and borderline pass students. Differentiating between borderline fail and pass students can be difficult and require very fine distinction.

There are several benefits of the borderline group method.

- Judgments are made on observations of actual student performances and not hypothetical students.
- It is easy to use, does not require any complex statistical procedures, and has higher face validity as it sets the passing score based on actual student performance.
- It utilizes the content experts time efficiently, as both the performance rating of the students and the standard setting happens simultaneously.
- It is a good method for situations with limited resources, statistical expertise, or experts as standard setting judges.

The borderline group method has some limitations.

- Utilizing the scores of borderline students only to set the passing standard results in the passing score based entirely upon the performance of the borderline students, irrespective of the entire cohorts performance.

- Students with a clear fail or pass performances are not taken into consideration by the borderline group method.
- If the student cohort is small or if the number of students identified as borderline is few in number, it is difficult to set the cutoff score.
- The validity and reliability of the passing score based on the few borderline students is questionable.

Borderline regression method

The borderline regression helps overcome some of the borderline group method by taking into account the performance of all students in the examination. Item checklist or rating-scale scores are regressed on the global-rating scores, and the equation is used to calculate the checklist or rating-scale score corresponding to the borderline grade as a passing score.

The general logistic regression equation used is as follows:

$$Y = bX + c$$

where

- b is the slope of regression function,
- c is the y-intercept or constant, and
- X and Y are the independent and dependent variables, respectively.

Using the above logistic regression equation, the passing score = intergrade discrimination (X) + constant, where X = point value on the global-rating scale on which the passing score is to be set, that is, corresponding to the borderline group.

The passing score is the rating-scale score corresponding to the borderline group or mid-way between the borderline pass and fail groups if two separate categories are used in the global-rating scale. Following a borderline regression method, a student marked as fail on a global rating may pass the exam if the overall performance score exceeds the passing score set by the method. For OSCEs, a student marked as pass on the global rating may fail the station, if the performance score on the rating-scale items does not meet the set standard.

Similar to the borderline group method, the judgments in the borderline regression method are made during the examination making it less resource-intensive and more acceptable.

A limitation of the borderline regression method is the assumption of a linear association between the item checklist or rating scores and the global grading. In addition, the passing score may be influenced by the extreme scores in each global grade and may affect the reliability and validity of the identified passing score.

Cluster analysis

Cluster analysis is an objective statistical technique to classify the data into categories of homogenous groups. The technique is used for classification purposes in many fields (social sciences, clinical medicine). Cluster analysis is mainly of two types, clustering or hierarchical model and partitioning or k-means model.

Using k-means cluster analysis the data can be categorized into a required number of homogenous groups. This method has been proposed and used as being more applicable for standard setting by the researchers in the field.[4] Cluster analysis identifies groups of similar performances in a cohort mathematically using concepts of distance (how far apart the two performances are) and similarity (how close the two performances are). Students with similar performances are grouped together forming clusters.

Standard setting through cluster analysis is more objective than other criteria-based standard setting methods. For the same reason, cluster analysis has been proposed to be used for evaluation and validation of other less objective standard setting methods requiring expert judgments like Angoff, Ebel, and borderline methods.

Combined norm- and criterion-referenced

Perhaps the best way of establishing such cutoffs is based on the performance of previous learners. This is a combination of criterion and norm-referenced grading. The absolute standards are established based on the normative performance of previous students. This method combines the advantages of both criterion and norm-referenced marking while avoiding the problems of each. The main drawback of this system, however, is that the assessors must have reliable and valid data on large numbers of previous learners. Most instructors probably use an "intuitive" method of setting standards as they develop a "feel" for what their learners are capable of or should be capable of. Obviously, such subjective approaches result in questionable standards of performance that are quite arbitrary.

Notwithstanding the above cautions, a percentage cutoff system that may be used as a general guideline is provided here for you. The guidelines should be used only as suggestions subject to change and revision by the instructor based on individual needs and circumstances. They should not be regarded as immutable standards.

$$A(A+, A-) = 85 - 100\%$$

$$B(B+, B-) = 70 - 84\%$$

$$C(C+, C-) = 59 - 69\%$$

$$D(D+, D-) = 50 - 58\%$$

$$F = 49\% \text{ and less}$$

TYPES OF SYMBOLS USED IN GRADING

There are numerous grading and marking symbols that have been used with varying degrees of success. Some of these have been used for a long time, while others are new. Despite the symbol system used, however, their main purpose is to communicate in a simple and understandable way—the achievement of the learner. Various grading symbols are discussed in turn as follows.

Letter grades

The most widely used symbol system is the traditional letter grade (A, B, C, D, F). Here, a letter grade is assigned for each subject to indicate the learner's achievement. While this system is concise, readily understandable, and familiar, it does have some difficulties. First, as we have seen, these letter grades lack universal meaning from teacher to teacher and from school to school. Second, the letter grade alone tells us nothing about other important educational matters such as effort, attitude, and interests. Third, the letter grade may have different meanings across subject matter itself. The grade B in histology, for example, may not reflect the same achievement as a B in biostatistics and epidemiology.

Numerous attempts have been made to improve the shortcomings of the traditional letter grade. This usually takes the form of using different symbols and reducing the number of categories. One system employs four categories, first class, second class, pass, and fail. Another attempt at improvement has been to use E (excellent), G (good), S (satisfactory), and U (unsatisfactory). Still another attempt at simplification has been to employ only two categories, S and U or P (pass) and F (fail).

These attempts are not really improvements over the letter grades, as they have the same problems and introduce new ones as well. Students and other learners tend not to like these systems as they are not as familiar as the letter grade. As well, the reduction of the number of categories reduces the reliability of the grades. As we saw in the discussion of reliability (Chapters 8 and 9), the reliability of an assessment or evaluation can be increased by increasing the number of items, questions, or categories in it. Reducing the number of categories in the grading system from five or more (A–F) to three or less (S, U) will substantially reduce the reliability of the grading system. For this reason, it is important to use a system with several categories (at least 5). Despite the shortcomings of the traditional letter grade system, it is likely to continue to be widely used in the foreseeable future.

Numerical grades

There are two generally used numerical-grading systems: (1) percentages and (2) numerals between 1 and 10. In the percentage system, the total achievement scores for the reporting period are summed and converted to a percentage value. This single number is then reported to indicate the quality of performance. To increase meaning, percentage ranges are frequently assigned adjective descriptors (90–100 = excellent, 80–89 = very good, etc.). Other adjectives descriptors for the above ranges are "first class", "second class", etc. In the second numerical system, a number between 1 and 10 is assigned with 1 indicating very poor and 10 indicating outstanding. The 1–10 numerical system is familiar in many countries such as Italy, France, England, India, and many others.

The main problems with these systems are their lack of familiarity and their deceptive nature. These numerical systems have not been used as widely as have the letter grade and therefore are not as widely known. Moreover, they are deceptive, because on the surface of it, they appear to be on an absolute scale of performance when this is not true. At best, these scales are ordinal but are interpreted as ratio or continuous scales. Does 100% indicate a complete knowledge of the subject matter? Does 50% indicate half knowledge? What does 7 mean? These numerical grades obviously offer no advantage over the letter grade especially when adjective descriptors are required to interpret them.

Pass-fail system

This system provides only two categories of grading, namely either a learner passes or fails a course. While there has been some enthusiasm for this system recently, and it is used at various levels of education from elementary to graduate school, it is currently used at some medical schools. It has never become widespread for at least three reasons. First, it is not as familiar as the letter grade system, which is generally preferred by students and the public. Second, it substantially reduces the information communicated to the learner. Did the pass indicate a borderline performance or an outstanding one? Did the learner who failed do so by a clear margin or was the performance within a standard error of measurement of the cutoff? How was the criterion for pass-fail established? Third, as we saw above, the system would be quite unreliable since it reduces the number of categories to the bare minimum (2).

For the above reasons, it is unlikely that this will ever become the preferred grading system although it has found some accepted use in specialized applications. Courses which are taken as electives, for example, and are not to be included in the grade point average calculation might profitably employ this system. Additionally, courses which are taught strictly as mastery learning could employ this grading system.

Checklists of objectives

In this scheme, a checklist of objectives or educational outcomes is used and each student is rated as to whether they have met the objective some rating to indicate the degree of performance on the objective. Table 16.1 is an example of paramedics using the checklist of objectives for assessing airway management proficiency. This method has the advantage of providing very specific and informative reports about the candidates' behavior and what they can and cannot do. Such information has obvious use for educational decision making and for undertaking remedial action.

The checklist assesses paramedics' progress on specific and relevant educational objectives rather than against peer performance or some numerical standard. Objective number I–57 "inserts laryngoscope to appropriate depth,", in intubation in Table 16.1, for example, communicates very specific information about the candidate's behavior as does objective number B-110, "Checks equipment for cuff leaks," in backup airway. This performance is not norm-referenced or based on some letter grade. It thus can be very useful for undertaking educational action if the learner is rated as "no" on this objective. By contrast, a C- on intubation might suggest that the paramedic is not doing well but would not provide any guidance or direction on remedial action.

Table 16.1 Airway management proficiency checklist instrument by subscale[5]

Item No.	Performance task	Yes	No
V-5	Inserts oropharyngeal (adjunct) airway		
V-7	Chooses correct adjunct airway size		
V-9	Inserts adjunct airway to proper depth		
V-11	Ventilates patient immediately (w/in 30 s)		
V-15	Ventilates patient at rate of 10–12/min		
V-16	Observes BVM technique for 30 s: Evaluates volumes		
V-19	Orients mask correctly		
V-20	Uses thenar eminence technique (E-C grip)		
V-21	Maintains C-spine precautions during BVM		
I-31	Uses straight-to-cuff stylette curvature technique		
I-33	Checks equipment for cuff leaks		
I-36	Positions head properly		
I-40	Grasps laryngoscope with left-hand		
I-47	Elevates mandibles from 45° to 90° w/laryngoscope		
I-55	Flips up epiglottis to expose larynx		
I-57	Inserts laryngoscope to appropriate depth		
I-58	Moves blade tip smoothly without shaking or jerking		
I-61	Maintains view until ETT has stopped advancing		
I-67	Passes ETT through cords with limited or no impingement		
I-68	Passes tube through cords (laryngoscope in mouth to tracheal placement) in 20 s		
I-70	Disconnects syringe IMMEDIATELY after inflating cuff of ET tube		
I-72	Listens over each lung		
I-75	Checks end-tidal CO_2-After ET Tube placement		
I-78	Checks pulse oximeter-After ET Tube placement		

(Continued)

Table 16.1 (*Continued*) Airway management proficiency checklist instrument by subscale[5]

Item No.	Performance task	Yes	No
I-80	Maintains control over ET tube placement		
I-81	Secures ET tube (with device)		
OI-84	Successfully intubates within one attempts		
B-106	Recognizes need for backup airway		
B-108	Identifies an appropriate backup airway device		
B-110	Checks equipment for cuff leaks		
B-114	Immediately inflates cuff, prior to ventilation		
B-117	Immediately disconnects syringe after inflating cuff		
B-119	Confirms proper placement by auscultation bilaterally over each lung-Backup airway		

B, backup airway; I, intubation; S, suction; V, ventilations.

Despite their obvious advantages, checklists of objectives have not flourished as the sole method of grading. The main reason for this is that learners still want to know the letter grade performance that meets what the objectives represents. A learner may be gratified that they have mastered 17 of the 20 objectives but will still want to know if this is an A or B performance. A second difficulty with checklists of objectives is that they can become overwhelmingly long and extensive with very specific objectives in every subject matter and skill domain. Evaluating every objective for each learner can become an onerous and unworkable task for instructors. Checklists of objectives are most useful and informative when they are used in conjunction with traditional letter grade systems. Here, they can be used to enrich and elaborate on the letter grade and communicate very specific information. These checklists work best when only a few of the most important objectives are included and evaluated.

Anecdotal records, narrative reports, and portfolios

Anecdotal records or narrative reports are detailed reports that contain statements about effort, attitudes, behavior, and achievement of each learner that are maintained in a portfolio or e-Portfolio (electronic version of the traditional paper portfolio). Narrative descriptions have the advantage of allowing for the instructors to include much more information in reporting the learner's performance than would otherwise be possible. Moreover, it allows the instructors to maintain detailed daily descriptions of important educational events of the student (e.g., dealing with a dying patient). These reports also tend to reduce norm-referenced comparisons and focus instead on a more comprehensive picture of the student.

Portfolios can be used to collect and evaluate evidence of medical students' competence across time. O'Brien et al.[6] developed a portfolio system at Northwestern University Feinberg School of Medicine for student assessments organized by competency domain. Five competencies were identified: professional behavior and moral reasoning, systems awareness and team based care, effective communication and interpersonal skills, continuous learning and quality improvement, and patient-centered medical care.

Subsequently, clinical faculty members set standards using expert judgment and holistic review to rate students' competency achievement: (1) progressing toward competence, (2) progressing toward competence with some concern, or (3) progressing toward competence pending remediation. With considerable effort, they rated 156 portfolios. An important finding in this study was that concerning student behaviors (e.g., professionalism transgressions) were identified early in the educational program, allowing intervention. Traditional letter or numerical grading systems may not detect these issues early enough for educators to intervene.

Anecdotal records, such as portfolios, have a number of problems associated with them. First, while students generally favor them as do instructors, course directors and administrators, students still want the traditional letter grades in the reports. Second, the collection of information and composing of the reports represents a tremendous amount of work for the instructors and students. If an instructor maintained a daily anecdotal record for each student in a rotation of 15 students, a great deal of time would be required to do this task. Also the amount of information that would accumulate over the course of a month or two would make summarizing and compiling the actual narrative report a huge undertaking. Third, most instructors, residents, or attending physicians have little or no training in making and recording behavioral observations. The reliability and validity of the information on the anecdotal record is accordingly poor. Generally, these records tend to be highly interpretive rather than strictly observational and thus lack validity. Fourth, instructors generally have many learners and generally tend to not to know them very well. Typically, the data collection and reporting is such an onerous task that it is unworkable. Finally, the anecdotal record/portfolio is probably most useful as an addendum to letter grade (or other) reporting systems. It enriches and elaborates the traditional mark. As a sole reporting system, however, it is doubtful if anecdotal records have much use.

DETERMINING GRADES

A final grade is usually a composite of a number of components. Several quizzes, tests, lab assignments, reports, clinical skills assessments, and so on may be combined to arrive at a total composite score which is used to determine the grade. It is usual for the course director to want some components of the grade to count more heavily than others in the final total. On the surface, it appears that the component with the largest maximum score will receive the greatest weight when the components are summed but this is not the case. If several components are merely summed, it is the standard deviation or the variance of the component that will result in differential weighting: the larger the variance, the greater the influence of the component.

Variance ratio equating

If four components with equal maximum scores and means are summed, for example, they may not contribute equally to the final total. The component with the largest variance will count most heavily. Ideally, in order to weigh each component equally, a course director should multiply each score in the distribution with the smallest variance by a ratio of the largest variance to the smallest. If two tests, for instance, both with means of 30 and maximum scores of 50 are summed, they may not weigh equally in the total. Suppose that Test 2 has a variance of 30 and Test 1 has a variance of 15. In order for Test 1 to contribute equally to the total, each score in Test 1 should be multiplied by 2 (variance of Test 2 divided by variance of Test 1; 30/15 = 2). Obviously, this procedure is very time consuming and would not generally be done by most instructors or course directors.

Range ratio equating

A less precise but acceptable approximation to the variance ratio equating is to use the range. In this case, the range is taken as an index of variability, and even though it is quite a crude index for this purpose, it is acceptable for most course use. Suppose that in the above example the minimum score on Test 1 was 20 and the maximum was 40 (range = 20), while on Test 2 the minimum was 7 and the maximum was 47 (range = 40). The multiplier for each score on Test 1, then, is the ratio of the two ranges (40/20 = 2). While in this method things are somewhat simplified because the range is much easier to compute than the variance, it still requires that every score be multiplied by some factor, in this case 2.

Combining letter grades

Converting each component to letter grades first and then combining them avoids the problems of both the variance and range ratio-weighting problems. The problem with this procedure is that it tends to reduce the reliability of the final grade because information is lost in determining letter grades for each component. Two learners may both receive a B, for instance, although one may be at the top of the range and the other at the bottom of the range. This loss of information tends to reduce the reliability of the final grades.

There is no definitive and yet simple method with which to combine components for a grade. You should be aware, however, that a simple adding-up of the various components may not weigh them equally because of the different variances of scores. You may wish to specifically weigh the scores by some weighting scheme based either on the variances, range, or some other predetermined values such as twice the value for the final exam compared to the mid-term test.

Grading assignments

Assignments such as reports, essays, problem solutions, book reviews, and other activities are not primarily assessment activities. Their primary purpose is for teaching and learning. That is, they have been assigned with the intention that learners should learn some important knowledge and skills as a consequence of doing the assignments. As we have seen, tests and other assessments are intended primarily as measurement instruments. It is these that should be used as the components for deriving grades. Strictly for purposes of reliability and validity, assignments ideally should not be included as components in the grade.

If assignments are not assigned a value or a mark, however, it is unlikely that learners will consistently do them and put as much effort into them as the teacher would like. If the assignments "don't count," they are not likely to be taken seriously by the learners. It is necessary, therefore, to assign some value to assignments. As a rule of thumb, assignments and homework should account for no more than 25% of the total value of the grade. This is because these are likely to lack reliability and validity for grading since they were not designed for that purpose. Keeping the value of the components that are low in validity and reliability to a maximum of 25% will tend to limit the extent to which they can reduce the reliability and validity of the final grade.

The primary problem with grading assignments is that the expectations of the instructors and the criteria by which the assignment will be evaluated are not clearly laid out and communicated before the assignment is done. Scoring criteria, just as *rubrics* in scoring essay tests, should be developed and guide the evaluation of the assignments.

Preparing and using a scoring guide or rubric can result in a number of benefits. First, grading can be done more efficiently because of a clear-cut set of criteria and expectations. Second, the feedback to students can include diagnostic statements indicating specific problems and deficiencies. Third, extraneous factors such as the halo effect, hawk-dove effect, and so on are less likely to influence the scoring since clear criteria are specified. Fourth, when the expectations and criteria are presented to the learners at the same time of the assignment, there is less possibility of misunderstanding and the nature of the assignment is made clearer. Expectations for the final product can be clearly indicated. Just as it is very important to prepare students about the nature of an upcoming test, it is important to prepare students about the requirements of the assignment.

NARRATIVE FEEDBACK CONFERENCE

The narrative feedback conference is generally used to complement the grade or mark. The conference offers a number of advantages. First, it enhances communication between the learner and the teacher. Second, it provides for the opportunity of some personal contact between students and instructors. Third, matters that are not reported or cannot be reported on the transcript can be discussed during the conference. Fourth, it provides an opportunity for the instructor to review some of their student's work and to comment on it. Fifth, it can further enhance educational engagement.

Notwithstanding the above strengths, there are a number of disadvantages with the conference. First, they are difficult to schedule for both instructors and students. Second, the conferences can be very time consuming. They can take up a great deal of valuable instructor classroom time. Third, some students, for a variety of reasons, will find difficulties in attending. These are frequently the students who would benefit most from such conferences. Fourth, in order for the conference to proceed well and to be productive, instructors require considerable counseling skills. Professors are rarely directly trained in counseling either in their own education or by continuing education courses.

There are a number of simple guidelines, however, that can be used to make conferences effective. Here are some Dos and Don'ts abridged from Hopkins et al.[7] (p. 327).

Dos
- Use a structured outline to guide the conference
- Review the learner's cumulative record
- Listen
- Maintain a positive and professional attitude
- Describe the learner's strengths but be honest about the problems
- Accept some responsibility for both achievements and problems
- Provide samples of the learner's work to discuss
- Conclude with a summary of the conference
- Reiterate what action the student and instructor have agreed to take

Don't
- Criticize other instructors, students, or the school
- Play amateur psychologist
- Discuss the conference with others except for relevant colleagues
- Gossip or do all the talking
- Argue, blame, or behave condescendingly

EXPLAINING THE MEANING OF TEST SCORES

Either during the conference or on some other occasion, instructors are frequently called on to interpret standardized test score results to learners (e.g., Step 1 scores or Surgery NBME shelf exam). As discussed in previous chapters, standardized test results produce several standard scores: z-scores, T-scores, stanines, percentile ranks, stanines, etc.

Most people have little understanding or appreciation of the meaning of standardized scores. Most people tend to think of test results as a percentage correct on the test. The instructor is faced with a difficult task, therefore, in helping learners fully understand standardized test score results.

Generally, the scores that are reported and interpreted are percentile ranks, T-scores and z-scores. The percentile rank is based on a reference group within age or year or a cohort. Criterion-referenced systems are based on absolute standards as we have seen. Together these two systems provide substantial information.

Class rank, while widely used in the past, particularly in medical school, is disappearing. It is a measure of how a student's performance compares to other students the class. A student may have a grade point average score better than 117 of his classmates in a class of 160. The class rank provides little pedagogically useful information that is not already included in the various assessments. Moreover, a rank of 15 in a highly pedagogically effective medical school does not mean the same as a rank of 15 in a less-effective school. The class rank has been largely used to publicly rank students ensuring that some will be higher than others. While some have believed that this will motivate students to increase their effort so as to improve their rank, there is no empirical evidence for this. On the contrary, this type of ranking is likely to cause hostile competition, exhaustion, and disengagement for many students. Class rank is being phased out of most medical schools and is considered archaic and counterproductive.

PUTTING IT ALL TOGETHER: DEAN'S LETTER AND MEDICAL STUDENT PERFORMANCE EVALUATION

The Medical Student Performance Evaluation (MSPE) is not a letter of reference. The purpose of the MSPE is to provide an authentic and objective summary of the student's personal attributes, experiences, and academic accomplishments based on verifiable information and summative evaluations. It is not to advocate for the student but rather to be an overall summative evaluation. Comparative assessments of the student's attributes, experiences, and accomplishments relative to their institutional peers should be included. The MSPE should primarily contain:

- Information about the student's medical school performance
- Brief summary of premedical experiences and achievements if relevant
- A summary letter of evaluation, not a letter of recommendation
- Information must be standardized, clear, concise, and transparent

Box 16.1 contains an abbreviated example of an MSPE as suggested by the AAMC.

REPORTING WORKPLACE-BASED ASSESSMENTS

Most health professionals now undergo assessment in the workplace as multi-source feedback (MSF), which has emerged as an important approach for assessing professional competence, behaviors, and attitudes in the workplace. Today, MSF tools are being used in the United States, Canada, and Europe (in the Netherlands and the United Kingdom) across a number of healthcare specialties. Data are collected using surveys or questionnaires from peers, coworkers, patients, and self-assessments.[8] Figure 16.1 contains an example of reports for MSF.

MSF is a means of providing healthcare professionals with relevant information about their practice to help them monitor, develop, maintain, and improve their competence through systematic feedback and reporting. The graphs in Table 16.1 are based on patient, colleague, and self-assessment data. The reports are based both on norm-referenced (means compared to group means) and criterion-referenced (five-point scale) basis reporting competencies such as communication, empathy, clinical competency, humanism, and so on. This provides professional development and enrichment (i.e., formative assessment) feedback to physicians about their performance and improves their practice.

BOX 16.1: Medical school performance evaluation example

Medical School Performance Evaluation
*Student: **Guglielmo Harvey***
October 1, 2018

IDENTIFYING INFORMATION

Guglielmo Harvey is a fourth-year medical student at School of Medicine in City, State/Province.

NOTEWORTHY CHARACTERISTICS

- Guglielmo has shown his commitment to regimented training, which began during his years of collegiate soccer and continues to this day.
- While in medical school, Guglielmo's commitment to serving his community was demonstrated through his service as a health educator for inner-city sixth graders, teaching them about the importance of healthy eating and exercise habits.
- Guglielmo has worked diligently on his community capstone research, which pertains to the complex relationship between the emergency department and the homeless

ACADEMIC HISTORY

- Date of expected graduation from medical school: 2018. Date of initial matriculation in medical school: 2014.
- No extension, leaves, or gaps in the educational program.
- Guglielmo was required to repeat the cardiovascular course in his M1 year, which he did successfully.
- Guglielmo was *not* the recipient of any adverse actions by the medical school or parent institution. (Adverse actions include: formal reprimand for unprofessional behavior, suspension due to failure to progress academically, and suspension due to egregious unprofessional behavior).

ACADEMIC PROGRESS

Professional performance

Guglielmo has met all the stated objectives for professionalism at School of Medicine. We have assessed all students' communication skills, adaptability, respect for patients and respect for the healthcare team, cultural competency, accountability, initiative, and composure under stress.

M1M2 curriculum

Graphs 1–4 summarize the final distributions of grades in the preclinical courses for Guglielmo as shown as follows.

(Continued)

BOX 16.1 (*Continued*): Medical school performance evaluation example

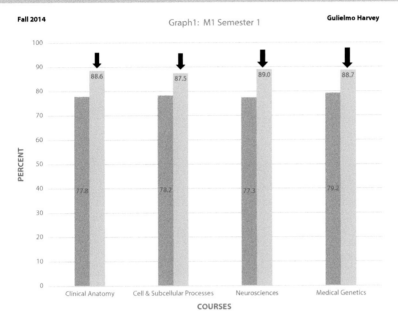

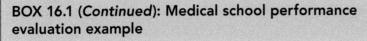

Fall 2014   Graph1: M1 Semester 1   Gulielmo Harvey

CLERKSHIPS

M3 required clinical clerkships

The required clerkships are graded honors/high pass/pass/fail. In order to earn a grade of Honors, students must receive honors on the shelf exam **and** on the clinical performance evaluation. Students receiving honors on the shelf exam **or** the clinical performance evaluation and passing all other components, receive the grade of High Pass. The **Grade Comparison** graphs summarize the final distribution of grades in the clerkships. Following are the unedited narrative evaluations of Guglielmo for performance on the:

INTERNAL MEDICINE: AUGUST 31, 2015–OCTOBER 22, 2015

Final Grade: Pass. Guglielmo performed well during his internal medicine clerkship. He was noted to be hardworking and eager to learn and improve and made important contributions to patient care. Faculty comments include: "Guglielmo is a strong student. His medical knowledge is above what is expected for his level of training. He was reliable and was actively engaged with our team and the care of the teams' patients. He showed enthusiasm the whole month that I worked with him." "Guglielmo has excellent written and verbal communications skills" and "I believe that he will make a terrific fourth-year medical student, eventually intern/resident."

(*Continued*)

BOX 16.1 (*Continued*): Medical school performance evaluation example

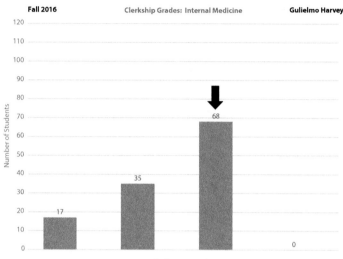

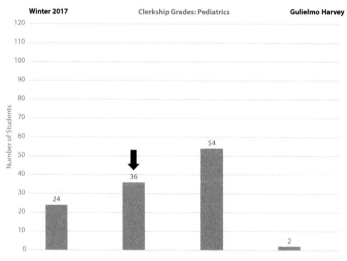

PEDIATRICS: OCTOBER 26, 2015–DECEMBER 17, 2015

Final Grade: High Pass. Some comments from the residents and faculty that Guglielmo worked with: "Good presentation, thorough, concise. Well-organized note." "Guglielmo did a great job in the clinic. He was engaged and has a nice demeanor with the kids. Nice to work with." "Well-organized. Professional and gets along with team members. Good

(*Continued*)

BOX 16.1 (*Continued*): Medical school performance evaluation example

presentation skills." "Always willing to help out. Positive attitude. Interested in learning and improving." "Guglielmo was an excellent student."

Organized presentations. Came to me for ideas for diagnosis when he had them. Excellent bedside manner with the kids and families." "Attentive to his patients, very helpful in developing and executing treatment plan." "Good history taking and presentation skills."

Good medical knowledge, patient interaction, and professionalism.

SUMMARY

Based on academic performance, Guglielmo has been placed in the **fourth quartile**** of the medical school class. The quartile ranking represents only academic performance. Please consider all aspects of this student's record in your evaluation. Guglielmo's narrative evaluations speak to his strong work ethic and positive attitude. He was consistently prepared and focused on learning and improving.

**Quartile placement is determined solely by final grades in courses and clerkships. Students are given 3 points for each grade of honors, 2 points for each grade of high pass, 1 point for pass, and –1 point for each failing grade. Every course in the M1–M3 year is counted equally with no weighting of courses or clerkships. USMLE scores are not considered in quartile placement. School of Medicine does not compute class rank.

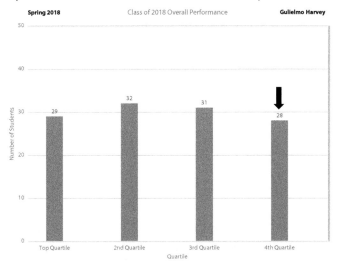

Associate Dean of Student Affairs

School of Medicine
email@schoolofmedicine

Assistant Dean of Student Affairs

School of Medicine
email@schoolofmedicine

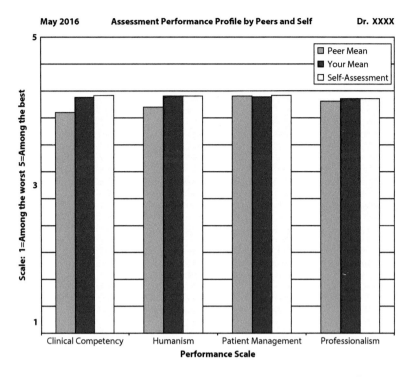

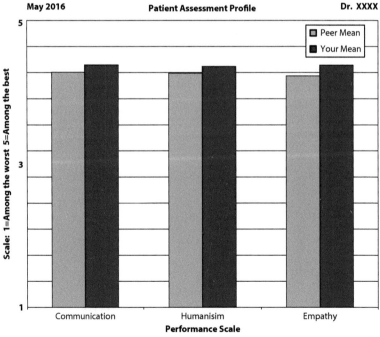

Figure 16.1 Examples of reports for workplace assessments.

Table 16.2 Guidelines for multiple grading and reporting systems

1. Involve all users in the development of the grading system. This should include student groups, professor, counselors, learners, and administrators. This will allow each group to feel "ownership" of the system and it will increase the likelihood that all will understand it
2. Keep the various components of the reporting separate. Report achievement separately with a letter grade and supplement these with checklists of objectives, assessment scores, and information
3. If learner aptitudes are to be assessed and reported, then valid instruments must be employed for this purpose. This cannot be based simply on instructor's subjective judgment
4. Strike a balance between detail and comprehensiveness of information and simplicity and brevity. Too much information and detail can confuse and overwhelm even the most earnest and dedicated student
5. There should be sufficient information on the report to indicate whether a student conference is warranted. The conference can then supplement the information summarized on the report

GUIDELINES FOR GRADING AND REPORTING SYSTEMS

As the main purposes of grading and reporting are to provide feedback to the learner, act as a source of accountability, and to reward and motivate learner efforts systems for this purpose should take various factors into consideration. Some of the most important ones are summarized in Table 16.2.

SUMMARY AND MAIN POINTS

This chapter dealt with grading, reporting, and standard setting, which are important elements of any educational enterprise if it is to remain effective. Grading and reporting have several purposes including feedback and accountability. Several types of marking systems are employed each representing some strengths and weaknesses. There are also several types of symbol systems used in reporting each having some advantages and disadvantages. The determination of the final grade involves weighting components differentially depending on the variance of the scores that they produce. Several norm-referenced and criterion-referenced standard setting and grading systems are described.

Assignments, while they are usually graded, should not figure heavily in the final grade since they are not primarily assessment devices and therefore lack reliability and validity. The Dean's Letter or MSPE brings all of the components together in an attempt to balance the detail of information required to report educational performance in the cognitive, affective, and psychomotor domains, with the need for brevity and understandability. The instructor–student conference can be an extremely useful activity to accomplish a variety of things including enhancing communication between teacher and student. The teacher may also have to interpret standardized test scores for students employing considerable skill and finesse.

1. The main purposes of grading and reporting are to provide feedback to the learner, act as a source of accountability, and to reward and motivate learner efforts. The main problem with grades is that they lack universal meaning across instructors, courses, and school.

2. Grading systems can be based on norm-referenced (grading on the curve) or on criterion-referenced bases. All of these systems have some problems associated with them.

3. The main and historically oldest symbols for grading are the letter grade, usually ranging from A to F. Substitutes have been attempted but have achieved little success because these usually involve reducing the number of categories (e.g., good, satisfactory, unsatisfactory).

4. Numerical grades (% or 1–10) have also met with limited success, as have pass/fail systems and checklists of objectives.

5. Norm-referenced grading this system is frequently called grading on the curve assuming that final achievement of a class is normally distributed and that marks can be derived based on the standard deviation and the mean of the distribution. Criterion based or absolute methods identify passing scores based on a predetermined level of expected competency of students in that phase or stage of learning and the content of the examination, irrespective of group or class performance.

6. A recent proposal that is gaining popularity is the anecdotal record, the narrative report or the portfolio. Because of the various problems associated with this system, it is likely to find only restricted and specialized use.

7. In order to determine final grades, various components must be combined in some fashion. Measurements that produce the highest variance in the scores will tend to influence the final grade disproportionately unless some weighting system is employed.

8. Assignments are primarily intended as learning devices and are not intended as measurement instruments. Their reliability and validity is likely to be low. Therefore, they should figure as little as possible in the total for the final grade as they will tend to reduce the validity of it otherwise. In order for learners to do assignments, however, it is necessary to assign them some value so that "they will count." Assignments in total should not exceed a value of 25% of the total course grade.

9. The Dean's Letter or Medical Student Performance Evaluation should employ multiple reporting systems dealing with the cognitive, affective, and psychomotor domains. There should be provisions for reporting learner achievement, effort, attitudes, interest, social and personal development, and other noteworthy outcomes. The wealth of information on the MSPE, however, should be balanced against the need for brevity and simplicity so that it can be readily understood.

10. The instructor–student conference has a number of advantages, in that it allows for enhanced communication between students and instructors and may engage the student further in their education. Scheduling and time problems are the biggest disadvantages of these conferences.

11. Professors are frequently called on to interpret standardized test score results to learners. When standardized test scores are used (e.g., z-scores; T-scores), they should always be interpreted in conjunction with another system such as percentile ranks.

BOX 16.2: *Advocatus Diaboli*: Alternative grading methods

Several alternative grading methods have been proposed.

IMPROVEMENT OR INDIVIDUAL GROWTH-BASED GRADING

This approach is an attempt to evaluate learner performance against themselves. That is, the improvement that the learner shows in a specified amount of time (e.g., at the beginning of the rotation and at the end) should be the bases for assigning the grade. Thus, a learner who shows marked improvement from September to November should receive an A even if her actual performance is average compared to her peers or an absolute standard. While such a system has appeal, the technical difficulties associated with this method are immense.

Measuring educational change involves the use of gain or growth scores. Even with highly reliable and valid instruments such as some standardized tests, gain scores are highly unreliable. Furthermore, when attempting to assess student growth, most assessors use informal, unsystematic, and subjective methods. Grading based on such procedures would become rather arbitrary and have little validity.

Even if some workable measurement system could be devised for reliably and validly assessing individual growth, there is no sound reason to grade an individual's performance based solely on their improvement or change. How can you justify assigning an A to a learner who has improved substantially but whose performance is average compared to his peers? Conversely, how can you justify assigning a C to a learner whose performance might be the best in the class but who has not improved since the beginning of the year?

In the individual growth system, you must also consider that it is very much easier for a learner to improve when their initial performance was poor than one whose initial performance was good. The learner beginning poorly has nowhere to go but to improve, while this is much more difficult for the learner giving a good initial performance. Finally, if learners begin to recognize that you are using this "growth" method of assigning grades, they may purposefully perform poorly initially in order to easily improve subsequently. Obviously, this would invalidate the entire system. The individual improvement method is so fraught with problems that it is generally unworkable and not recommended as a system of assigning grades.

(Continued)

BOX 16.2 (*Continued*): *Advocatus Diaboli*: Alternative grading methods

EFFORT-BASED GRADING

In this method, learners who expend great effort in their studies are assigned high grades, while those who put in less effort are assigned poor grades. This system, however, confuses the primary purpose of grading which is to summarize and communicate achievement in a subject matter, content area, or procedural skills. While effort is an obviously important educational objective, it should be assessed and reported separately from achievement. The grade should reflect achievement per se and not other extraneous factors such as effort, attitude, and study habits. Indeed, grading systems are most meaningful and valid when these elements are reported separately. There is no pedagogical, measurement, or theoretical basis on which to base a grading system on effort.

ACHIEVEMENT AND APTITUDE-BASED GRADING

In this system, there is an attempt to judge learner's academic attainment based on their aptitude or potential. Learners who are performing up to their potential might receive marks in the average to good range (C, B), those working below their potential might receive marks in the poor to fail range (D, F), and those above their potential receive marks in the excellent to outstanding range (A). This system has appeal for instructors and others alike because it avoids the criticisms of the other grading systems (criterion-referenced, norm-referenced, growth, effort). Proponents of this system argue that each learner should be judged according to what they can do instead of what others do or based on some external standards of performance.

As appealing as this idea is, it is completely unworkable in practice. The main problem is that the instructor must know the learner's aptitude or potential in order to judge the merit of their performance. The only valid way that a learner's potential might be estimated is through standardized test scores and aptitude scores. These data are frequently not available for most learners. Moreover, estimating potential requires different test scores for different subjects as aptitude varies across subject matter. Even with valid test scores available, the technical difficulties in judging achievement relative to potential are large. Instructors who attempt to use such a system frequently "intuit" or guess at a learner's potential. The resulting grading system, of course, lacks any validity whatsoever.

REFLECTIONS AND EXERCISES

1. Summarize the main functions and purposes of grading and reporting.
2. What are some of the main problems of grading and reporting?
3. What are the main advantages and disadvantages of the various grading systems? Discuss at least four grading systems.
4. Notwithstanding attempts with substitutes, letter grades have remained the predominant mode of marking. What are the reasons for this?
5. Describe the limitations of the various reporting systems that have been used as substitutes for the letter grade (i.e., numerical grades, pass/fail, narrative reports, letters, checklists of objectives).
6. How should various components be combined into a total score with which to assign some final grade?
7. How should an instructor handle assignments in the final grade? What are the reasons behind these decisions?
8. Design an ideal MSPE. What are the main reporting systems that should be employed?
9. What are the main functions of the instructor–student conference?
10. Summarize the do's and don'ts of the instructor–student conference.
11. What are the pitfalls that an instructor should be aware of in interpreting standardized test scores for learners? How should these be handled?

REFERENCES

1. Alexander EK, Osman NY, Walling JL, Mitchell V (2012) Variation and imprecision of clerkship grading in U.S. medical schools. *Acad. Med.* 87: 1070–1076.
2. Lefroy J, Hawarden A, Gay SP, McKinley RK, Cleland J (2015) Grades in formative workplace-based assessment: a study of what works for whom and why. *Med. Educ.* 49: 307–320.
3. Ebel RL, Frisbee DA (1986) *Essentials of Educational Measurement* (4th ed.). Toronto, ON: Prentice Hall.
4. Violato C, Marini A, Lee C (2003) A validity study of expert judgment procedures for setting cutoff scores on high-stakes credentialing examinations using cluster analysis. *Eval. Health Prof.* 26: 59–72.
5. Way DP, Panchal AR, Finnegan GI, Terndrup TE (2017) Airway management proficiency checklist for assessing paramedic performance. *Prehosp. Emerg. Care* 21(3): 354–361.
6. O'Brien CL, Sanguino SM, Thomas JX, Green MM (2016) Feasibility and outcomes of implementing a portfolio assessment system alongside a traditional grading system. *Acad. Med.* 91(11): 1554–1560.

7. Hopkins K, Stanley J, Hopkins K (1990) *Educational and Psychological Measurement and Evaluation*. Englewood Cliffs, NJ: Prentice Hall.
8. Emke AR, Cheng S, Dufault C, Cianciolo AT, Musick D, Richards B, Violato C (2015) Developing professionalism via multisource feedback in team-based learning. *Teach. Learn. Med.* 27(4): 362–365.

Glossary of Terms

Ability: the level of a person on a domain, trait, or competence in areas such as intelligence, reading, clinical reasoning, or cognitive, psychomotor, or physical functioning.

Accommodation (testing): a change in the standard procedures for administering the assessment for students with disabilities or special abilities (e.g., visual impairment, attention deficits).

Accommodation (Piaget): accommodation occurs by restructuring, elaborating, or discarding the schema as a result of assimilation. Meaningful improvement in learning, therefore, results when the schemas or cognitive structures are altered.

Achievement Test: a test designed to measure the extent to which a person has acquired certain knowledge and/or skills that have been taught in school as part of some other planned instruction or training. National Board of Medical Examiners (NBME) subject matter tests ("shelf exams") in specialty areas such as pediatrics, psychiatry, internal medicine, and so on are examples of achievement tests.

Adaptive Test (Computer-Adaptive Test): a form of testing in which items are selected for administration to the test-taker based on the psychometric properties and content of the item because of the test-taker's responses to previous items.

Aggregation: the compilation of the results of students for the purpose of reporting.

Alternate Forms: two or more versions of a test that is parallel or equivalent because they measure the same constructs in the same ways.

Analytic Scoring: a scoring method in which performance is assessed for specific traits, dimensions, and/or domains.

Answer Choice: all options available for a student to select from a multiple-choice item.

Aptitude Test: measures the ability of a person to develop skill or acquire knowledge. IQ tests are examples of an aptitude test for measuring general academic ability.

Assessment: systematic methods of obtaining information (usually quantitative) using instruments about people, objects, or programs.

Assimilation (Piaget): the process by which material is taken into and subsumed in cognitive structures. Assimilation takes information through sensory input and attentional selection. This information is fit into existing schemas until the schemas no longer can hold new information.

Average: more formally, the central tendency of a set of scores—such as the arithmetic mean, median, and mode. "Average" is considered an imprecise, slang term among testing experts.

Battery: a set of standardized tests designed to be administered as a unit.

Benchmark: a value of what students are expected to learn at various developmental levels or points in time (e.g., 1st year university, 3rd year university). They are used to indicate a student's progress.

Bias: source of systematic error of the measurement. This often refers to tests that differentially affect the performance of different groups of test-takers (e.g., sex, ethnic, or age).

Ceiling Effect: the upper limit of a variable that can be measured effectively; a ceiling effect on a test indicates that it is probably too easy.

Central Tendency: the tendency for scores in a distribution to cluster around the center of the distribution; the mean and median are measures of central tendency.

Chance Level: the probability of random guess correctly at the answer on a question. For example, for a four-response option MCQ item, each examinee has 25% chance level of correctly selecting the answer.

Checklist: a list of characteristics or behaviors used by an examiner as a guide for evaluating performance, by noting the presence or absence of each item. Each item is dichotomously scored (yes or no).

Classical Test Theory (CTT): the historically oldest psychometric theory (before generalizability and item response theory) that postulates that an individual's observed score is the sum of a true score plus error. Many standard procedures for test construction and the evaluation of a test's reliability and validity are based on CTT.

Classroom-Based Assessment ("homemade tests"): assessments developed, administered, and scored by instructors or course directors to assess student's performance on a topic.

Coefficient Alpha (Cronbach's Alpha): an internal consistency measure of reliability; very widely used to report scale and test reliability.

Coefficient of Determination: the correlation coefficient squared (r^2) and an indicator of the variance accounted for in y by x.

Cognitive Assessment: measures a person's ability to perform various mental activities involved in the processing, acquisition, retention, conceptualization, and organization of sensory, perceptual, and verbal information.

Cohort: a group of people with a common demographic (e.g., age).

Completion Rates: the percent of test-takers completing the entire test or the percent of test-takers completing a specific percent of the number of items.

Composite Score: derived by combining one or more scores according to a pre-specified weighting.

Computer-Based Testing (CBT): any test that is delivered via computers.

Confidence Interval: the interval between two values that a value is thought to exist. The confidence level is usually 68%, 90%, or 95%, indicating the probability that the interval will contain true score. Confidence intervals are constructed using the observed score and the standard error of measurement (S_e).

Consequential Validity: see Validity.

Construct: a hypothetical concept or trait inferred from multiple evidences and used to explain observable behavior patterns (also referred to as a latent variable). Examples of constructs are intelligence, introversion, neuroses, conscientiousness, and creativity.

Constructed-Response Item: items that require examinees to create or construct the responses or answers. These are also referred to as open-ended items that include essays and short-answer questions.

Construct-Related Validity: see Validity.

Construct Validity: see Validity.

Content Validity: see Validity.

Correlation: the degree of relationship (or strength of association) between two variables. A correlation of zero indicates lack of any relationship. The most commonly used statistic for correlation is Pearson's product–moment r (Pearson's correlation coefficient). Other correlations are Spearman's rho which is based on rank-order between two variables and the biserial correlation.

Correlation Coefficient: a statistic that indicates the strength of the relationship between two variables. This coefficient, r, ranges in value from -1 to $+1$. A correlation of $+1$ or -1 indicates a perfect (positive or negative) relationship, while a correlation of 0 (zero) indicates the complete absence of a relationship.

Criterion: a standard, guideline, or rule by which a judgment or decision may be based.

Criterion-Referenced Interpretation: the interpretation of performance compared to an absolute standard.

Criterion-Referenced Test (CRT): a test where performance is compared to an absolute standard irrespective of the norm group performance.

Criterion-Related Validity: see Validity.

Cronbach's Alpha (also Coefficient Alpha): an internal consistency measure of reliability which is the most general reliability coefficient.

Cutoff Score: a specified point on a scale such that cuts scores above or below that point. This usually sets pass/fail scores.

Decile: divides a distribution into ten equal groups, each containing one-tenth (10%) of the data.

Diagnostic Test: a test used to identify specific areas of strength or weakness and identify learning difficulties.

Difficulty Index: the difficulty of an item is the percentage or proportion of people who got the item correct. The difficulty index (*P*) is usually expressed as a proportion such as $P = 0.72$ (72% got it correct).

Discrimination Index: item discrimination is the extent to which an item distinguishes or "discriminates" between high-test scorers and low-test scorers. Positive D indicates discrimination in the correct direction. The point-biserial is commonly used for item discrimination, D.

Distractor: an incorrect response option for a multiple-choice question. Distractor effectiveness refers to the ability of distractors in attracting responses.

Distribution: tabulations of scores into frequencies. Common distributions include histograms and frequency polygons. There at four important types of frequency polygons in test data analysis: normal, skewed, bimodal, and rectangular.

Equating: a procedure or process where scores from various assessment methods are converted to a common scale or metric for equating them.

Equivalent Forms: see Alternate Forms.

Error of Measurement: the difference between an observed score (actual score received) and the true score.

Extended-Response Item: a constructed-response question that requires an extended essay response.

Face Validity: see Validity.

Factor: a hypothetical variable that is not directly measurable. In psychometrics, a factor is a statistical dimension identified by factor analysis.

Factor Analysis: a collection of methods used for exploring the correlations between a number of variables seeking the underlying clusters or subsets called factors or latent variables. It addresses the number of factors that are needed to summarize the pattern of correlations in the correlation matrix. It is a method of data reduction.

Factor Loadings: correlations of the items to the factor derived in factor analysis.

Factor Scores: a linear combination of item scores and factor score coefficients calculated in a factor analysis.

Field Test: a pilot test to check testing procedures, such as administration directions, responding, scoring, and reporting of the results.

Floor Effect: the lower limit of scores on a test; the lowest possible scores.

Formative Assessment: assessment that provide feedback during the educational sequence. It is not intended for evaluation purposes (e.g., pass/fail).

Frequency: the number of times that a value or interval of values occurs in a distribution of scores.

Frequency Distribution: important frequency distributions for statistics include histograms and frequency polygons. There at four important types of frequency polygons in test data analysis. These include the following distributions: normal, skewed, bimodal, and rectangular.

Generalizability Theory (G-theory): focuses on the principle of generalizing from a sample of observations to a universe of observations from which the observations were randomly sampled. The reliability of an observation depends on the universe about which the inferences are to be made. A given score may generalize to several different universes; it may vary in how reliably it allows inferences about these universes.

Generalizability Coefficient (Ep^2): a coefficient that can range from 0 to 1 and provides information about the dependability of the scores generalized to a universe of interest.

Growth: for an individual or group, the amount of change or difference between two test scores.

High Stakes Test: a test that has important consequences for candidates, programs, or institutions. Health professions licensing or certification tests are high stakes.

Histograms: a histogram is a method of graphing and displaying data to indicate the shape of a distribution. It is particularly useful when there are a large number of observations.

Holistic Scoring: a scoring method based on a judgment of overall performance using specified criteria or scoring rubrics. Holistic scoring is usually used with essay tests to determine a grade, A, B, etc.

Homoscedasticity: uniform variance across measured variables.

Intelligence Test: a psychological design to measure an intelligence or level of cognitive functioning (verbal reasoning, abstract reasoning, memory, etc.).

Intercorrelations: a matrix of correlation coefficients, calculated between two or more sets of scores for the same sample.

Internal Consistency: the degree of cohesion among the items of a test.

Interpolation: a process of estimating missing values of scores between two values.

Interquartile Range: the distance between the lower quartile and upper quartile; the upper quartile minus the lower quartile.

Inventory: a self-report questionnaire that elicits information about a person's opinions, interests, attitudes, preferences, personal characteristics, motivations, and typical reactions to situations and problems.

IQ Test: Intelligence Quotient (IQ) expressed as the ratio of an examinee's mental age to his/her chronological age times 100.

Item Analysis: statistical analyses of test questions to determine the item difficulty, item discrimination, and distractor effectiveness.

Item Characteristic Curve (ICC): a graphical function that represents the examinee's ability as a function of the probability of getting the item correct. An item's location is defined as the amount of the latent trait needed to have a .50 probability of getting the item correct. The trait level is labelled ability (θ) with mean = 0 and a standard deviation = 1. Like z-scores, the values of θ typically range from −3 to +3. Up to 3 parameters may be represented on the graph: (a) the slope, or discrimination, (b) the difficulty of the item, or θ value, and (c) the guessing parameter of the item (lower asymptote).

Item Difficulty: the percentage or proportion (P) of test-takers who got the item correct.

Item Discrimination: the extent to which an item on a test differentiates high scorers from low scorers. In Classical Test Theory, item discrimination indices generally range from 0.0 (little or no differentiation) to +1.0 (high differentiation). Negative discriminations indicate the item may be mis-keyed or is working backwards.

Item Response Theory (IRT): also known as latent trait theory, and can be used for the design, analysis, and scoring of tests, questionnaires, and assessments' measuring abilities, attitudes, or other variables. IRT is based on mathematical modelling of candidates' response to questions or test items.

KR20: a reliability computation was invented by Frederick Kuder and Marian Richardson in 1937. It is a shortcut computation which fortunately avoids the necessity of calculating correlations at all. It measures the internal consistency of a set of dichotomously scored items (i.e., "1 = correct" or "0 = wrong"), based on a single administration of the test.

Longitudinal: data of growth or change over time of an individual or group.

Mastery Level: the cut score for a criterion-referenced or mastery test. Test-takers who score lower than the cut score or "below the mastery level" are considered not to have mastered the test material, while those scoring at or above the cut score, or "above the mastery level", are considered to have demonstrated mastery of the test material. The method of setting the score designated as representing "mastery" can vary and is often subjectively determined.

Mastery Test: a criterion-referenced test designed to assess if examinees have mastered a domain of knowledge or skill. Mastery is achieved by superseding a cutoff score (i.e., passing score).

Mean: the arithmetic "average": the sum of scores in a distribution divided by the number of scores.

Measurement: the assignment of numbers to observations in a systematic manner as a way to quantify properties or characteristics of learners or other people.

Median: the middle point (score) in a distribution of ranked-ordered scores that divides the group into two equal parts, each part containing 50% of the data. The median is the 50th percentile.

Medical Student Performance Evaluations (MSPE): also known as the Dean's Letter, the MSPE should employ multiple reporting systems dealing with the cognitive, affective, and skills domains. There should be provisions for reporting learner achievement, effort, attitudes, interest, social and personal development, and other noteworthy outcomes. The wealth of information on the MSPE, however, should be balanced against the need for brevity and simplicity so that it can be readily understood.

Mode: the score that occurs most frequently in a distribution of scores.

Multiple-Choice Item: items that require candidates to select a response from possible choices in selecting the answer to the question posed. MCQ (multiple-choice question) is a commonly used acronym.

Normal Distribution: a theoretical distribution that characterizes many human traits, physical characteristics, and psychological constructs (e.g., height, ear length, intelligence, etc.). It has a distinctive bell-shaped curve where scores are distributed symmetrically about the center; there are an equal number of scores above as in below the mean, with most scores concentrated around the center.

Norm Group: a standardization sample or norm-referenced peer group.

Norm-Referenced Interpretation: interpretation of scores based on a norm or peer group. Norm-referenced interpretations can be for individuals (i.e., student norms) or for institutions (e.g., school norms). Standard scores such as percentile ranks, stanines, z-scores, T-scores, etc. are used for this interpretation.

Norm-Referenced Tests (NRTs): standardized tests or assessment instruments with scores that are interpreted based on a norm-group (i.e., reference group). The Medical College Admission Test, Dental College Admission Test, Law School Admission Test, Intelligence Tests are examples of such NRTs.

Norms: statistics or data that summarize the distribution of test scores for norm or peer groups. Norms are typically developed using representative samples (i.e., the standardization sample or norms group) of the group.

Number Attempted: the number of items that an examinee attempts to answer on a test or the number of examinees that attempted a particular item.

Objective: a statement of some desired educational outcome. These are stated in terms of what learners can do after some pedagogical event (e.g., a course).

Objective Structured Clinical Exam (OSCE): consisting of several stations, the OSCE concentrates on skills, clinical reasoning, and attitudes; to a lesser degree basic knowledge. Content checklists and global rating scales are used to assess observed performance of specific tasks. Candidates circulate around a number of different stations containing various content areas from various health disciplines. Most OSCEs utilize standardized patients (SPs), who are typically actors trained to depict the clinical problems and presentations of real issues commonly taken from real patient cases.

Objective Structured Performance Exam (OSPRE): similar to the OSCE, this examination type can assess skills in surgery together with communication and professionalism as well as skills in sigmoidoscopy, colonoscopy, laparoscopy, and epidural anesthesia. Multi-station OSPREs can assess skills in excision of a skin lesion, central line and chest tube insertion, enterotomy closure, tracheostomy, laparoscopic tasks, and so on. The OSPRE is intended to assess all levels of performance (e.g., Miller's Pyramid) for specified competencies.

Objective Test: a test or assessment that can be scored routinely according to a predetermined key, eliminating the judgments of the scorers. Objective tests such as MCQs have keyed responses that can be scored mechanically or by computer.

Oblimin Rotation: the method for a non-orthogonal (oblique) solution in factor analysis. The factors are allowed to be correlated with each other. While there are other rotation methods, they are not widely applicable in medical education.

Open-Ended Items: see Constructed-Response Item.

Percent Correct (PC): percentage of the total number of marks that are received on a test or other assessment. This is derived by dividing the raw score by the total number of points possible and multiplying by 100.

Percentile: the score in a distribution at or below which a given percentage of scores fall, based on the standard normal curve. For example, the 65th percentile means that 65% of all scores fall below this point. This is a common way of reporting individual results on standardized tests.

Percentile Rank (PR): percentile ranks range in value from 1 to 99, and indicate the relative standing of a candidate relative to a peer group (i.e., norms group). The PR indicates the percent of people in that group who obtained lower scores.

Pilot Test: a test administered to a representative sample of examinees for purpose of testing some aspects of the test such as instructions, time limits, item response formats, or item response options.

Point Biserial: a correlation between a dichotomous variable and a continuous variable such as the total test score. It is commonly used for item discrimination in item analyses.

Power Test: a test that has no time limit or, more likely, has a time limit to ensure that each examinee has time to complete the test. Most classroom tests are of this type, where speed is not a factor.

Population: *all* of the objects (people, fish, rats, trees, rocks, test scores, or anything else that can be measured) in the set that is of interest. All American medical students can be defined as a set, for example, and called a population. Then at least one, or all but one, of the medical students constitutes a subset or sample of the population. Populations are usually very large and samples are usually small by comparison.

Predictive Validity: see Validity.

Proctor: a person who supervises candidates during the administration of an examination and is responsible for the distribution and collection of test materials, managing time, and supervising behavior during the test to ensure that there is no cheating.

Profile: a graphic presentation of data for individuals or groups summarizing the results of tests, assessments, and other performance. This type of display is useful for identifying relative strengths and weaknesses and is used in the *Medical Student Performance Evaluations* (e.g., Dean's letter).

Prompt (Stimulus): information on a test item that activates prior knowledge and requires analysis to respond. A prompt may be a case history, graph, x-rays, photograph, lab data, or any combination of these.

Protocol: a code prescribing conventions governing the collection of information and data such as assessments or test scores.

Psychometric: measurement of psychological and educational characteristics such as abilities, aptitudes, knowledge, skills, constructs, and traits. It is also a field of study that focuses on the construction and validation of assessment instruments such as question-naires, tests, raters' judgments, and personality tests. This work is based on measurement theories particularly classical test theory, generalizability theory, item response theory.

P-value (Item Difficulty): an item's difficulty, calculated as the proportion that answered a test item correctly. The values range from 0.0 to 1.0.

Quartile: scores in a distribution are divided into four equal groups, each containing 25% of the data.

Random Error: non-systematic measurement error; a variable that has no relationship to any other variable probably due to random events.

Range: the difference between the two extremes (maximum score − minimum score); indication of the spread or variability of the scores.

Rasch: an item response theory (IRT) model used to analyze data from assessments. It is a special case of a 1-parameter model.

Rating Scale: an instrument used for assessing the performance of tasks, skill levels, pro-cedures, processes, and products that indicate the degree of behavior. Rating scales state the criteria and provide selections to describe the quality or frequency of the performance. The 5-point scale is preferred because it provides the best all-around psychometrics.

Raw Score (RS): the sum of the number of questions answered correctly. Raw scores typi-cally have little meaning by themselves and are transformed to percentages or standard scores or pass/fail for criterion-referenced tests.

Readability: refers to the difficulty level of reading of test items. Several different formu-lae provide the readability of a text: the total number of words, average sentence length, number of sentences, length of words, amount of empirical data, difficulty of graphics (e.g., ECG, x-rays). The readability index is an indicator of difficulty.

Readiness Test: a prognostic test that is used to predict a student's future success or academic risk for undertaking or engaging in a new learning activity such as clinical rotations.

Reference Population: the population of test-takers represented by the test norms.

Regression: simple regression refers to the situation of one dependent variable (y) and one independent variable (x). The regression equation is $Y' = \beta_1 X_1 + c$. Frequently, there are several independent variables so as to improve the predictive validity of the dependent variable. The multiple regression equation is $Y' = \beta_1 X_1 + \beta_2 X_2 + \cdots + \beta_k X_k + c$.

Regression to the Mean: the tendency of extreme scores on one test to be less extreme on a second-related test. Extreme scores will tend to regress to the mean on subsequent measurements.

Reliability: consistency of measurement either through test–retest or through internal consistency. Reliability is typically expressed as a reliability coefficient or by the standard error of measurement derived by that coefficient.

Reliability Coefficient: a statistic, often expressed as a correlation coefficient (r_{xx}) that reflects the degree of measurement error of a test. Other common coefficients are KR 20, KR21, Cronbach's alpha, and Ep^2. The closer the value of the coefficient to 1.0, the greater is the reliability of the test.

Representative Sample: see Sample.

Rubric: a scoring guide used to evaluate the quality of constructed responses. Rubrics employ specific criteria to evaluate performance. They consist of a fixed measurement scale and detailed description which focus on the quality of performance with the intention of including the result in a grade.

Sample: a subset of selected sampling units (e.g., people, examinees, items) from a larger specified set, the population. A random sample is a selection of entities from the population such that each unit has an equal probability of being selected. There are many other types of sampling procedures including stratified, quota, snowball, and so on.

Scale Score (SS): a transformation of the raw score to scale scores that provide a continuous scale across different levels and forms of a test. This permits direct comparison of different groups of examinees, regardless of the time of year tested and the level/form administered such as NBME subject matter exams (e.g., pediatrics, surgery) taken either in the Fall or Spring with resulting difference in performance.

Scaling: the process of creating a scale or a scale score.

Selected-Response Item: a type of item format, most commonly the multiple-choice item, which requires the test-taker to select a response from a group of possible choices.

Short-Answer Item: an item test format that requires a short response: a few words, phrase, or a number as an answer.

Speediness: time limits imposed for the completion of a test. A measure of speediness is the percent of test-takers completing the test.

Speed Test: a test in which time is a relevant aspect of performance. It is measured by the time to perform a specified task. Memory tests on aptitude or intelligence test batteries as sometimes speeded as a measure of "speed of processing."

Split-Half Reliability Coefficient: an internal consistency, reliability coefficient obtained by correlating scores on two halves of a test. The Pearson's r is then adjusted via the Spearman–Brown formula, providing an estimate of the reliability of the total test.

Standard Deviation (SD): a measure of the degree of dispersion of a set of scores. Each score is deviated around the mean, these deviations are squared and summed and divided by the number of scores. Take the square root and the result is the deviations scores standardized or the "standard deviation."

Standard Error of Measurement (S_e): indicates the amount of error in a score or the standard deviation of the errors of measurement. The S_e is estimated from group data using the reliability and the standard deviation for a set of test scores. The S_e is often used in the construction of a confidence interval around a test score.

Standardization: the process of maintaining a constant testing environment according to a strict protocol. In test development, it is establishing scoring norms based on the test performance of a representative (i.e., standardization sample) for which the test is intended for future use.

Standardization Sample: the sample from the population that the resulting test scores are used in the development of norms.

Standardized Test: a test designed to be administered, scored, and interpreted according to a prescribed set of rules or instructions. It has known psychometric qualities (e.g., norms, reliability, validity evidence).

Standard Score (SS): derived scores that are transformations of raw scores. Well-known fundamental standard scores are z-scores (mean = 0.0 and standard deviation = 1.0). Standard scores permit the direct comparison of candidates from different tests.

Standard Setting: the procedure used in the determination of the cutoff scores for an assessment. Various techniques are available for this including the Angoff and Ebel procedures. The latter is commonly used in setting cutoff scores in OSCE stations.

Shelf Exams: slang term for the clinical subject matter examinations (e.g., surgery, internal medicine, psychiatry) developed by the National Board of Medical Examiners and taken by third-year medical students typically during the relevant clinical rotation.

Stanine: a "standard-nine" scale. Stanines are normalized standard scores, ranging in value from 1 to 9, with a mean of 5 and a standard deviation of 2.

Stem: the question (e.g., essay) or statement (MCQ) of a problem statement.

Subject Area: a body of content derived from related disciplines and organized for curriculum and testing.

Subjective Test: an assessment (e.g., extended essay) where subjectivity from the scorer is inherent in the score or grade assigned to the response.

Summative Assessment: a measure of student performance at the completion of instruction. Summative assessment, in contrast to formative assessment, is used primarily for evaluation purposes (e.g. grades).

Systematic Error: a consistent measurement error that is not related to test performance (such as cultural differences); also known as a bias.

Technology-Enhanced Item (TEI): items that capitalize on computer-based functionality (hot-spots, drag-and-drop, creating graphs and plots, categorize, fill in the blanks, etc.) to create specialized interactions for collecting response data.

Test Battery: see Battery.

Test Modification: altering the content, format, and/or administration procedure of a test in order to accommodate test-takers who are unable to take the original test under standard test conditions (e.g., signing for hearing impaired, a braille version of a test). Such modifications may require special norms and interpretation of test scores.

Test–Retest Reliability: the same test is administered a second time to the same group after a short time interval and correlating the two sets of scores.

Table of Specifications (TOS): a detailed description for a test that *specifies* the number and proportion of items for each content and process, often called a blueprint. Additionally, the TOS specifies the format of items, responses, scoring rubrics, and procedures.

True Score: in classical test theory, X (observed score) = T (true score) + e (error). In item response theory, the true score is the error-free value symbolized by theta, a construct of examinees' "true" ability. In generalizability theory, it is the universe scores that are estimated by the observed scores.

T-Score: a normalized standard score, with mean = 50 and a SD = 10.0. *T*-scores are a direct transformation of z-scores ($T = 50 + 10z$) and ranges about 3 SDs above and below the mean (20–80).

Validity: the extent to which a test measures what it is intended to measure. It is based on the accumulated data and evidence to support the theory and the purposes of a test.

- **Face Validity**—it has to do with appearance: Does the test appear to measure whatever it is supposed to measure? Face validity provides an initial impression of what a test measures but can be crucial in establishing rapport, motivation, and setting classroom climate.
- **Content Validity**—content validity involves sampling or selecting. The domain of measurement must be clearly defined and detail the cognitive processes involved employing levels of *Bloom's Taxonomy* (knows, comprehends, applies, analyzes, synthesizes, evaluates, creates). Enhancing content validity may be achieved most directly through the use of a table of specifications (TOS). A well-designed and carefully developed TOS will provide a sound plan for a test. The closer is the match between the test's accuracy in sampling of the content and learning outcomes, the higher is the content validity.
- **Criterion-Related Validity**—is when performance on a test correlates with performance on some other criterion. There are two sub-categories of criterion-related validity: (1) predictive and (2) concurrent. Predictive validity refers to how current test performance correlates with some future performance on a criterion and thus involves the problem of prediction. Concurrent validity refers to how test performance correlates concurrently (at the same time) with some criterion.
- **Construct Validity**—is about the truth or correctness of a construct and the instruments that measure it. A construct is defined as an entity, process, or event which is itself not observed and can be measured only indirectly. Establishing the validity of constructs also requires determination of the validity of relevant instruments. Establishing construct validity is a complex process.

- **Consequential Validity**—this focuses on the consequence that the use of the test and score interpretations have upon candidates, selection and screening, instruction, and the curriculum.
- **Ecological Validity**—the situation approximates the real-world that is being examined.

Validity Coefficient: a correlation that is interpreted within the context of validity. Interpretations can be aided further by using the coefficient of determination (r^2) and then determining the percentage of variance that is accounted for in the criterion by the test. The percentage of variance accounted for is derived by multiplying the coefficient of determination by 100 ($r^2 \times 100$ = percent of variance accounted for).

Variability: the degree of spread or dispersion of a set of scores.

Variance: a statistic that summarizes the degree of spread or dispersion of a set of scores. Each score is deviated around the mean, these deviations are squared and summed and divided by the number of scores to result in the variance. The greater the dispersion of the scores, the larger is the variance.

Varimax Rotation: the most common rotation option in factor analysis is an orthogonal rotation of the factors to maximize the variance extracted that is accounted by that factor. A varimax solution yields results which make it as easy as possible to identify each variable with a single factor.

Weighting: a process of assigning weights to a score usually in the process of assigning grades.

z-Score: a standard score expressed as standard deviation unit. For a normal distribution, it has a mean of 0.0 and a standard deviation of 1.0. A z-score indicates the amount that a score (X) deviates from the mean as a standard deviation (SD) unit.

Index

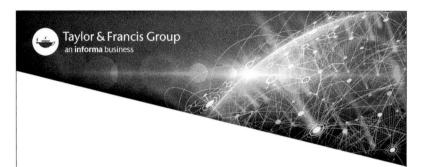